LEGAL AND ETHICAL ISSUES FOR HEALTH PROFESSIONS

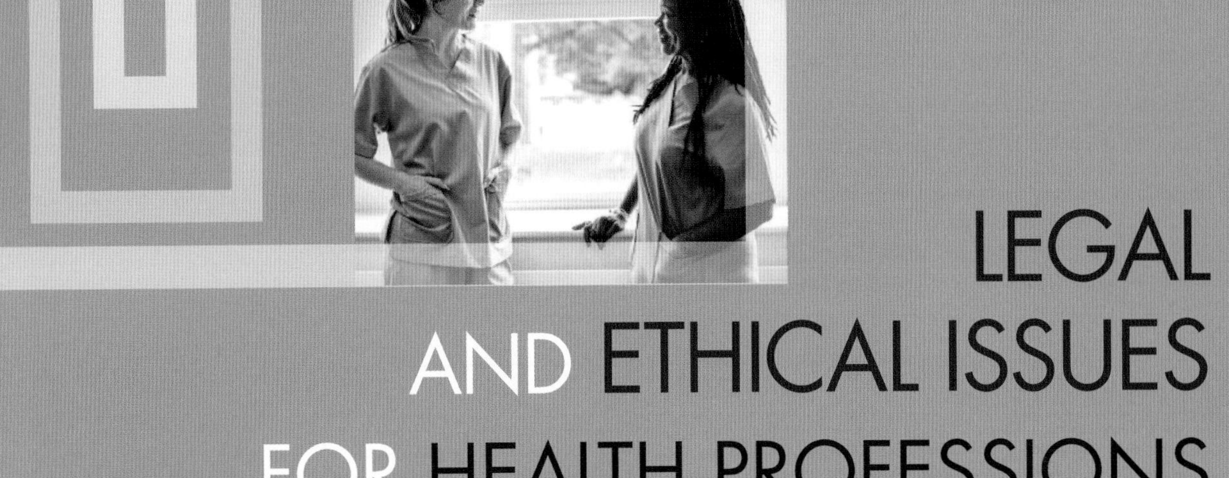

LEGAL AND ETHICAL ISSUES FOR HEALTH PROFESSIONS

FIFTH EDITION

JAIME NGUYEN, MD, MPH, MS, BA
Director of Healthcare Programs
Penn Foster College
Scranton, PA

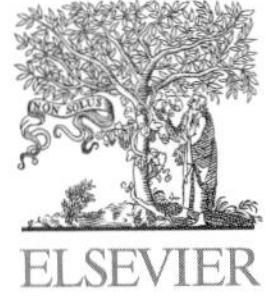

ELSEVIER

Elsevier
3251 Riverport Lane
St. Louis, Missouri 63043

LEGAL AND ETHICAL ISSUES FOR HEALTH PROFESSIONS, FIFTH EDITION ISBN: 978-0-323-82750-8

Senior Content Strategist: Luke Held
Senior Content Development Manager: Somodatta Roy Choudhury
Senior Content Development Specialist: Vasowati Shome
Publishing Services Manager: Deepthi Unni
Project Manager: Nayagi Anandan
Design Direction: Brian Salisbury

Printed In India

Last digit is the print number: 9 8 7 6 5 4 3 2 1

CONTRIBUTORS

Linda Bartolomucci Boyd, BA, RDA, CDA
Professor/Emeritus,
Registered Dental Assisting Program,
Diablo Valley College,
Pleasant Hill, CA

Cheryl Fassett, CPC, CPB, CPPM, CPC-I
Practice Manager,
Riverside Associates in Anesthesia, PC,
Binghamton, NY

James J. Mizner, Jr., MBA, BS, RPh
President & CEO,
Panacea Solutions Consulting,
Reston, VA

REVIEWERS

Wendy C. Craven, AS, CMA (AAMA)
Adjunct Instructor of Medical Assisting,
Forsyth Technical Community College,
Winston-Salem, NC

Chad Hensley, MEd, RT (R)(MR)
Clinical Coordinator,
University of Nevada Las Vegas,
Las Vegas, NV

Debra G. Herring, MAT, RT (R)(M)
Program Coordinator/Instructor,
Radiological Technology Program,
Meridian Community College,
Meridian, MS

Anna B. Hilton, BS, CMA (AAMA)
Program Coordinator,
Forsyth Technical Community College,
Winston-Salem, NC

PREFACE

This fifth edition of *Legal and Ethical Issues for Health Professions* is a comprehensive, user-friendly textbook and reference that focuses on legal and ethical issues for future healthcare professionals. With an approachable writing style, abundant case studies, and comprehensive information, this textbook offers accessible and relevant content to prepare students for real-life issues that they will face as healthcare professionals.

The beginning chapters introduce students to the basic principles of law and ethics, including the legal system and the bases of ethics, morals, and values. By providing this foundation, students will gain a better understanding of how these laws, ethics, and standards are applied in the healthcare setting and how healthcare professionals comply with them, which are discussed in the next section of the textbook.

New to the fourth edition is the addition of Chapter 12 on "Birth and Life," which complements Chapter 13 on "Death and Dying." Chapter 12 reviews many of the current and often controversial ethical and bioethical issues regarding birth and life. These issues include family planning, reproductive health, abortion rights, organ donations, and autonomy and the ability to consent to specific populations, such as minors and those with mental health issues and physical disabilities.

In each edition, Chapter 14 on "Key Trends in Healthcare Law and Ethics" is updated to address and discuss topics and issues currently affecting the healthcare industry. The chapter will review the role of public health in the United States, including the history of vaccines and vaccine mandates. Other topics discussed in the chapter include the growing awareness and public consciousness of the meanings of sex and gender, transgender, gender identity, and being biologically male or female vs. identifying as either or none at all. This group often faces health disparities due to societal stigma, discrimination, denial of their civil and human rights, and a general lack of visibility in the healthcare system. Healthcare professionals must work toward creating a more inclusive environment and exploring ways to improve accessible healthcare and services to marginalized and vulnerable patient populations.

FEATURES

This new edition contains many helpful features, with up-to-date information, applicable questions that require critical thinking, and real-life, relatable scenarios. These valuable learning aids include the following:

- **Key Terms** are identified and defined at the beginning of each chapter, providing students with a valuable terminology overview for each chapter.
- **Chapter Objectives** are listed at the beginning of each chapter, thus providing both students and instructors with definitive evaluation tools to use, as each chapter's content is covered.
- **Discussion Boxes** provide topical discussion questions that will generate beneficial classroom dialogue and promote critical thinking about topics related to the real world of healthcare professions.
- **Relate to Practice Scenarios** are designed to assist students in responding to realistic situations and real-life ethical dilemmas that they may encounter in the workplace.
- **Self-Reflection Questions** are placed at the end of every chapter to provide students with pertinent questions that can be used to analyze and evaluate various legal and ethical issues.
- **Internet Activities** are positioned at the end of every chapter to provide students with additional topics to research and investigate.
- **Additional Resources** are listed at the end of some chapters to offer students a chance to take their learning a step further.
- **Chapter Review Questions** accompany every chapter and greatly enhance the learning value of the textbook by providing appropriate topic-specific questions so that students can test their retention of each chapter's content.
- **Case Discussions and Case Studies**, available under "Appendices," are activities that include actual legal cases and common scenarios that students may encounter in their future health careers. They are followed by several thought-provoking, situational-type questions to encourage critical thinking, personal reflection, and classroom discussion.

APPENDICES

The fifth edition provides three helpful appendices to encourage classroom discussion. Appendix A includes case discussions, which are legal and ethical scenarios. Appendix B contains case studies, which are actual legal cases. Appendix C details different state laws pertaining to state retention laws for medical records.

EVOLVE RESOURCES

The Evolve site (http://evolve.elsevier.com/healthprofessions/legalissues/) includes all instructor materials (TEACH Lesson Plans, TEACH PowerPoint slides, TEACH Answer Keys, and Test Banks, which are for instructors only) and a practice examination for students.

ACKNOWLEDGMENTS

I would not be who I am and where I am without my family. Much love, thanks, and respect to my parents, who instilled in me the importance of education, intellectual curiosity, and having a strong work ethic. This textbook is my tribute to their love of literature and pursuit of knowledge. I am grateful to Sandra Arch for always serving as my sounding board, walking dictionary and thesaurus, and for being everything that I am not.

I thank Elsevier for giving me this opportunity to share my knowledge and experience and to help educate future healthcare professionals. Also, a big thank you to all the authors who contributed to this textbook.

Jaime Nguyen, MD, MPH, MS, BA

CONTENTS

1

The U.S. Legal System

CHAPTER OBJECTIVES

1. Describe the three branches of the federal government in the United States.
2. Define law and the sources of law.
3. Explain the different types of law in the United States.
4. Explain key laws affecting healthcare professionals.
5. Demonstrate understanding of the various levels of the U.S. court system.
6. Describe the trial process in a lawsuit.

KEY TERMS

Administrative law Establishes laws between citizens and government agencies and provides certain power to the agencies to enforce these laws and regulations.

Admissions of fact Discovery technique that asks the opposing party (in writing) to admit or deny any material fact or the authenticity of documents to be introduced into evidence at trial.

Amendment An official or formal change made to a law, contract, constitution, or other legal document.

Appellate court A court that hears appeals from lower court decisions; sometimes called court of appeals.

Assault A threat or attempt to inflict offensive physical contact or bodily harm on a person that puts the person in immediate danger of or in apprehension of such harm or contact.

Battery Bodily harm or unlawful touching of another. In the medical field, treating the patient without consent is considered battery.

Burden of proof The legal responsibility and requirement to prove a claim is true.

Civil lawsuit A noncriminal lawsuit for damages, usually based in tort, contract, labor, or privacy issues.

Common law Law of precedents built on a case-by-case basis and established by citing interpretation of existing laws by judges in previous suits. Also known as "judge made law."

Criminal law State or federal government law covering violations of a written criminal code or statute.

Defendant Person or entity sued.

Discovery Process of gathering information in preparation for trial.

Executive branch President of the United States or the governor of an individual state. Can propose laws, veto laws proposed by the legislature, enforce laws, and establish agencies.

Federal court Court having jurisdiction over cases in which the U.S. Constitution and federal statutes apply; these can be federal district courts (trial courts), district courts of appeals, or the U.S. Supreme Court.

Felony Serious crime punishable by relatively large fines and/or imprisonment for more than 1 year and, in extreme cases, death.

***In personam* jurisdiction** A court's power to adjudicate cases filed against a specific individual, as opposed to *in rem* jurisdiction, which concerns property disputes.

***In rem* jurisdiction** A term that delineates the court's jurisdiction over property or things, including marriage, rather than over persons.

Interrogatory Pretrial set of written questions that must be answered in writing under oath and returned within a given time frame.

Judicial branch Federal constitutional court system; one of the three parts of the U.S. federal government; interprets legislation and determines its constitutionality and applies it to specific cases. May overrule cases presented on appeal from lower courts.

Jurisdiction Authority given by law to a court to try cases and rule on legal matters within a geographical area and/or over certain types of legal cases.

Law The foundation of statutes, rules, and regulations that governs people, relationships, behaviors, and interactions with the state, society, and federal government.

Legislative branch The U.S. House of Representatives and Senate and any similar state legislature that develops statutory law.

Malpractice The failure of a professional to meet the standard of conduct that a reasonable and prudent member of the profession would exercise in similar circumstances; it results in harm.

Medical law Laws that are prescribed to pertain specifically to the medical field.

Misdemeanor Lesser crime punishable by usually modest fines or penalties established by the state or federal government and/or imprisonment of less than 1 year.

Negligence The failure to use such care as a reasonably prudent and careful person would use under similar circumstances; an act of omission or failure to do what a person of ordinary prudence would have done under similar circumstances.

Ordinance Statutory law passed by local or city governments or councils.

Plaintiff The person or entity bringing a suit or claim.

Res ipsa loquitur In Latin: "the thing speaks for itself." Legal doctrine that there is clear proof that the defendant had the responsibility (duty) to the patient and that the injury would not and could not have occurred without the negligence of the defendant.

Standard of care Basic skill and care expected of healthcare professionals in the same or similar branch of medicine; based on what another medical professional would deem to be appropriate in similar circumstances.

Stare decisis In Latin: "to stand by the things decided" or to adhere to a decided case; condition in which, once a court rules, that decision becomes law for other cases. Also known as precedent.

State supreme court Highest court in any given state in the U.S. court system.

Statute Written laws enacted by the state or federal legislative branch.

Statute of limitations Defense against a tort action; requires that a claim be filed within a specific amount of time of discovering that a wrong has been committed.

Statutory law Written laws, usually enacted by a legislative body, that include regulatory, administrative, and common laws.

Tort A wrongful act, not including a breach of contract or trust, that results in injury to another's person, property, reputation, or the like, and for which the injured party is entitled to compensation.

Writ of certiorari Order a higher court issues to review the decision and proceedings in a lower court and determine whether there were any irregularities.

INTRODUCTION

All healthcare providers and professionals have a primary responsibility to provide high-quality patient care and to prevent and manage diseases and conditions, while respecting patient privacy, maintaining confidentiality, and communicating responsibly in fulfillment of this role. To ensure patient protection, healthcare professionals are bound by a variety of laws and regulations and by a wide range of legal and ethical responsibilities to their patients, employers, and society. These myriads of laws that affect healthcare professionals and their conduct can be complex and difficult to understand.

This chapter provides an overview of the legal system and reviews major legal concepts and terms. By understanding the sources of laws, the different types of law, and what constitutes medical negligence, healthcare professionals will be better able to conduct themselves in a manner that is legal and compliant. In addition, they will be more capable of making sound decisions concerning their role in providing quality patient care and in protecting themselves and their employers from negligence and lawsuits.

Branches of Government

Before understanding the laws and the legal system in the United States, it is important first to understand the system of government and structure of the legal system. In the United States, there are three branches of government that provide the basic sources of law. They are the legislative, executive, and judicial branches. This structure of government exists in both the federal and state government.

The first branch—the legislative branch—consists of the House of Representatives and the Senate and any similar state legislature (Fig. 1.1). This branch of the government develops and enacts statutory laws, which are written laws and that vary from regulatory, administrative, and common laws. These laws are codified and binding on all citizens in the country or that state if passed by the state's government. For example, the legislative branch of the United States, commonly referred to as Congress, passed the Medicare and Medicaid bills in the Social Security Amendments of 1965, which dramatically affected health care by expanding health services to low-income families, pregnant women, people with disabilities, and people who need long-term care in the United States. Written laws enacted by the legislative branch are called **statutes**.

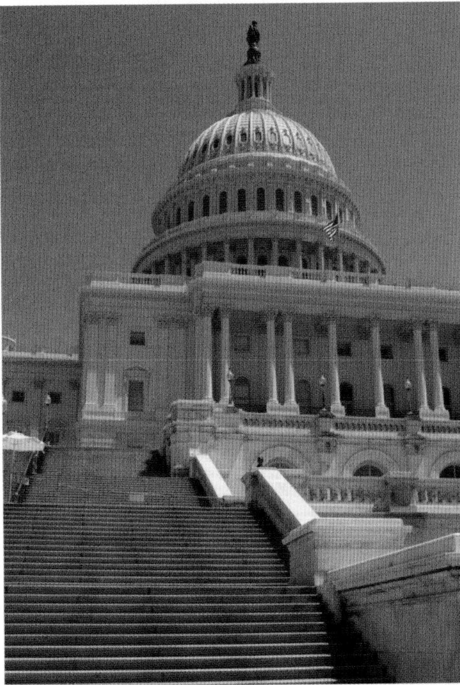

Fig. 1.1 Steps leading up to the U.S. Capitol where the Senate and House of Representatives meet. (Copyright © qingwa/iStock/Thinkstock.com.)

The second branch of government is the executive branch. The leader of the executive branch may vary but is commonly the head of state or head of government, such as the President of the United States or the governor in each state. The president or a state governor proposes legislative action to be taken by individual legislators, either vetoes or approves laws agreed on by the legislature and enforces laws. The executive branch may also establish administrative law, which codifies interactions between citizens and government agencies and provides certain power authority to the agencies to enforce these laws and regulations. An example of an administrative law is the passage of the Occupational Safety and Health Act of 1970, which includes the Occupational Safety and Health Administration (OSHA), that enforces the rules and regulations of almost all industries and workplaces, including healthcare facilities (Fig. 1.2). In addition,

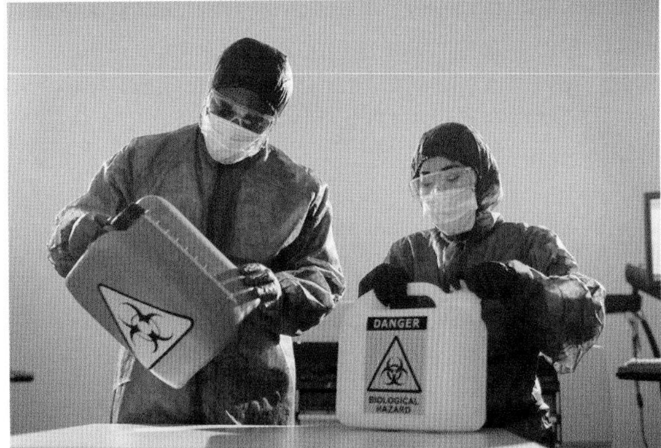

Fig. 1.2 An administrative law enacted OSHA, the agency that enforces the rules and regulations of almost all industries and workplaces. (iStock.com/SeventyFour.)

once the legislature creates a statute, it empowers the appropriate agency in the executive branch to implement rules and regulations to meet the intent of the statute.

Finally, the third branch is the judicial system, which is comprised of the court system. The judicial branch is responsible for interpreting laws, resolving legal disputes, punishing those who violate the law, making decisions in civil cases, and determining the innocence or guilt of a person based on criminal laws. The judicial branch also enacts common law, or case law, which is the law that develops from the decisions made by courts. Previous court decisions are considered precedent and binding on all lower courts. In Latin, this doctrine is called ***stare decisis***, which means to stand by things decided or to adhere to decided cases. The court system and the trial process will be discussed in further detail later in this chapter.

Checks and Balances

The three branches of government are critical in ensuring a separation of power. Each branch serves as a "check and balance" for the other branches of government to ensure that political power is not concentrated in one particular branch (Box 1.1). For example, the legislative branch may propose and pass statutes and can override the veto of the president or a governor. A governor or the president can propose that legislative action be taken and veto legislation, appoint or nominate individuals to certain courts, and enforce laws. The courts interpret the laws and can declare a law passed by the legislature as unconstitutional. This oversight provides the necessary "checks and balances" for each branch to ensure that power and responsibility are shared and that no one branch becomes too powerful. Box 1.2 lists examples of checks and balances in the U.S. government.

BOX 1.1 Checks and Balances in the United States

Executive branch: president or governor can veto legislation and enforces the laws

Legislative branch: proposes and passes legislation and can override the president or governor

Judicial branch: interprets legislation and can overrule laws and actions of the executive branch

BOX 1.2 Current Examples of Checks and Balances

- In September 2016, Congress overrode a veto by President Barack Obama over the issue of families of 9/11 victims being allowed to sue Saudi Arabia.
- In January 2021, the House of Representatives voted to impeach Trump for incitement of insurrection. The Senate voted to acquit him by a vote of 43–57, with conviction requiring two-thirds vote.
- In January 2021, Congress overturned President Donald Trump's veto of a $740 billion defense spending bill.

WHAT IS THE LAW?

The term ***law*** refers to any collection of statutes, rules, and regulations that govern people, relationships, behaviors, and interactions with a state, society, or nation. Laws are often created by an authority, such as the federal, state, city, or local government. In addition, there are even recognized international laws agreed on by a group of nations through treaties and resolutions, such as the Geneva Convention, which is an international humanitarian law that regulates conduct during war and times of conflict.

Laws are created and written to provide guidance, structure, and instruction on how to act and what is expected of us as members of a society. Laws are also meant to provide order in negotiating conflicts among individuals, corporations, states, and other entities. The goal of law is to resolve disputes without violence and to protect the health, safety, and welfare of individual citizens.

Laws in the United States are often based on long-held tenets, customs, and beliefs. However, society changes and becomes more complex with advancements in technology and changing demographics, political climate, morals, and social norms. As a result, laws are constantly having to evolve and adapt to meet these changes, challenges, and shifts in our society (Fig. 1.3). For example, in the early 21st century, laws were amended or changed to recognize and protect various groups in society, such as laws on antimiscegenation (forbidding interracial marriages) and same-sex marriages.

A specialized field of law is medical law. Medical law is a specific body of laws that the rights and responsibilities of healthcare professionals and their patients. The primary areas of focus for medical law include confidentiality;

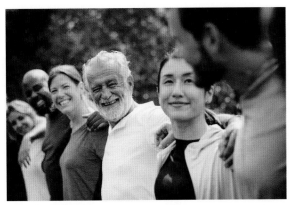

Fig. 1.3 Laws are constantly having to evolve and adapt to meet the changes, challenges, and shifts in our society. (iStock.com/Rawpixel.)

negligence and other torts related to medical treatment, especially regarding medical malpractice; and criminal law and ethics. Unlike law, medical law is generally more steadfast and slower to adapt to changes.

DISCUSSION

The passage of the Affordable Care Act (ACA) in 2010 by the United States federal government is one of the most important healthcare reform laws passed by the U.S. federal government in 2010. It increased health insurance coverage for the uninsured and implemented reforms to the health insurance market. However, since its passage, various states, private entities, and even individuals have challenged parts or all the ACA in state and federal court. The U.S. Constitution does not set forth an explicit right to health care.

1. Should every U.S. citizen have the right to health care?
2. Should the federal or state government be responsible for ensuring that?

Sources of Law

Laws originate or are created from a variety of sources. In the United States, the four primary sources of law are:

- Constitutional law,
- Statutory law,
- Administrative law, and
- Common (or case) law.

Constitutional Law

Constitutional law is the fundamental law of a country. Constitutional law specifically addresses the relationship between individuals and their government and not between individuals or businesses. In the United States, the basis of constitutional law is the Constitution of the United States of America, enacted in 1789. The Constitution outlines the federal government's structure and powers and establishes basic law in the United States. In addition, each state has its own state constitution that establishes basic law for the people of the respective state. State constitutions are often modeled after the U.S. Constitution; however, the U.S. Constitution would take precedence over a state's constitution if a conflict should arise.

Constitution and Bill of Rights

The Constitution and the Bill of Rights are two historical documents that guarantee certain fundamental freedoms and rights to individuals in the United States. As a result, many existing laws have been created to protect and enforce these freedoms and rights, such as the fundamental rights to privacy, equal protection, and freedom of speech and religion. The supreme law of the United States is the Constitution, which establishes shared powers between federal and state governments.

The constitutional basis for federal involvement in health care is found under the provision for the general welfare and regulation of interstate commerce. The states have the power to regulate health care through their power and enforcement to protect the health, safety, and welfare of their citizens. This includes the regulation of the education and licensure of nurses, pharmacists, physicians, chiropractors, physical therapists, and other healthcare professionals.

DISCUSSION

Although laws are often believed to be permanent, laws may change by **amendment**, which is an official or formal change made to a law, contract, constitution, or other legal document. For example, the Constitution provides that an amendment may be proposed either by Congress with a two-thirds majority vote in both the House of Representatives and the Senate or by a constitutional convention called for by two-thirds of the State legislatures.

1. What current laws would you want to amend? Why?
2. Why should laws be allowed to be amended?

Statutory Law

Statutory laws, or statutes, are written by federal and state legislatures. City governments or councils may enact similar statutory laws called **ordinances**. Statutes begin as bills introduced by legislators at the state or federal level, by either the Senate or the House of Representatives. Once the bill passes one of the houses, it becomes an act and then goes to the other house for review and approval. For example, if the Senate originates and approves a bill, it will then go to the House of Representatives, where the act can be amended or approved. Once approved by both houses, the act will be signed by the heads of each house: the Speaker of the House of Representatives and the president pro tempore of the Senate or Vice President of the United States. Finally, the act needs to be signed by the chief executive to become a public law or statute which would be the President of the United States for federal acts and the governor of the respective state for state acts.

Administrative Law

Both state and federal governments authorize administrative agencies to make administrative laws. These governmental administrative agencies may make rules and laws, adjudicate, prosecute, supervise, investigate, and enforce regulations. For example, the U.S. Food and Drug Administration (FDA) is an administrative agency that is authorized to pass rules and regulations governing the sale and use of a wide range of products, including certain foods, pharmaceutical products, medical devices, and tobacco products. The FDA's authority to regulate and enforce is based on the laws set forth in the Federal Food, Drug, and Cosmetic Act, an administrative law enacted by Congress.

Common (or Case) Law

Common laws are made by the courts, or the judiciary branch, and are often based on previous court decisions or interpretation of a law that are then applied to current cases, rather than resulting from specific legislation, such as a statutory law. Because they are established from court decisions and are on a case-by-case basis, common laws may also be referred to as case laws.

Common laws are based on precedents, or rulings from earlier cases that are now applied to subsequent or current cases when the facts or situations are similar. However, each time a common law is applied, it must be reviewed to ensure that it is still relevant and has not been overturned (reversed) by an existing law. Further, the precedent or application of a common law to a case depends mainly on the court in which it is decided. For example, a higher court is not bound to follow the precedents established by the lower courts in its jurisdiction. However, lower courts must follow the precedents of all higher courts having jurisdiction over them.

DISCUSSION

In response to the COVID-19 pandemic, New York City Mayor Bill de Blasio mandated the vaccine to all its employees and students. Mayor Blasio relied on legal precedent that gave states and local governments the right to uphold compulsory vaccination laws. The legal precedent is from a 1905 U.S. Supreme Court case, Jacobson v. Massachusetts, that allowed states the power to require the smallpox vaccine.

1. The use of the legal decision from Jacobson v. Massachusetts is based on which kind of law?
2. If the federal government passed a mandate, would state and local governments need to follow this mandate?

TYPES OF LAW

In general, there are two main categories of law: criminal and civil. Criminal law protects the rights of the state or government, whereas civil laws protect the private rights of person or a person's property (Box 1.3). The following sections take a closer look at the distinctions between these two types of law.

Criminal Law

Criminal law is concerned with violations against society based on the criminal statutes or codes. The remedies or punishments for violating state or federal criminal laws are monetary fines, imprisonment, and capital penalty (death). Violations of criminal laws are called crimes. **Misdemeanors** are lesser crimes punishable usually by monetary fines established by the state but may also include imprisonment of 1 year or less. **Felonies** are more serious crimes punishable by larger fines and/or imprisonment for more than 1 year or, in some states, death. In many states, a felony conviction

BOX 1.3 Examples of Criminal and Civil Laws

Criminal law: theft, assault, robbery, trafficking in controlled substances, murder

Civil law: tort, contract, labor, or privacy issues; landlord/tenant disputes; divorce proceedings, child custody proceedings, property disputes, personal injury

for a healthcare professional may also include the revoking of a license to practice in his or her profession. A healthcare professional may also be prosecuted for a crime for practicing without a license, falsifying information in obtaining a license, or failing to provide life support for a patient.

There are also the related felonies called assault and battery. An assault is the threat of bodily harm that reasonably causes fear of harm in the victim. If the victim has not actually been physically harmed or touched, but only threatened or an attempt was made to harm, the crime is an assault. Battery is the actual unconsented physical contact on another person. Healthcare professionals may be at risk of a charge of assault and battery, for example, if they treat a patient without consent. Likewise, unlawful restraint of a patient against his or her will by a healthcare professional without legal authority or justification will constitute false imprisonment and is a violation of both criminal and civil law.

APPLY THIS

Mr. Garrison is seen for a routine medical visit and consents to the physician's removal of several skin lesions on the patient's arm. During the procedure, the physician, Dr. Huang, ends up having to remove deeper tissue than he originally expected, which leaves the patient with scarring. Mr. Garrison is upset with the scarring on his arm and that he was not made aware of the possible risks before the procedure. He decides to sue Dr. Huang.

1. Can Dr. Huang be criminally charged for this offense? If so, what would be the charge?
2. How could this have been avoided?

Civil Law

Civil laws are laws that protect the private rights of a person or a person's property. Civil laws include the areas of contracts, property, negligence and malpractice, labor, privacy issues, and family law. A violation of civil law may lead to a civil lawsuit by the victim, which is a case brought to the courts to hold a party responsible for a wrongdoing.

Civil lawsuits against healthcare professionals often include allegations of failure to provide care that meet the standard of care, resulting in harm or injury to the patient. Penalties in civil law are almost exclusively monetary, which the court decides on for damages (Box 1.4). In some cases, the court may order a

BOX 1.4 Remedies for Violations of Law

- Civil remedies: usually monetary award
- Criminal remedies:
  1. Misdemeanors: lesser fines and jail time of less than 1 year
  2. Felonies: major fines and jail time of more than 1 year, or the death penalty (in some states)
- Administrative remedies:
  1. Monetary fines
  2. Required education
  3. Loss of license to practice

healthcare professional to stop performing an act until a full hearing is held on an issue to prevent further harm from occurring that money cannot remedy, such as stopping a physician from practicing medicine.

A wrongdoing or violation of civil law is called a tort. The term tort comes from the Latin word *tortus*, meaning to twist or to be twisted. A tort is a private and civil wrong causing an injury. There must always be a violation of some duty owed to the plaintiff, and generally such duty must arise by operation of law and not by mere agreement of the parties.

Negligence and Malpractice

The most common tort against healthcare professionals is for negligence. Negligence does not require a specific intent to harm someone and is not a deliberate action but is the result of an individual or party failing to act in a reasonable way where a duty was owed. There are four basic elements in negligence:

- Duty of Care: One party has a legal obligation to act in a certain manner toward the other.
- Dereliction of Duty: Also called a breach, this is a failure to use reasonable care in fulfilling the duty.
- Direct Cause: The failure in the duty leads to harm suffered by the injured person.
- Damages: The harm or injury can be remedied by monetary compensation.

Malpractice is an act of negligence and describes an improper or illegal professional activity or treatment, often used regarding a healthcare professional causing an injury to a patient. The negligence might be the result of errors in diagnosis, treatment, postoperative care, or a violation of patient confidentiality. Malpractice requires proof of a breach of a standard of care, and the breach must cause damage or harm. In general, the standard of care in a medical malpractice case is defined as the

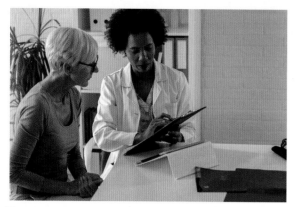

Fig. 1.4 To minimize risk of medical malpractice, healthcare professionals must demonstrate standard of care. (iStock.com/Lordn.)

type and level of care an ordinary, prudent, healthcare professional, with the same training and experience, would provide under similar circumstances (Fig. 1.4). In other words, the critical question in a medical malpractice case is—"Would a similarly skilled healthcare professional have provided me with the same treatment under the same, or similar, circumstances?" Negligence torts and medical malpractices will be discussed in further detail in later chapters.

> **APPLY THIS**
>
> A hospital's policies and procedures require that all bedridden patients must be turned every 6 h to prevent bedsores. Is it a form of negligence if you decide not to turn a patient because the patient was sleeping and you did not want to disturb her?

THE COURT SYSTEM

Now that we have discussed the law, types of law, and violation of the law, this section will describe how these laws are enforced to protect an individual or a party. As discussed earlier, the court system in the United States interprets and applies the law in the name of the state and federal government. It decides whether a person committed a crime and what the punishment should be. The court system also provides a mechanism for the resolution of disputes, which includes monetary damages, imprisonment, and, in extreme cases, capital punishment.

The United States has a two-court system: state and federal. Depending on the dispute or crime, cases will be in either state courts or federal courts. Both state and federal courts generally follow the same three levels and divide most cases into the following sequence: (1) trial courts, (2) appellate (appeals) courts, and (3) the supreme court. Most medical malpractice lawsuits, excluding Medicare fraud, which would go to federal court, are tried in the state courts because they often violate state regulations or laws.

Cases in which the Constitution and federal statutes are violated or applied are heard in federal district courts (trial courts), district courts of appeals, or the U.S. Supreme Court. When a lawsuit is not connected in some way to federal constitutional issues, such as divorce or a traffic violation, it is tried in a state court. Each state has its own constitution that often mirrors the U.S. Constitution.

State Trial Courts

State courts are divided into district or municipal trial courts, state courts of appeals, and the supreme court. In some states, there may be courts with limited jurisdiction over specific types of case, such as family or probate cases, juvenile cases, divorce, child custody, and housing or land issues.

State courts primarily address crimes and civil cases that do not exceed a certain monetary sum established by the state legislature. These cases often involve no jury and are often handled quickly. It is in this court that negligence, medical malpractice, elder abuse, major crimes, and other civil wrongs are tried.

Courts of Appeals

Once a trial is completed or a verdict given in a case in the court of general jurisdiction or in one of the specific courts, the verdict may be appealed to a higher court, usually called an appeals court or appellate court. There are both state and federal appellate courts.

Courts of appeal do not rehear cases in their entirety or the facts, as done by the jury or the judge during the trial (Fig. 1.5). Instead, courts of appeals typically address whether a lower court made any errors in interpreting the law. An appeal may only raise an issue of law.

If the appeals court decides a case and no further appeal is taken, the appellate decision is binding on all lower courts in the state. The decision of the court of

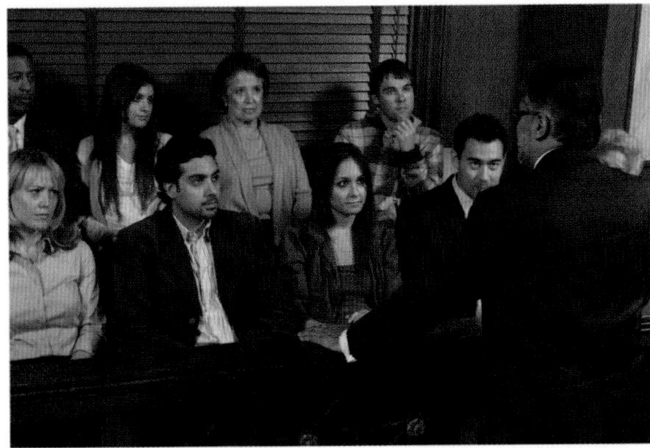

Fig. 1.5 The jury and judge do not rehear the facts of a case during an appeal but only address if an error in interpreting the law occurred. (Copyright © IPGGutenbergUKLtd/iStock/Thinkstock.com).

appeals will usually be the final word in the case, unless the case is sent back to the trial court for additional proceedings, or the parties ask the supreme court to review the case.

State Supreme Courts

The supreme court is the highest court in any jurisdiction. To request a review of an appeal, the party must submit a ***writ of certiorari*** to the supreme court. The supreme court, however, does not have to grant a review. The supreme court typically will agree to hear a case only when it involves an important legal principle or when two or more courts of appeals have interpreted a law differently. The ruling by the supreme court is binding on all lower courts.

Federal District Court System

The structure and procedural sequence are nearly identical since the state court systems are generally modeled after the federal court system. There are 94 judicial districts organized into 12 regional circuits. Each circuit has a U.S. court of appeals.

In the federal court system, if a case that has been decided in a district court undergoes appeal, the appeal is then decided in the regional circuit court of appeals. After the regional circuit court, the only appeal for a federal case is through the U.S. Supreme Court, which may or may not agree to review the case. Federal courts will hear and decide on cases that involve federal law, such as constitutional rights, taxes, intellectual property, or cases between residents of two different states or countries. Some cases may be pursued only in federal courts (e.g., bankruptcy, admiralty).

The Supreme Court of the United States

The Supreme Court of the United States is the highest court in the U.S. judicial system and has the power to decide appeals on all cases brought in federal court or those brought in state court but dealing with federal law. The members of the U.S. Supreme Court are referred to as justices and are nominated by the President of the United States and confirmed by the Senate for a life term. There are nine justices on the court—eight associate justices and one chief justice. The chief justice chooses the cases that the U.S. Supreme Court hears (Fig. 1.6).

As discussed earlier, the party appealing either a federal circuit court's decision or a state supreme court's decision on a federal question files a *writ of certiorari.* The U.S. Supreme Court chooses very few cases to hear. The cases that are chosen must involve a question of substantial importance. Box 1.5 lists landmark cases heard by the U.S. Supreme Court. Once the U.S. Supreme Court decides a case, it is binding on all state and federal courts.

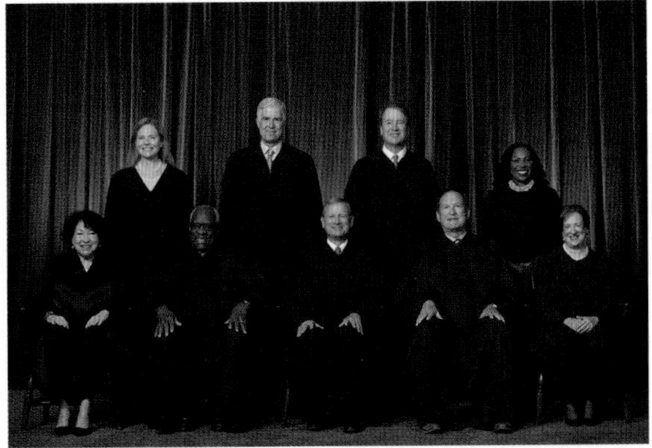

Fig. 1.6 The Supreme Court as of June 30, 2022. Front row, left to right: Associate Justice Sonia Sotomayor, Associate Justice Clarence Thomas, Chief Justice John G. Roberts, Jr., Associate Justice Samuel A. Alito, Jr., and Associate Justice Elena Kagan. Back row, left to right: Associate Justice Amy Coney Barrett, Associate Justice Neil M. Gorsuch, Associate Justice Brett M. Kavanaugh, and Associate Justice Ketanji Brown Jackson. (Credit: Fred Schilling, Collection of the Supreme Court of the United States, https://www.supremecourt.gov/about/justices.aspx.)

BOX 1.5 Landmark U.S. Supreme Court Cases

- *Brown v. Board of Education* (1954): Do racially segregated public schools violate the Equal Protection Clause? The overturning of "separate but equal" doctrine by the court helped lay the ground for the civil rights movement and integration across the country.
- *Miranda v. Arizona* (1966): Are police constitutionally required to inform people in custody of their rights to remain silent and to an attorney? The now famous "Miranda warnings" are required before any police custodial interrogation can begin if any of the evidence obtained during the interrogation is going to be used during a trial; the court has limited and narrowed these warnings over the years.
- *Roe v. Wade* (1973): Does the Constitution prohibit laws that severely restrict or deny a woman's access to abortion? Roe has become a centerpiece in the battle over abortion-rights, both in the public and in front of the court.
- *Regents of the University of California v. Bakke* (1978): Can an institution of higher learning use race as a factor when making admissions decisions? The decision started a line of cases in which the court upheld affirmative action programs.

APPLY THIS

A registered nurse is responsible for taking a patient's vital signs every 4h. Today, however, the nurse was assigned several new patients, which doubled his patient caseload. As a result, he did not have time to check on his last patient and decided to copy the patient's vital signs taken 4h earlier.

1. Could the registered nurse be held legally responsible if the patient suffers any injuries?
2. What are some possible legal repercussions if this patient suffers injuries from the registered nurse's failure to act in this case?

The Trial Process and Lawsuits

To try a specific case, the court must have **jurisdiction** over the case. Jurisdiction can be *in personam* or *in rem*. ***In personam* jurisdiction** means in Latin "against the person"; in other words, the court has jurisdiction over the person. For example, the major trial court's jurisdiction is based on county, parish lines, or other such divisions, and the case must be tried in the county or parish in which the incident leading to a lawsuit occurred. The plaintiff may have the option of presenting the case in his or her own county or parish, depending on the rules of procedure for that state. In certain instances, the plaintiff may have to file a case where the defendant lives, such as in collection of money owed.

***In rem* jurisdiction** means in Latin "power about or against the thing," specifically that the court has jurisdiction over the property or thing itself rather than over the people involved. The court determines the right to the specific property. For example, during a divorce proceeding, the court would supervise the sale and division of monies, property, or assets of the home.

In addition, filing a lawsuit must be timely. It must be filed within the **statute of limitations**—a claim filed within a specific amount of time of discovering that a wrong has been committed. Statutes of limitations vary by state and the type of offense (Box 1.6). At the federal level, the majority of crimes have limits on when the government can bring someone to court. The main category of crimes that do not carry a time limit is capital offenses—those that could involve the death penalty. Most federal crimes have a statute of limitations of 5 years, with some crimes having more extended time limits (Box 1.7).

The person or entity bringing the lawsuit is called the **plaintiff**, for example, the patient who brings a complaint against the hospital or healthcare provider. The person or entity who is sued and defending against the allegations is the **defendant**. In a court case citation, the

BOX 1.6 Examples of State Statute of Limitations

- Medical malpractice in New York is 30 months and 3 years in South Carolina.
- In Massachusetts, crime, such as theft or receiving stolen goods, is 6 years, and robbery is 10 years.
- In Virginia, personal injury and fraud lawsuits are 2 years.

BOX 1.7 Statutes of Limitations for Federal Crimes

- Theft of artwork: 20 years
- Arson: 10 years
- Nonviolent terrorist offenses: 8 years
- Kidnapping or child abuse: the longer of 10 years or the victim's life

BOX 1.8 How to Read a Case Citation

Plaintiff's name v. Defendant's name, volume number, name of reporter, series number, page number (court name, year).

plaintiff is listed first in the caption and the defendant is listed after the versus *(v.)*, such as *Alexis and Brett Kyle v. Alexandra Hospital.* Box 1.8 describes how cases are named.

In most cases, responsibility rests on the plaintiff to prove his or her case, as opposed to the defendant. For violations of criminal law, the government must bring charges or file a claim against an individual or individuals. The government has the burden of proof, which is the legal responsibility and requirement to prove the claim is true and must present enough evidence to prove guilt beyond a reasonable doubt.

For violations of civil laws, the party that files a lawsuit against another party has the burden of proof. The burden of proof in civil law must prove a "preponderance of evidence," or must produce evidence beyond the balance of probabilities. In the case of negligence, the case may be decided by a judge to be ***res ipsa loquitur***, which means in Latin "the thing speaks for itself." ***Res ipsa loquitur*** is a doctrine of law in which one is presumed to be negligent if he or she had exclusive control of whatever caused the injury, even though there is no specific evidence of an act of negligence, and without negligence the accident would not have happened. It indicates that the defendant had the responsibility or duty to the plaintiff and that the injury would not and could not have occurred without the negligence of the defendant.

Pretrial Discovery

Before trial, both parties have strategies for gathering information in preparation for the trial; this is called the discovery process. These discovery strategies include the following:

1. Interrogatories are written questions that must be answered in writing under oath, sent by one party to another. They are part of the discovery process to prepare for mediation, settlement, or trial.
2. **Requests for production of documents** are submitted to the opposing party to produce specified documents or items that are pertinent to the issues of the case, such as medical records or policies and procedures.
3. Admissions of fact ask the opposing party (in writing) to admit or deny any material fact or the authenticity of documents to be introduced into evidence at trial.

CONCLUSION

This chapter provides a brief introduction to the terms and concepts of the law and legal system in the United States. Many of the concepts discussed in this chapter will be discussed and further explored in more detail in subsequent chapters, especially about how these laws directly affect healthcare professionals and the delivery of patient care.

APPLY THIS

A 75-year-old patient at a licensed, long-term care facility suffers from diabetes, dementia, coronary artery disease, and immobile decubitus ulcers (bedsores). She is unable to walk, talk, or feed herself. Her physician prescribed a daily whirlpool bath as a medical treatment for the decubitus ulcers. The facility does not have a whirlpool, so the patient was given regular daily baths instead. A certified nursing assistant (CNA) prepared a bath for the patient and placed her in hot water that was 128°F, which subsequently caused severe burns. As a result of the burns, the patient developed a bacterial infection and died 3 days later of sepsis. A wrongful death lawsuit was brought against the long-term care facility. The parties settled before the trial for $1.5 million.

4. Who would have been named in this lawsuit?
5. How could the patient's death have been prevented? How could a safer environment have been provided?
6. Define and describe the four elements of negligence in this case.

Source: Strine v. Commonwealth of Pennsylvania et al., 894 A.2d 733 (Pa. 2006).

CHAPTER REVIEW QUESTIONS

1. Which of the following is not a branch of the government?
   A. appeals
   B. executive
   C. judicial
   D. legislative
2. The highest court is the
   A. criminal court.
   B. state court.
   C. appeals court.
   D. supreme court.
3. One of the four elements of negligence is
   A. dereliction of duty.
   B. deliberate act.
   C. the defendant.
   D. standard of care.
4. A law that has the court's decision based on a verdict from a previous case is called a(n)
   A. administrative law
   B. common law
   C. constitutional law.
   D. statutory law.
5. The purpose of the *checks and balances* system in government is
   A. to allow the executive branch to veto any laws and prevent their passage.
   B. to ensure laws are passed in a timely manner.
   C. to avoid any one branch from having too much power.
   D. to allow one or two branches the power to pass laws.
6. The statute of limitations refers to
   A. the amount of time it takes to go to trial.
   B. the amount of time someone must file a lawsuit.
   C. the sentencing given in a lawsuit.
   D. the amount of time a defendant must respond to a plaintiff.
7. The civil cases seen in courts are suits that may involve
   A. criminal acts.
   B. kidnapping.
   C. theft.
   D. negligence.
8. The term ________ means that a specific legal issue was settled in another similar case, setting a precedent.
   A. *res ipsa loquitur*
   B. malpractice
   C. tort
   D. *stare decisis*
9. *In rem* jurisdiction means the court has jurisdiction over
   A. civil law cases.
   B. malpractice cases.
   C. property.
   D. appeals only.
10. The Latin term for wrongdoing or violation of civil law is
    A. *res ipsa loquitur.*
    B. *writ of certiorari.*
    C. *tortus.*
    D. *stare decisis.*

SELF-REFLECTION QUESTIONS

1. Discuss the purpose and goals of the law.
2. Discuss examples of why laws must change and adapt to society.
3. Discuss how the various sources of law might affect one another.
4. Describe the differences among civil, criminal, and administrative law.
5. Discuss why statutes of limitations are important.

INTERNET ACTIVITIES

1. Determine the statute of limitations for medical malpractice lawsuits in your state.
2. Investigate the medical practice acts for your state online and review procedures for licensing.

ADDITIONAL RESOURCES

http://www.findlaw.com

http://www.lexisone.com or www.lexisnexis.com/community/portal/ (To research cases a fee is charged. Other information from the site is still free.)

http://www.usa.gov

http://www.definitions.uslegal.com

http://www.uscourts.gov

https://www.uscourts.gov/about-federal-courts/educational-resources

https://www.archives.gov/research/alic/reference/law.html

2

Basis and Principles of Ethics

CHAPTER OBJECTIVES

1. Define ethics and explain the different branches of ethics.
2. Examine the importance of ethics in health care.
3. Understand the differences between ethics, morals, and values.
4. Describe the importance of a code of ethics for healthcare professionals.
5. Describe the difference between standards of practice and standards of care.
6. Relate specific ethical theories to healthcare situations.
7. Apply one of the ethical decision-making models to a specific ethical healthcare dilemma.
8. Explain the function of an ethics committee and risk management.

KEY TERMS

Accreditation Process of officially recognizing a person or organization for meeting the standards and qualification in an area based on preestablished industry criteria.

Code of ethics Standards of behavior, initiated by an employer or organization, defining the acceptable conduct of its members/employees (also called *code of conduct*).

Common ethics Also called group ethics, a system of principles and rules of conduct accepted by a group or culture.

Duty-based ethics (deontology) Philosophy of ethics that focuses on performing one's duty to a group, individual, or organization.

Ethics Branch of philosophy that relates to principles, rules, and standards that govern a person's behavior and decisions.

Integrity Unwavering adherence to an individual's values and principles with a dedication to high standards.

Justice-based ethics Ethical philosophy based on all individuals having equal rights.

Medical ethics A field of ethics that specifically addresses how to handle issues arising out of the care of patients and focuses on the healthcare professional's duty to the patient.

Medical practice acts Laws defined by each state that regulate the licensing and medical laws for that state and define the scope of practice for licensed and unlicensed individuals in the healthcare field.

Morals Standards of right and wrong.

Personal ethics A type of ethics determined by what an individual believes about morality and right and wrong.

Professional ethics A type of ethics that aims to define, clarify, and criticize professional work and its typical values.

Rights-based ethics Philosophy of ethics based on the theory of the rights of each individual (autonomy).

Standard of care Basic skill and care expected of healthcare professionals in the same or similar branch of medicine; based on what another medical professional would deem to be appropriate in similar circumstances.

Standards of practice Officially sanctioned description of the specific procedures, actions, and processes that are permitted for a licensed or unlicensed professional; based on the specific state's laws for education and experience requirements, plus demonstrated competency. Established by the state's laws, licensing board, and/or agency regulations.

Utilitarianism Ethical theory based on the greatest good for the greatest number (also known as cost–benefit analysis).

Values Principles that individuals choose to follow in their lives.

Virtue-based ethics Ethical theory or philosophy that relies on the principle that individuals share and will hold as their governing principle the values of moral behavior and character.

INTRODUCTION

As members of a society, we generally understand how to act and behave in terms of right and wrong, moral and immoral, and good and bad. This is all based on ethics. The study of ethics is also a necessary part of preparing for a career in the healthcare field. Healthcare professionals often face dilemmas that the general population may not encounter, such as illness and death. These situations will require critical thinking, the ability to be objective, and an understanding of the laws and ethics that govern their profession.

Most healthcare professionals are accountable to a healthcare provider or a hospital, but this does not exclude them from personal responsibility. Understanding the laws and standards of practice will help every healthcare professional make legal and sound decisions when confronted with an ethical situation or dilemma.

WHAT IS ETHICS?

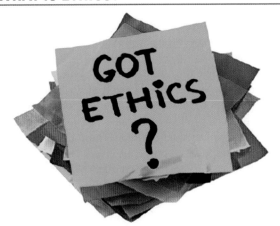

(Copyright © marekuliasz/iStock/Thinkstock.com.)

Ethics is often difficult to define, although many people associate ethics with their feelings or personal beliefs. However, ethics may be very different from these. In fact, often behaving ethically may contrast with an individual's feelings or beliefs and even with what is considered lawful.

The word "ethics" comes from a Greek term meaning "duty." In general, **ethics** are the rules, standards, and moral principles that govern a person's behavior and on which the person bases decisions on. Ethics is concerned with questions of how individuals in a society should act by defining right and wrong and appropriate conduct to serve the greater good (Box 2.1).

Ethics encompasses several different facets. One aspect is **morals**, which describes the goodness or badness or right or wrong of actions. Similarly, **values**, or an individual's ethics, refer to one person's moral principles or what an individual believes is right or wrong. Values govern a person's decisions, with a goal of maintaining one's integrity or conscience. An individual's values may be influenced by concepts of honesty, fidelity, equality, compassion, responsibility, humility, and respect for life.

There may be circumstances in which a proposed action is not necessarily against a code of ethics or ethical standard, but it may be an **integrity** issue, which may challenge one's personal values. Integrity is based on one's personal values or moral principles, which may be of higher or different standards than those outlined in a particular principle or law. In ethics, integrity is the honesty and truthfulness of one's actions. For example,

BOX 2.1 Importance of Ethics

- Ethics is a basic requirement for human life.
- It helps in decision-making regarding course of action.
- It helps promote harmony and teamwork.
- It helps enhance public image and credibility.
- It assists in complying with laws and regulations.
- It helps in organizing goals and actions.
- It is the basis for long-term success.

a nurse may be strongly opposed to abortion, but the facility where the nurse is employed may legally perform abortions. This would then become an integrity issue for the nurse but not one for the facility.

DISCUSSION

Which of the following qualities do you think are the most important in the healthcare field?

- Honesty
- Fidelity
- Integrity
- Justice
- Respect
- Empathy
- Sympathy
- Responsibility
- Fairness
- Sanctity of life
- Equality
- Compassion
- Humility

TYPES OF ETHICS

There are many types and fields in ethics, including personal, common, and professional. **Personal ethics** determines what an individual believes about morality and right and wrong. It includes one's personal values and moral qualities and is influenced by family, friends, culture, religion, education, and many other factors. Personal ethics has an impact on areas of life such as family, finances and relationships and may change during one's life. An example of one's personal ethics may be for a person to believe in the death penalty but support a woman's right to an abortion.

Common ethics, also called group ethics, is a system of principles and rules of conduct accepted by a group based on ethnicity, political affiliation, or cultural identity. An example of common ethics is for a person who is religious to believe all abortion and the death penalty is bad and all life should be preserved.

Professional ethics is a type of ethics that aims to define, clarify, and criticize professional work and its typical values. Professional ethics sets the standards for practicing one's profession and can be learned only through education, training, or on the job. It involves attributes such as commitment, competence, confidence, and contract. Professional ethics is often used to impose rules and standards on employees in an organization or members of a profession. Examples of professional ethics are in employee handbooks, code of ethics, and the Hippocratic Oath taken by physicians.

MEDICAL ETHICS

As discussed in Chapter 1, the law provides a standard by which to measure an individual's actions and to punish those who would violate it. Many actions punishable by law are also considered morally wrong, such as murder and theft. However, the law does not effectively address other ethical or moral offenses, such as adultery or gambling. Thus, a healthcare professional's actions and behaviors should not rely solely on the law but also on ethical and moral decision making.

A healthcare professional's conduct and behavior are based on the branch or field of ethics called **medical ethics**. Medical ethics is the morals, moral principles, and moral judgments that healthcare professionals use to determine whether an action should be allowed based on "right and wrong." In addition to examining facts, medical ethics uses moral analysis to assess the obligations and responsibilities of healthcare professionals on various issues and challenges related to health care and medicine. It specifically addresses how to handle ethical issues arising from the care of patients and focuses on the healthcare professional's duty to the patient.

The basic principles of medical ethics are:

- *Autonomy*
  The capacity to think, decide, and act on one's own free will and initiative. The patient's decision-making process must be free of coercion or coaxing. Healthcare professionals should help patients come to their own decisions by providing full information.
- *Justice*
  The principle that ethics should be based on what is consistent and fair to all involved. Patients in similar situations should have access to the same care. Healthcare professionals must consider four main areas when evaluating justice: fair distribution of scarce resources, competing needs, rights and obligations, and potential conflicts with established legislation.
- *Beneficence*
  The general moral principle of doing the "most good" or doing what is best for patients. This must consider the patients' pain, their physical and mental suffering, the risk of disability and death, and their quality of life. What is best for the patient may be in agreement or disagreement with the health

professional's clinical judgment and the patient's wishes (see Autonomy).

- *Nonmaleficence*
  This is the principle of "do no harm" to the patient or to the fewest number of people in society. It is difficult for healthcare providers to always apply successfully the "do no harm" principle because, for example, most treatments involve some degree of risk or adverse effects.

As we continue in our discussion of medical ethics, consider how these basic principles are applied and how they can often agree or disagree with one another.

APPLY THIS

A medical assistant is working in a family practice clinic when a patient requires an immunization. The physician takes the medical assistant aside and explains that it is a particularly busy day because the nurse has called in sick. The physician asks the medical assistant to administer the injection so she can proceed to the next patient. The medical assistant explains that it is not within the scope of practice in the state for her to administer an injection. The physician insists, saying she will take that responsibility.

1. What should the medical assistant do?
2. Is this an ethic or legal dilemma? Or both?

Codes of Ethics

Almost all businesses and professional organizations have a code of ethics. A code of ethics or code of conduct consists of all the obligations that an employer expect their employees to respect and follow when carrying out their duties. It includes the core values of the organization and profession, as well as the behavior that should be adopted. Usually, a healthcare organization or clinic's code of ethics will include policies on treating patients with dignity and respect and respecting patient confidentiality. To practice competently and with integrity, all healthcare professionals must have regulation and guidance within the profession. Any violation of the code of ethics may result in sanctions, corrective action, and even termination of employment.

Medical Codes of Ethics

As discussed earlier, many professions have their own code of ethics, including health care. One of the first and most known medical code of ethics is the Hippocratic Oath, written in 400 BC by Hippocrates, a Greek physician, who is considered "the father of medicine" (Fig. 2.1). The Hippocratic Oath is traditionally taken by new physicians whereby they pledge to prescribe only beneficial treatments, according to their abilities and judgment; to refrain from causing harm or hurt; and to live an exemplary personal and professional life.

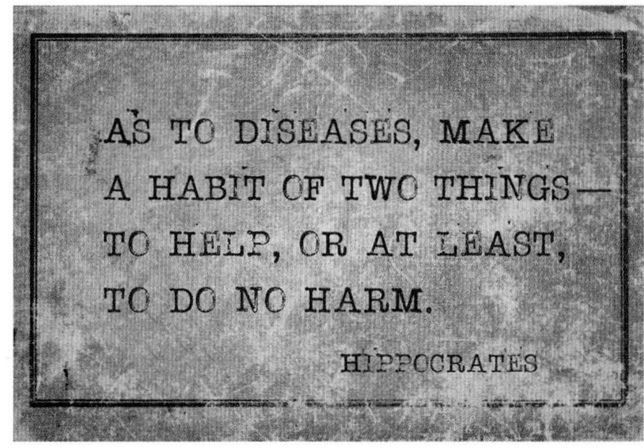

Fig. 2.1 Hippocrates is considered the "father of medicine" and the medical code of ethics for physicians is named after, the Hippocratic Oath. (iStock.com/yuriz.)

In 1847, the American Medical Association (AMA), which is the country's largest physician group and currently representing more than 240,000 members, adopted its own more encompassing and more contemporary code of medical ethics for physicians called the *Code of Medical Ethics.* The AMA's *Code of Medical Ethics* is periodically reviewed and updated, with the newest edition adopted in June 2016 to better reflect the changing demographics, technological advancements, and new laws and regulations.

Ethics in the nursing profession can be traced back to the 19th century. The first formal code of ethics to guide the nursing profession was developed in the 1950s. Developed and published by the American Nurses Association (ANA), it guides nurses in their daily practice and sets primary goals and values for the profession. Its function is to provide a statement of the ethical obligations and duties of every individual who enters the nursing profession. It provides a nonnegotiable ethical standard and is an expression of nursing's own understanding of its commitment to society. The code of ethics has been revised over time, and the current version represents advances in technology, societal changes, expansion of nursing practice into advanced practice roles, research, education, health policy, and administration, and builds and maintains healthy work environments (Box 2.2).

BOX 2.2 The Code of Ethics for Nurses

Provision 1. The nurse practices with compassion and respect for the inherent dignity, worth, and unique attributes of every person.

Provision 2. The nurse's primary commitment is to the patient, whether an individual, family, group, community, or population.

Provision 3. The nurse promotes, advocates for, and protects the rights, health, and safety of the patient.

Provision 4. The nurse has authority, accountability, and responsibility for nursing practice; makes decisions; and takes action consistent with the obligation to provide optimal patient care.

Provision 5. The nurse owes the same duties to self as to others, including the responsibility to promote health and safety, preserve wholeness of character and integrity, maintain competence, and continue personal and professional growth.

Provision 6. The nurse, through individual and collective effort, establishes, maintains, and improves the ethical environment of the work setting and conditions of employment that are conducive to safe, quality health care.

Provision 7. The nurse, in all roles and settings, advances the profession through research and scholarly inquiry, professional standards development, and the generation of both nursing and health policy.

Provision 8. The nurse collaborates with other health professionals and the public to protect human rights, promote health diplomacy, and reduce health disparities.

Provision 9. The profession of nursing, collectively through its professional organization, must articulate nursing values, maintain the integrity of the profession, and integrate principles of social justice into nursing and health policy.

In addition to the AMA and ANA, other healthcare professions and professional organizations have established their own code of ethics, including the American Association of Medical Assistants (AAMA) for medical assistants and the American Academy of Professional Coders (AAPC) for medical billers and coders. (See Additional Resources for further information on examples of the Hippocratic Oath and other codes of ethics.)

Standards of Practice and Standards of Care

Similar to a code of ethics, many healthcare professions have established their own set of ethical and professional principles in a **standard of practice**. Standards of practice, sometimes called *scope of practice,* refer to the professional activities defined under state law. They describe the procedures, actions, and processes that a healthcare practitioner is permitted to undertake in keeping with the terms of his or her professional license. The standards of practice are limited by the provisions of the law required for education, experience, and demonstrated competency.

Healthcare professionals, such as physicians, nurses, pharmacists, social workers, dietitians, physical therapists, and emergency medical technicians (EMTs), all have standards of practice guidelines that are determined by **medical practice acts** established in each state. These medical practice acts establish and govern licensing boards, determine requirements for education and training, and define the scope of practice for healthcare professionals in their respective field. Working within the guidelines of the scope of practice can protect the professional from liability. Conversely, if a healthcare professional acts outside the scope of practice of his or her profession or field, that professional would be considered legally liable if any personal harm or injury occurs.

Different from the standard of practice is the **standard of care**. The standard of care sets minimum criteria for job proficiency and establishes basic requirements for skill and care commonly used and expected of the healthcare professional of that same or similar branch of medicine. It establishes what another healthcare professional would deem to be appropriate in similar circumstances. For example, it would be a standard of care that a nurse would use a new needle every time she performs an injection on a patient. This is a practice that would commonly be practiced or expected, and that a "reasonable person" in that profession would do. Often, standard of care is used to determine medical liability and malpractice lawsuits.

APPLY THIS

On a particularly busy day at the clinic, a medical assistant is performing a patient intake for a new patient. He decides to skip over parts of the medical history, including the section on drug allergies. On a follow-up visit, the patient is prescribed penicillin for an infection. A few days later, the patient calls the clinic complaining of a rash, hives, itchiness, and a swollen lip, most likely a reaction to the penicillin.

1. What did the medical assistant do wrong?
2. Was this a violation of the standard of practice, standard of care, or both?

ETHICAL DECISION MAKING

Now that we have discussed what ethics is, how we do practice it? Because ethics is not based on feelings, religion, or even the law, how do we know how to act ethically? How can we make the best ethical decisions? The next sections will discuss the different types of ethical models and theories for ethical decision making and how they can be incorporated into the healthcare profession.

Ethical Theories

Most ethical theories are based on common or group ethics principles. Philosophers have developed these theories over the years to explore their effects on individual and group behavior. In fact, many of these theories are the basis for many of our current laws and regulations.

Although there are several different theories on ethics, most fall into one of the following categories: utilitarianism (teleology), duty-based ethics (deontology), rights-based ethics, justice-based ethics, and virtue-based ethics (see the below box).

ETHICAL THEORIES

Utilitarianism (teleology)	The greatest good for the greatest number
Duty-based ethics (deontology)	The obligation of the individual to fulfill his or her responsibilities
Rights-based ethics	Based on an individual's rights
Justice-based ethics	No special advantages or disadvantages to certain individuals
Virtue-based ethics	Actions are based on the individual's character

Utilitarianism (Teleology)

One of the most known ethical theories is **utilitarianism**. This is a type of consequence-focused theory known as teleology, or that duty or moral obligation from which what is good or desirable needs to be achieved. Thus, utilitarianism bases the decision making on the greatest good for the greatest number. This theory is based on either the greatest benefit to the general population or the best total outcome and not on the process. It is also referred to as "the ends justifying the means." It therefore does not always consider the "means," or the method or process, but instead the general outcome: What will benefit the greatest number of people?

The utilitarian model is often used in a cost–benefit analysis, which is a systematic approach that takes into consideration the cost of resources vs. the overall benefit. Utilitarianism is used to determine the most efficient use of resources—the best value for the least number of resources—and looks beyond individual effects to overall benefits. For example, this theory may be used in determining the allocation of organ donations. Owing to high need and shortage of organ donations, policies must be developed to evaluate and decide who should be placed on an organ waiting list vs. those who are not eligible.

DISCUSSION

A neurology practice is interested in investing in a new piece of equipment, an electromyogram (EMG) machine, which would be used for nerve conduction testing. The new EMG machine would cost $20,000. The practice estimates that with the machine it would be able to perform 20 EMGs per month and charge $500 for each testing. However, the practice budgeted to give raises to its five employees this year, which be $90,000.

1. Based on the utilitarianism theory, what would be the best option?
2. What would be the cost–benefit analysis to purchasing the machine vs. giving raises to the employees instead?

Duty-Based Ethics (Deontology)

The **duty-based ethical** theory is based on the duty of an individual to a society, group, or organization. It focuses solely on the obligation of the individual to perform his or her responsibility, no matter what the circumstances. The general principles include impartial thinking with respect to individuals as not being the "ends justify the means" but absolute rules that should be obeyed. In other words, it is the duty of an individual to adhere to universal rules and regulations, regardless of circumstances.

The problem with the duty-based ethical theory is that not all "duties" are defined that simply—it does not take into account the conflicting duties that may arise. For example, a nurse is responsible for taking vital signs of each of her patients every 4 h, a duty she must perform regardless of the situation. However, one day, one of the nurse's patients has a cardiac arrest and the nurse must perform cardiopulmonary resuscitation and spends the next several hours making sure the patient is stable. As a result, the nurse misses the 4-h timeframe and has violated her duty to take vital signs for the rest of her patients. This theory is based on impartial judgment and does not take into consideration the consequences. Thus, as we see, it may cause additional dilemmas if duties are conflicting.

Rights-Based Ethics

The rights-based ethical theory is based on the individual's rights. The emphasis is on the individual and does not always take the consequences to the general population into consideration. For example, the right of free speech and the right to bear arms are upheld by the U.S. Constitution. These laws protect the individual's rights, although they may conflict with the rights of a society—upholding an individual's right to bear arms vs. the need for gun control regulations to keep firearms out of the hands of irresponsible, dangerous, or mentally unstable individuals. Under this principle, the individual's rights must be respected even when this may be contradictory to society's rights.

DISCUSSION

Under the First Amendment to the U.S. Constitution, an individual has the right to freedom of religion and to practice that religion. However, in the healthcare setting, there may be situations in which the religious rights of the patients and/or the family members may conflict with the healthcare provider's medical advice and recommended treatment.

1. How does a physician handle a case in which a child needs a blood transfusion to save his life, yet the parents' religious beliefs do not allow blood transfusions?
2. Using the rights-based ethical model, should the physician respect the religious beliefs of the parents and allow the child to die?
3. Or does the physician respect the child's right to life, despite parental beliefs?

Justice-Based Ethics

The justice-based ethical theory is based on the idea that "justice is blind"—all individuals should be treated with impartiality, and no individual should have advantages over or disadvantages relative to other individuals. John Rawls, the philosopher who wrote extensively on the theory of justice, believed that the justice-based theory would prevent unfairness and injustice under social contracts. One individual should not have a greater chance over another. For example, a person should not be placed higher on an organ donor list over another person just because that person has more money or resources (Fig. 2.2).

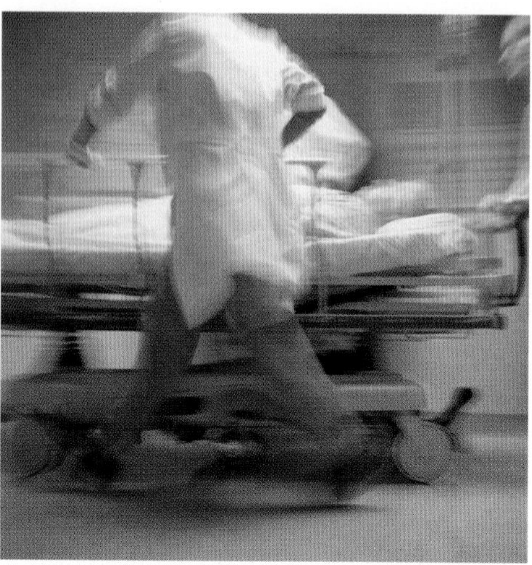

Fig. 2.2 Justice-based ethics is meant to prevent injustice under social contracts, such as the distribution of organ donations. One individual should not have a greater advantage over another. (Copyright © Ryan McVay/Digital Vision/Thinkstock.com.)

DISCUSSION

More than 32 countries, including the United Kingdom, Germany, and France, have some form of universal health care, sometime referred to as *socialized medicine*. Under this system of health care, all citizens of a country are provided medical and hospital care by means of public or government funds. Thus, theoretically, all individuals are treated equally, and no individual can gain advantage over another based on income, age, race, or employment status. Central to this system of health care is the belief in fairness and justice for all. However, the idea of universal health care is controversial.

1. Is it the government's responsibility to care for its citizens, including providing health care? What role should it have?
2. Do we have a moral or ethical obligation to provide health care to everyone as needed?
3. Is it fair or unfair for the healthy, rich, or employed to be burdened or help pay to support the unhealthy, poor, and unemployed?

Virtue-Based Ethics

The virtue-based ethical theory places an emphasis on the characteristic traits and qualities of individuals. This theory places less emphasis on the rules people should follow and instead focuses on helping people develop good characteristic traits, such as kindness, generosity, honesty, and integrity. These character traits will, in turn, allow an individual to make the correct decisions.

Ethical Decision-Making Models

After our discussion on ethical theories and principles, how do we put them to practice so they can help in our decision making? Ethical decisions should not be based on emotions. Ethical dilemmas should be decided on according to logic and facts, weighing the alternatives and the consequences, and keeping an objective mind. The following models are commonly used to evaluate and resolve ethical dilemmas.

The Seven-Step Decision-Making Model

The seven-step decision-making model was developed by the philosopher Michael Davis, who believed that relying on a model or guide will result in stronger "moral reasoning skills." A key feature of Davis' approach is his emphasis on identifying multiple options for responding to ethical dilemmas. There are many different versions of the seven-step decision-making model, but all have the same objective: to identify the facts of the dilemma and to use this guide to assess all the viable options in a thorough and objective manner.

1. Determine all the facts of the situation—what, when, where, who, and why.
2. Determine the exact ethical issue involved.
3. Determine the rules, laws, principles, or values that are involved.
4. List all viable options or courses of action.
5. Determine all the advantages and disadvantages of each option.
6. Determine all the possible consequences and who would be affected by the options.
7. Determine which decision is best and act on that decision.

Depending on the situation, these steps may all be done by one individual or by a group of individuals. For example, some hospitals may have an ethics committee that would work together to evaluate a situation. One member of the committee may have just one of these steps to complete, and then all members involved would convene to determine the best course of action. This may be accomplished in collaboration with a risk management team or a quality assurance team, which will be discussed later in this chapter.

Dr. Bernard Lo Clinical Model

The second ethical decision-making model is one developed by Dr. Bernard Lo, a physician who has written extensively on ethical issues concerning end-of-life care, stem cell research, oversight of human participants research, the doctor–patient relationship, and conflicts of interest. Dr. Lo's model is designed to take into consideration both the patient's and healthcare provider's points of view. The steps in the model include the following:

1. Gather information—Patient's mental status, comorbidities, assessments from the other healthcare professional for the patient, and other issues that might complicate the patient's case.
2. Clarify the ethical issue—What is the ethical issue and what does it involve? What principles should be employed used, and what are the ramifications of the possible courses of treatment?
3. Resolve the dilemma—List all available options and discuss with all the patient's healthcare professionals; negotiate the best viable options. If the patient is mentally competent, include the patient in the decision-making process.

Blanchard–Peale Model

According to Kenneth Blanchard and Norman Vincent Peale, authors of The Power of Ethical Management, answering the following three questions sequentially will help you determine if a decision is ethical:

1. *Is it legal?*
   Will it be violating criminal or civil law or company policy? Will I be violating any code of conduct?
2. *Is it fair and balanced?*
   Is it fair to all parties concerned both in the short-term as well as the long-term? Does it or can it result in a win-win situation?
3. *How does it make me feel?*
   Will it make me proud? Would I feel good if my family or others knew about it?

Answering yes to any or all the questions is not a guarantee that an ethical decision will be reached.

However, you should feel more confident that you have made a good-faith effort to make an ethical decision.

ETHICS COMMITTEES AND QUALITY ASSURANCE

Ethics Committees

Most hospitals and large medical facilities have an ethics committee comprised of physicians, nurses, social workers, chaplains, and members of the community. Ethics committees are used to address and resolve difficult ethical issues (Fig. 2.3). Some members of the ethics committee do not generally see or speak with the patients themselves, so they can focus solely on the facts involved in the situation. This helps them make ethical determinations on the issues or cases presented to them based on logic and the codes and standards, as opposed to emotions.

In addition to facilitating decision-making in individual cases (as a committee or through the activities of individual members functioning as ethics consultants), many ethics committees assist ethics-related educational programming and policy development within their institutions (Box 2.3).

APPLY THIS

Is it ethical for an ethics committee to make a life-and-death decision for patients without even interviewing them? Why or why not?

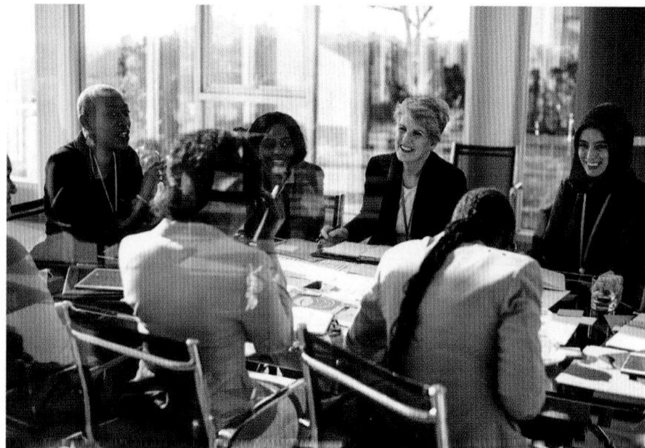

Fig. 2.3 Many healthcare organizations have ethics committees to address and resolve difficult ethical issues. (Istock.com/Rawpixel.)

Risk Management and Quality Assurance

Almost all clinics, hospitals, and large healthcare facilities have a risk management or quality assurance team or department. These departments are created to evaluate and prevent situations that may result in ethical dilemmas and legal issues. They evaluate patient satisfaction, patient complaints, and treatment outcomes. These departments focus on the prevention and quality assurance and recommend improvements for noncompliant healthcare facilities (Box 2.4).

Accreditation

Another method of quality assurance in establishing and maintaining a standard of practice is **accreditation**. Accreditation is a process of officially recognizing

BOX 2.3 Issues for Healthcare Ethics Committees

- advance directives
- do not resuscitate processes
- patient refusal of services
- "Baby Doe" guidelines
- withholding life sustaining treatment
- patient–caregiver confidentiality
- medical futility
- admission and discharge considerations
- family communications
- nutrition and hydration
- organ donation

BOX 2.4 Healthcare Risk Management Examples

- Evaluate and audit records for completeness, accuracy, and compliance to prevent any situations of insurance fraud and billing abuse
- Use of hand sanitizer to minimize the risk of spreading infections to patients
- Color-coded signs and walkways so visitors can navigate through the building without entering dangerous or hazardous areas
- Developing harassment-related training and policies to staff to ensure codes of conduct
- A cybersecurity system to protect confidential health data from being compromised or manipulated

a person or organization for meeting the standards in an area based on preestablished industry criteria. Accreditation is generally performed by an external body to evaluate services and operations of an institution or program to determine whether applicable standards and regulatory regulations are met. If standards and regulations are met, accredited status is granted by the appropriate agency.

Many healthcare facilities and organizations maintain voluntary participation with accreditation organizations, which routinely examine the organization or facility to verify that the standards of care and procedures of the organizations are in compliance. Although there are many different accrediting bodies, the most common one for hospitals, laboratories, nursing homes, and ambulatory health clinics is The Joint Commission (TJC). TJC accredits more than 21,000 healthcare organizations and programs in the United States. In addition to TJC, there are other healthcare accreditation organizations, such as the Accreditation Commission for Health Care, Inc., the Community Health Accreditation Program, and the Healthcare Facilities Accreditation Program.

DISCUSSION

According to the Organ Procurement and Transplantation Network, there are approximately 107,000 people who need a life-saving organ transplant with only 39,000 transplants were performed in 2020. Often, an ethics committee must decide who is placed on the waiting list for an organ donation and who will not be.

1. Who do you think should be included on the ethics committee in this decision? How should they decide?
2. What factors or qualities should the committee consider to qualify a person for an organ transplant?

CONCLUSION

All members of the healthcare profession, in whatever capacity they are working, must understand their responsibility to themselves, their employers, and their patients. They must uphold the highest standards of ethical behavior and professionalism. Using the described ethical models and principles and putting them into practice will alleviate a considerable degree of emotional stress and aid the healthcare professional in making the best possible decisions.

CHAPTER REVIEW QUESTIONS

1. An example of utilitarianism would be the
   A. decision of which patients should receive immunizations if supplies are limited.
   B. decision of employees' rights in a work resolution.
   C. decision of what was fair in a given work resolution case.
   D. decision in a malpractice suit of responsibility in the case.
2. Almost all professions and organizations have standards of behavior for their employees called
   A. applied ethics.
   B. code of ethics.
   C. medical ethics.
   D. medical law.
3. What does an ethics committee handle?
   A. Decisions on possible violations of codes of ethics
   B. Decisions on workplace rights
   C. Decisions on hiring practices
   D. Legal decisions on scope of practice
4. What are values?
   A. Principles by which an individual chooses to live
   B. Moral guidelines for the workplace
   C. Manners and etiquette
   D. Workplace hiring guidelines
5. What is autonomy?
   A. An individual's right to make decisions for one's own life
   B. Group ethics guideline
   C. Accreditation
   D. Risk management principle
6. A person knows it is illegal to steal but steals food because she is hungry. Which types of ethics is this?
   A. common ethics
   B. professional ethics
   C. personal ethics
   D. group ethics

7. The basic principles of medical ethics include all the following *except*
   A. do no harm
   B. justice
   C. autonomy
   D. standard of care
8. The concept that a "reasonable person" in a particular profession would be expected to do or act is called the
   A. standard of care
   B. standard of practice
   C. medical practice act
   D. Scope of practice
9. In the Blanchard–Peale Model for ethical decision making, which of the following questions do you not need to ask?
   A. Is it legal?
   B. What are my options?
   C. Is it fair?
   D. How does it make me feel?
10. A nurse is assigned to do her first rounds with her patients before lunchtime. She is running late and decides to skip her lunch to complete her rounds. This is an example of
    A. duty-based ethics
    B. rights-based ethics
    C. justice-based ethics

SELF-REFLECTION QUESTIONS

1. What kinds of ethical situations would be particularly challenging or difficult for me to encounter?
2. What would I do if my best friend became my co-worker and I witnessed him or her doing something unethical at work?
3. Which of the principles of ethics is the most important to me?
4. Which of the ethical theories do I find most agreeable?
5. Using an ethical dilemma you create, select one of the two decision-making models discussed in this chapter to determine the best course of action.

INTERNET ACTIVITIES

1. Research several different codes of ethics models that apply to your field and develop your own model.
2. Research online the different versions of the Hippocratic Oath and discuss why there are different versions.
3. Research one of the nations that provide universal health care. Compare the similarities and differences between that healthcare system and the U.S. health-care system.

ADDITIONAL RESOURCES

Organ Procurement and Transplantation Network—Ethics Committee https://optn.transplant.hrsa.gov/

https://optn.transplant.hrsa.gov/about/committees/ethics-committee/

The Hippocratic Oath: https://www.nlm.nih.gov/hmd/greek/greek_oath.html

https://www.ascensionhealth.org/components/com_filesandlinks/uploads/96_clinical_ethics.pdf

The American Medical Association's code of Medical Ethics: https://www.ama-assn.org/delivering-care/ethics/code-medical-ethics-overview

National Commission for Health Education Credentialing's Code of Ethics: https://www.nchec.org/code-of-ethics

BIBLIOGRAPHY

Lo, B. (2009). *Resolving ethical dilemmas: A guide for clinicians* (4th ed.). Philadelphia: Lippincott Williams & Wilkins.

Peale, N. V., & Blanchard, K. (1988). *The power of ethical management* (1st ed., p. 27). New York: William Morrow.

3

Bioethical Issues in Health Care

CHAPTER OBJECTIVES

1. Define the term bioethics.
2. Discuss bioethical issues involved in clinical trials.
3. Describe the ethical principles in medical research.
4. List the different types of genetic testing.
5. Describe ethical considerations for healthcare professionals in issues of gene therapy and stem cell research.
6. Explain what genetic discrimination is and what defines it.

KEY TERMS

Bioethics A field of ethics that examines the ethical, social, and legal issues that arise from advances in medicine, medical research, and science.

Chromosomes Threadlike structures in the center of the cell (nucleus) that transmit the genetic information about the person.

Clinical trials A type of medical research that involves patients or human subjects.

Clones Duplicate cell reproduced artificially from a natural, original single cell.

Conflict of interest An occurrence when self-interest affects an individual's professional obligations to one's patients, organization, and/or profession.

Control group Also called nontherapeutic group, test subjects in a research study who do not receive any treatment or, in some cases, are given a placebo. In testing, it is the principle of the constant that remains the same to evaluate the changes of a given experiment.

Double-blind study In testing, one group receives the placebo and the other group receives the new agent, which prevents either group from knowing who is receiving the real drug or the placebo.

Experimental group In testing, the group that receives the new, researched treatment agent.

Gene therapy Process of splicing or infusing genes to replace malfunctioning genes. Alteration of the DNA of body cells to control production of a particular substance.

Genetic discrimination A type of discrimination when people treat others differently because of their genetic information.

Genetic testing A type of medical test that identifies changes in genes, chromosomes, or proteins.

Human Genome Project Medical research program, sponsored by the federal government, established to map and sequence the number of genes that are within the 23 pairs of chromosomes (i.e., the 46 chromosomes) with the goal of advanced life-saving or disease-preventing treatments.

Informed consent A process when a detailed, listing and covering all possible risks and potential prognoses to patients or participants for having a treatment or procedure performed and the alternatives available.

Placebo Nontherapeutic drug or agent given to a control group (commonly referred to as a "sugar pill").

Stem cells Cells of the body that can control the production of specialized cells by becoming other types of cells as needed during growth or healing.

INTRODUCTION

Currently, much of our media exposure and knowledge concerning ethics in health care and medical research seems like science fiction. In fact, debates over controversies in ethics in this field often parallel science fiction discussions. As technology and medical research advances, they bring with them not only important discoveries but also challenges to the rights and privacy of their subjects. Ethical issues, such as cloning, stem cell research, eugenics, and advances in reproduction, are controversial issues that we are having to address now that were not even a part of our national dialogue a few decades ago.

BIOETHICS

Bioethics, or biomedical ethics, is a field of ethics that examines the ethical, social, and legal issues that arise from advances in medicine, medical research, and science. Bioethics is concerned about the determination of the rightness or wrongness of the discoveries and developed technologies in science, as well as the incorporation of human rights and values to health and life. As we discussed professional ethics and the importance of organizations having a code of ethics in Chapter 2, ethics also serve the aims or goals of research and apply to people who conduct scientific research or who work to advance medicine.

There are many reasons to have and adhere to bioethics in medical and scientific research. Bioethics ensures that researchers and research can be held accountable to the public. There are many federal policies and standards that must be met to prevent misconduct, conflicts of interest, and animal care and use and human subjects' rights in clinical trials. This is particularly necessary when the research is funded by public money.

Bioethics is important to ensuring the quality and integrity of the research and to prevent occurrences of fabrication and falsifying or misrepresenting research data. The research and findings that result from medical and scientific research must be valid and have integrity.

Bioethics also promotes moral and social values. This includes social responsibility, human rights, animal welfare, compliance with the law, and public health and safety. Researchers and research that do not adhere to the standards of bioethics may result in false and invalid data, harm or death to human and animal subjects, and loss of public trust in science and information.

MEDICAL AND SCIENTIFIC RESEARCH

Medical and scientific research is conducted to aid and support the development of knowledge in the field of medicine and science that can then be utilized to advance health care and improve a patient's quality of life. The knowledge gained from medical research can lessen the impact of our greatest diseases and disorders, including diabetes, cancer, and heart disease. It can provide valuable information about diseases and risk factors, outcomes of treatment, and healthcare costs and use. It can help determine efficacy and adverse effects of medical interventions, which is crucial for comparing and improving the use of drugs, vaccines, medical devices, and diagnostics.

For a life-saving drug to be used in the United States, the drug must be tested in clinical trials. **Clinical trials**, or clinical research, is a type of medical research that involves patients or human subjects. Clinical trials are research studies performed in people that are aimed at evaluating a medical, surgical, or behavioral intervention. They are the primary way that researchers find out if a new treatment, like a new drug or diet or medical device, is safe and effective in people. Often a clinical trial is used to learn if a new treatment is more effective and/or has less harmful side effects than the standard treatment. Other clinical trials test ways to find a disease early, sometimes before there are symptoms, while others test ways to prevent a health problem. A clinical trial may also look at how to make life better for people living with a life-threatening disease or a chronic health problem.

Clinical trials often recruit a few hundred to a few thousand patients, before being approved by the U.S. Food and Drug Administration (FDA). Thus, guidelines to include ethical principles must be in place so that medical research can be conducted.

To safeguard human rights and upholding ethical standards, many different professional associations, government agencies, and universities have adopted specific codes, rules, and policies relating to bioethics in medical and scientific research (Box 3.1).

BOX 3.1 Codes and Policies for Research Ethics

- National Institutes of Health (NIH)
- National Science Foundation (NSF)
- Food and Drug Administration (FDA)
- Environmental Protection Agency (EPA)
- Nuremberg Code
- World Medical Association's Declaration of Helsinki

Ethical principles in medical research should include the following:

- obtain informed consent from potential research participants
- minimize the risk of harm to all participants
- protect participants' anonymity and confidentiality
- give participants the right to withdraw from the research

Obtain Informed Consent

One of the most important concepts in health care is **informed consent**. Informed consent is to list and cover all possible risks and potential prognoses to patients or participants for having a treatment or procedure performed and the alternatives available. Specifically, in medical research, informed consent means that participants should understand that they are taking part in research and what the research requires of them.

Information should include the purpose of the research, the methods being used, the possible outcomes of the research, and any associated demands, discomforts, inconveniences, and risks that the participants may face. Participants in any medical research should be taking part without being coerced and deceived and with full knowledge.

Minimize the Risk of Harm

Although there may be the risk of unintentional harm in participating in medical research, great lengths should be taken to do no harm or minimize harm and discomfort to participants. All research using human and animal subjects raises ethical concerns because participants in research undergo risks of potential harm primarily, if not solely, for the benefit of others. Balancing benefit and risk of harm is an essential part of the design of any medical research.

Possible harms that may occur to participants are physical harm; psychological distress and discomfort; and invasion or violation of privacy, anonymity, and confidentiality. Where there is the possibility that participants could be harmed or put in a position of discomfort, there must be strong justifications for this.

DISCUSSION

No medical research or clinical trial is free of risk or adverse effects. There is always an element of risk involved, but the patients or subjects of the study should be fully informed of the risks and give full written consent. This is an example of the utilitarian theory of reasoning—that is, the greatest good for the greatest number would outweigh the risks involved for the study's subjects.

1. Based on the other ethical theories discussed, would the decision to enroll in a clinical trial be different than the utilitarian theory?
2. What risk would you be willing to take knowing that the clinical trial could help find a cure for cancer or other life-threatening diseases?

Protecting Privacy and Confidentiality

Protecting the privacy, anonymity, and confidentiality of participants in medical research is critical. Many clinical trials require participants to share personal information, including past and present health information.

Patient information that has been collected must be protected in terms of the storage of data, its analysis, and in any step or process in the clinical trial. This may mean removing identifying information from the patient information, such as their names and address, securing any information in computer systems, and only allowing authorized users to access patient information.

Provide the Right to Withdraw

There are many different types and designs for clinical trials. To maintain the integrity and objectivity of any research using human subjects, some clinical trials withhold information from patients. Participants may not know if they are in the experimental group or **control group**. Participants in the control group or nontherapeutic group receive a **placebo**, or a harmless pill with no therapeutic effect. Participants in the **experimental group**, or treatment group, receive the new, researched treatment agent (Fig. 3.1). This is called a **double-blind study**, because the participants do not know whether they are receiving the placebo or the new agent (Box 3.2).

Double-blind trials, also called double-masked studies, are considered the most ideal and produce more objective results since the researchers and the participant are both unaware and are less likely to affect the outcome. This helps to ensure that the subjects will not have any preconceptions of the effects of the drug and

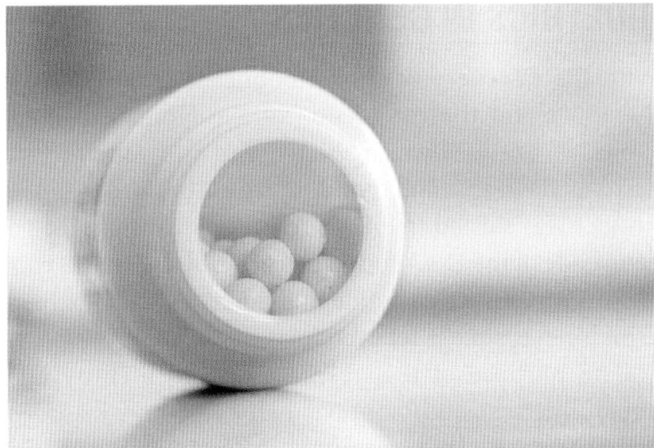

Fig. 3.1 In a double-blind study, patients may receive no drug (the control group), the new trial drug, or a placebo. (Copyright © simplytheyu/iStock/Thinkstock.com.)

provide more objective data. However, ethical dilemmas may arise in therapeutic research, for example, participants receiving the placebo and going extended periods of time with no treatment.

BOX 3.2 Types of Clinical Trials

- Non-randomized controlled trials—a trial where the participants are assigned to the experimental group by a method that is not random. The investigator defines and manages the alternatives.
- Randomized controlled trials—a trial where the participants are randomly selected for one or another of the different treatments under study.
- Single blind—a study in which one party, either the investigator or participant, is unaware of what medication the participant is taking; also called single-masked study.
- Double blind—a clinical trial design in which neither the participant nor researchers know which participants are receiving the experimental treatment or placebo.

Participants should always have the right to withdraw at any stage from the research process. When a participant chooses to withdraw from the research process, they should not be pressured or coerced in any way to try and stop them from withdrawing.

DISCUSSION

One of the most controversial biomedical research studies in the United States was the Tuskegee Syphilis Study. Between 1932 and 1972, the U.S. Public Health Service, along with the health departments from six different states, conducted a clinical study to investigate the natural progression of untreated syphilis in rural Black men. Working in collaboration with Tuskegee University, a historically black college in Alabama, more than 600 impoverished Black sharecroppers from Macon County, Alabama, were recruited under the guise of receiving free medical services.

Of the recruited men, 399 had contracted syphilis before the study began, and 201 did not have the disease. For participating in the study, these men were given free medical care, meals, and free burial insurance. However, none of the infected men were ever told they had the disease and never received treatment, even though, by 1947, penicillin was found to be effective in treating syphilis. Local Black and White physicians were recruited to not treat the men in the study. Furthermore, these men were told that the study was going to last only 6 months, but it lasted 40 years. The study continued until 1972, when a whistleblower's leak to the press resulted in its termination that year. The Black men subjected to the study included numerous men who died of syphilis, 40 wives who contracted the disease, and 19 children born with congenital syphilis.

The Tuskegee Syphilis Study brought up many ethical issues that had lasting effects even to the present time. The study highlighted issues of lack of informed consent and economic exploitation based on race and poverty. As a result of the Tuskegee Syphilis Study, the federal government established the National Commission for the Protection of Human Subjects of Biomedical and Behavioral Research, the Office for Human Research Protections, and the Behavioral Research and the National Research Act, which created the Institutional Review Boards that review the methods proposed for research to ensure that they are ethical and that the human subjects provide informed consent.

In addition, in 1973, the surviving patients sued and received a $10 million settlement, which was payable to patients and their more than 6000 heirs. Even though women were not included in the study, many women contracted syphilis from men who participated in the study's syphilitic group. Thus, infected wives, ex-wives, widows, and offspring received lifetime medical and health benefits.

1. What difference would it have made if these men had participated with informed consent, or full knowledge of the trial and their participation in it?
2. Why should the study have been discontinued after the discovery of penicillin as a treatment for syphilis?
3. In the chapter on ethics, we learned that ethical medical behavior should always be governed by the principles of autonomy, beneficence, nonmaleficence, and justice. How did this study fail to address these principles?

CONFLICT OF INTEREST

In medical research, it is important to verify if there is any **conflict of interest**. A conflict of interest occurs when self-interest affects an individual's professional obligations to one's patients, organization, and/or profession. This is most common with physicians since they often become involved in partnerships with different industries to conduct research and clinical trials. Physicians and any healthcare professional having dual commitment such as these must be mindful of the conflicts such engagement poses to the integrity of the research and the welfare of human participants. For example, if a pharmaceutical company will profit from the sale and production of the product being tested, no employee or no one affiliated with the company or its shareholders should be enrolled as a subject in the clinical trials. Other examples of conflicts of interests that may occur in health care are:

- accepting company gifts of various kinds, including meals and drug samples,
- acting as promotional speakers or writers on behalf of companies, and
- having a financial interest in a medical product company whose products they prescribe, use, or recommend.

It is important for every healthcare organization to prevent conflicts of interest by establishing, implementing, and enforcing a policy that addresses conflict of interest. The policy should be appropriately detailed and include examples of conflicts of interest. This should include self-reporting of questionable business relationships and receiving any gifts or payments; declining financial compensation that is in excess of the research effort and does not reflect fair market value; or, if a research relationship exists, refraining from initiating any financial relationship until the research relationship ends.

BIOETHICS IN GENETICS

With the discovery of deoxyribonucleic acid (DNA) in the 1950s and the completion of the Human Genome Project in 2003, advances in genetics and gene therapy have made leaps and bounds. The **Human Genome Project** was started to enable researchers to map the genetic code of the DNA found on each cell and the 23 pairs of **chromosomes** that define individuals. The entire blueprint for everyone is referred to as the *human genome*.

The purpose of this research was to identify and, hopefully, treat and/or prevent diseases and disorders that are genetically transmitted. Alterations in the normal sequence may result from mutations and may lead to diseases and disorder, such as diabetes, sickle cell anemia, cystic fibrosis, heart disease, and various cancers. Understanding the genetic code may allow researchers to prevent the transmission of certain genetically based diseases. As a result, current medical research in genetics focuses on predicting and diagnosing disease and conditions and developing medical treatments.

GENETIC TESTING AND SCREENING

Genetic testing, or genetic screening, is a type of medical test that identifies changes in genes, chromosomes, or proteins. The results of a genetic test can confirm or rule out a suspected genetic condition or help determine a person's chance of developing or passing on a genetic disorder (Fig. 3.2). There are more than 77,000 genetic tests that are currently in use, with many more being developed.

Genetic testing has potential benefits, whether the results are positive or negative for a gene mutation. Test results can provide a sense of relief from uncertainty and

DISCUSSION

Wakefield Study

In 1998, Andrew Wakefield, MD, was a gastroenterologist and medical researcher who published his study, along with 12 coauthors, in *The Lancet* that claimed there was a link between the administration of the measles, mumps, and rubella (MMR) vaccine and autism. However, soon after the study's publication, 10 of the 12 coauthors retracted their interpretation of the data that there was a link between the MMR vaccine and autism. Furthermore, Wakefield failed to disclose his financial ties and conflict of interest, with his study being funded by lawyers representing lawsuits against vaccine-producing companies.

Wakefield's study and his claim that the MMR vaccine might cause autism resulted in a decline in vaccination rates in the United States, United Kingdom, and Ireland, and a corresponding rise in measles and mumps, resulting in serious illness and deaths, and contributed to the public's distrust of all vaccines.

1. What bioethical code or rule did this violate?
2. Why was the Wakefield study not considered valid?

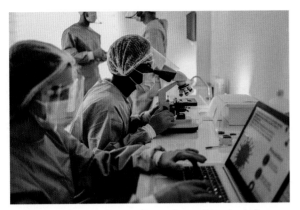

Fig. 3.2 Genetic testing can be performed to check for gene mutations, which may help people make informed decisions about managing their health care. (iStock.com/DisobeyArt.)

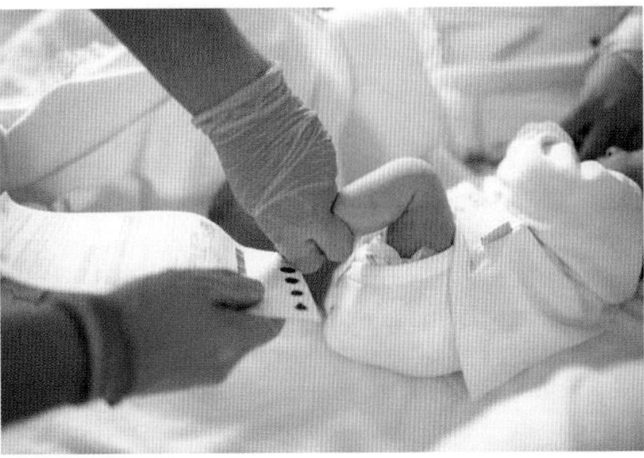

Fig. 3.3 Newborn screening for PKU is performed with a heel stick where a blood is taken from a small puncture in the newborn's heel.

help people make informed decisions about managing their health care. For example, a negative result can eliminate the need for unnecessary checkups and screening tests in some cases. A positive result can direct a person toward available prevention, monitoring, and treatment options. Some test results can even help people make decisions about having children.

Newborn Screening

Some available genetic tests are used in newborn screening, which is used just after birth to identify genetic disorders that can be treated early in life. Millions of babies are tested each year in the United States. In fact, although this may vary by state, every newborn is required to be tested for a group of genetic disease that would not have been otherwise found at birth (Box 3.3). For example, all infants in the United States are tested for phenylketonuria (PKU) as part of their newborn screening within 24–72 h after birth. PKU is an inherited metabolic disorder and results in the inability to break down the amino acid phenylalanine. Phenylalanine is essential for infant growth; however, if there is too much as in the case with PKU, there will be a buildup of phenylalanine, which may affect the infant's brain, causing seizure, developmental delays, and intellectual disability. As a result, being able to screen newborns for PKU as soon as possible will allow for early diagnosis and treatment, which will require the newborn to be on a special diet that is low in protein (Fig. 3.3).

BOX 3.3 Common Genetic Screening Test for Newborns

- Phenylketonuria (PKU)
- congenital hypothyroidism
- congenital adrenal hyperplasia
- sickle cell disease
- hemoglobin SC disease
- beta thalassemia
- cystic fibrosis
- severe combined immunodeficiency (SCID)
- spinal muscle atrophy (SMA)

Prenatal Testing

Prenatal testing is used to detect changes in a fetus's genes or chromosomes before birth. This type of testing is offered during pregnancy to help determine if there is an increased risk that the baby will have a genetic or chromosomal disorder. There are many types of prenatal screening methods during pregnancy, including blood tests, amniocentesis, and ultrasound scans.

In some cases, prenatal testing can lessen a couple's uncertainty or help them make decisions about a pregnancy. However, it cannot identify all possible inherited disorders and birth defects.

Carrier Testing

Carrier testing is used to identify people who carry one copy of a gene mutation that, when present in two copies, causes a genetic disorder. This type of testing is offered to individuals who have a family history of a genetic disorder and to people in certain ethnic groups with an increased risk of specific genetic conditions, such as cystic fibrosis, hemophilia, and sickle cell disease. If both parents are tested, the test can provide information about a couple's risk of having a child with a genetic condition.

Carrier testing can be performed on the mother and father and done before or during the pregnancy. However, genetic disorders can occur in families with no history of genetic disorders.

Based on an individual's genetic screening, parents can decide whether to conceive a child or not. Unfortunately, some genetic screening cannot be done until the fetus is in the second or third trimester and then the decision to continue the pregnancy full term or to terminate the pregnancy may become an ethical and legal issue.

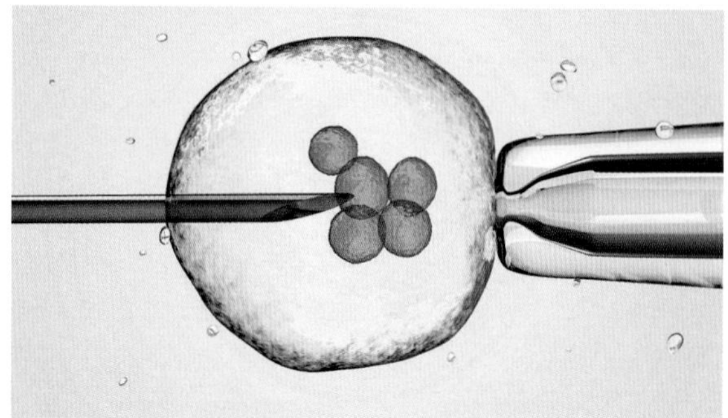

Fig. 3.4 Stem cells can be cloned, or be developed into many different types of cells, and used in genetic research. (iStock.com/The-Lightwriter.)

GENE THERAPY

Another area of focus for medical research is on gene therapy, which is an experimental technique that uses genes to treat or prevent disease. **Gene therapy** is a type of therapeutic technology that hopes to rid the population of various diseases and disorders. Specifically, gene therapy seeks to alter genes to correct genetic defects and, thus, prevent or cure genetic diseases. Using gene therapy technology, mutated genes that cause diseases can be replaced with a healthy or normal copy, can be inactivated to prevent the abnormal function, or a new gene can be introduced in the body to combat a disease.

Gene therapy's approach is different from traditional medical approaches, which may only treat symptoms but not the underlying genetic problems. There are different types of gene therapy, but the most common is to use a vector, usually a virus, to deliver a specific gene inside the cells. Once the new gene is inside, the cell incorporates and uses it to produce new genetic material and protein molecules, which may have been missing or defective to cause the disease or condition.

Although gene therapy is a promising treatment option for a number of diseases, the FDA has approved only a limited number of gene therapy product to be available in the United States. However, hundreds of gene therapy products are in clinical trials for genetic conditions, cancer, and HIV/AIDS.

STEM CELL RESEARCH

Another area of medical and scientific advancement and controversy is stem cell research. Stem cell research and therapy focus on duplicating or growing stem cells from human embryos and other tissues to either promote healthy cells or grow specific types of cells to study diseases or conditions. **Stem cells** are unique cells in that they have the ability to divide indefinitely and can be developed into many different types of cells, called **clones**, particularly during early life when growth and development are underway (Fig. 3.4). Thus, stem cells can theoretically provide essential replacement cells. In some types of cancer, stem cells may be able to extend a patient's life expectancy. For example, a single stem cell can be cloned to become a specialized cell, such as red blood cells for treatment of leukemia.

In studying these cells, researchers found a way to obtain stem cells from human embryos, called *human embryonic stem cells.* Because these embryos were created through in vitro fertilization under laboratory conditions for research purposes and were then destroyed (with donor consent) when no longer needed, their use can be highly valuable but controversial. Until recently, the only way to get stem cells for research was to remove the inner cell mass of an embryo. Thus, destroying a human embryo can be unsettling to many people, even if it is only 5 days old, and raises many ethical and moral issues.

In the United States, the question of when human life begins has been highly controversial and closely linked to debates over abortion, which will be further discussed in later chapters. Some people, however, believe that an embryo is a person with the same moral status as an adult or a live-born child. As a matter of religious faith and moral conviction, they believe that "human life begins at conception" and that an embryo is therefore a person. According to this view, an embryo has interests and rights that must be respected. Many other people have a different view of the moral status of the embryo, for example that the embryo becomes a person at a later stage of development than fertilization, such as after birth or after it takes its first breath.

Few people, however, believe that the embryo or blastocyst is just a clump of cells that can be used for research without restriction. Many hold a middle ground that the early embryo deserves special respect as a potential human being but that it is acceptable to use it for certain types of research provided there is good scientific justification, careful oversight, and informed consent from the woman or couple for donating the embryo for research.

Currently, stem cell research is legal in the United States but with restriction on its use. State laws may vary regarding research on stem cells, with some states restricting research on aborted fetuses or embryos unless permitted with consent of the patient.

GENETIC DISCRIMINATION

There are deep ethical implications to having this knowledge about the human genome and what we will or are doing with it. The manipulation of our own nature may seem to break certain traditional limits. Many people have a sense of uneasiness about the process, and concerns about altering human nature itself. For example, how do researchers determine which disorders or traits warrant gene therapy? Few would argue that diseases that cause suffering, disability, and, potentially, death are good candidates for gene therapy. However, there are genetic "diseases," such as achondroplasia, which causes dwarfism, that may be present in an otherwise healthy individual. Could the widespread use of gene therapy make society less accepting of people who are different? Who decides which traits are normal or acceptable and which constitute a disability or disorder?

Another concern in this age of increased genetic information is the idea of ownership. Who owns the information obtained from the sequencing of genes and other pieces of DNA? Who will have access to it? Can genes be patented in order to protect proprietary research protocols, drugs, and treatments arising from the information?

There are many ethical issues with knowing people's genetic information. There are concerns about privacy and confidentiality and how scientists, researchers, the healthcare system, employers, health insurance companies, and other interested parties may use this information. Knowing people's genetic information and that there may be a genetic mutation that causes or increases the risk of an inherited disease or disorder may lead to genetic discrimination. **Genetic discrimination** occurs when people treat others differently because of their genetic information. This includes information about one's genetic tests and the genetic tests of family members and any information about any disease, disorder, or conditions. For example, an insurance company can refuse to cover an individual who is known to have the genetic mutation for a chronic disease. Or an employer may refuse a worker's compensation if they believe the employee's genetic mutation was the cause of the accident or predisposed them to the injury.

As a result, in 2008, Congress passed the Genetic Information Nondiscrimination Act. The Genetic Information Nondiscrimination Act (GINA) prohibits specific types of genetic discrimination, specifically discrimination in health insurance and employment. It prohibits group health plans and health insurers from denying coverage to a healthy individual or charging that person higher premiums based solely on a genetic predisposition to developing a disease in the future. It also forbids employers from using individuals' genetic information when making hiring, firing, job placement, or promotion decisions. GINA protects a person's genetic information revealed when seeking genetic testing or participating in a research study. It also protects a person's family medical history, including a family member's genetic information. GINA is enforced by the U.S. Equal Employment Opportunity Commission.

However, GINA does not include life insurance, disability insurance, or long-term care insurance. Furthermore, the law does not protect people from genetic discrimination where an employer has fewer than 15 employees. GINA also does not alter the provision of the Americans with Disabilities Act, "under which an employer, after a conditional offer of employment, lawfully requires an individual to sign an authorization to disclose all of his or her health records."

GINA hopes to not only protect people's civil rights and ensure privacy and confidentiality, it also hopes to advance medical research. If people feel safe and protected from genetic discrimination, they may more likely be willing to participate in genetic research and share their genetic information with scientists and researchers.

DISCUSSION

The BRCA1 and BRCA2, which stand for Breast Cancer gene 1 and 2, respectively, are genetic mutations found to increase lifetime risk of developing breast cancer in women with these mutations. This information could potentially be used by health insurance companies to deny coverage to women who test positive for these mutations or to increase their cost of insurance coverage. The recently passed Genetic Information Nondiscrimination Act of 2008 makes such a move illegal and makes discrimination in the workplace based on genetic traits also unlawful.

1. What are some other benefits and disadvantages to knowing you carry a genetic mutation for a disease?
2. Should employers be able to increase the insurance payments from employees with chronic conditions that may require expensive medical treatment?

CONCLUSION

We have seen medicine evolve from application of leeches for bloodletting to being able to grow cells and tissues from stem cells. The future will hold even more amazing discoveries that will prolong and enhance life. As we learn more about genetics and make new advances in procedures, treatments, and disease prevention, ethical and moral issues will arise. Keeping in mind the basic principles of ethics and ethical decision making, the future can hold astounding cures and treatments for patients who a decade ago would have died.

CHAPTER REVIEW QUESTIONS

1. What is a double-blind test?
   - **A.** All participants receive the same drug.
   - **B.** All participants must sign waivers.
   - **C.** No participants are paid for participation.
   - **D.** None of the participants or evaluators knows who is receiving the real drug or the placebo.
2. What do we mean by a nontherapeutic group?
   - **A.** Participants do not benefit from the research done.
   - **B.** Participants benefit from the research done.
   - **C.** No actual participants are involved in the research.
   - **D.** Research focuses only on equipment.
3. Which of the following is not an ethical principle in medical research?
   - **A.** Allow patients to withdraw from the clinical trial.
   - **B.** Ensure there is no harm done to the patient.
   - **C.** Attaining informed consent from the patient.
   - **D.** Protecting patient privacy and anonymity.
4. Telling a patient about the benefits and risk of enrolling in a clinical trial is called
   - **A.** informed consent.
   - **B.** conflict of interest.
   - **C.** consent.
   - **D.** conscience clause.
5. The group in a clinical trial that receives a treatment with no therapeutic value is called the
   - **A.** experimental group.
   - **B.** blind group.
   - **C.** placebo group.
   - **D.** therapeutic group.
6. A nurse works as a researcher in a clinical trial. He forgets to mention that his wife works for the pharmaceutical company that is conducting the trial. This is an example of a
   - **A.** discrimination.
   - **B.** conscience clause.
   - **C.** informed consent.
   - **D.** conflict of interest.
7. Which of the following is not true of gene therapy?
   - **A.** It can alter genes and correct a defect.
   - **B.** It can treat symptoms but not the underlying genetic problems.
   - **C.** The technology replaces mutated genes, in some cases, by introducing a healthy or normal gene with a virus.
   - **D.** It can be used in an adult or newborn to identify genetic mutations that may lead to a disease or condition.

8. Testing for phenylketonuria (PKU) is what kind of screening?
   A. Carrier screening
   B. Prenatal screening
   C. Newborn screening
   D. Gene therapy
9. A man and a woman are considering starting a family. The man knows he is a genetic carrier for cystic fibrosis, an inherited disease. The woman decides to be tested for the gene for cystic fibrosis. This is an example of
   A. carrier screening.
   B. prenatal screening.
   C. newborn screening.
   D. gene therapy.
10. Which of the following is *not* an example of genetic discrimination?
    A. A new employee is told her premium, which is what she will pay for her health insurance policy, will be 25% higher than her coworkers because her medical records show a diagnosis of sickle cell disease.
    B. A worker injures himself after falling off a tall ladder and files for worker's compensation. The employer's insurance company denies the claim and tells the worker, since he has Ehlers-Danlos syndrome, which affects his joints, that was the actual reason for his fall.
    C. A man was terminated from his job after his employer found out he is a gene carrier for Huntington's disease, a neurological disease that manifests later in life.
    D. A person tries to enroll in a paid clinical trial but is rejected because of a family history of heart disease. However, he believes he can be treated by the drug that is being tested.

SELF-REFLECTION QUESTIONS

1. Will the high costs of genetic testing and gene therapy make it available only to the wealthy?
2. Could the widespread use of gene therapy make society less accepting of people who are different or with disabilities or disorders?
3. Who should decide which traits are normal and which constitute a disability or disorder and can be changed by gene therapy?
4. As discussed, use of stem cells in research and in medical technology is controversial. What if their use could save thousands of people's lives? When do you think it should be widely permitted?

INTERNET ACTIVITIES

1. Research the Nuremberg Trials and discuss its significance in bioethics and medical research.
2. Look up a case called *The Radiation Experiment* and discuss it with others in your class.
3. Research the diseases stem cells are being used to research.
4. Discuss the different phases of clinical trials. Discuss the bioethical issues that may arise at each phase.

ADDITIONAL RESOURCES

https://www.genome.gov/about-genomics/policy-issues/Genetic-Discrimination#gina

https://www.nia.nih.gov/health/what-are-clinical-trials-and-studies

https://www.fda.gov/patients/learn-about-drug-and-device-approvals/drug-development-process

https://www.emedicinehealth.com/is_stem_cell_research_illegal_in_the_united_states/articleem.htm

https://history.nih.gov/display/history/Nuremberg+Code

https://www.briandeer.com/mmr/lancet-paper.htm

https://www.cdc.gov/tuskegee/timeline.htm

https://www.pbs.org/independentlens/stemcell/bioethics.html

BIBLIOGRAPHY

National Institutes of Health (NIH), U.S. Department of Health and Human Services (DHHS). (2012). *Research ethics and stem cells*. Available from: http://stemcells.nih.gov/info/pages/ethics.aspx.

U.S. Equal Employment Opportunity Commission. https://www.eeoc.gov/youth/genetic-information-faqs#Q5.

U.S. Equal Employment Opportunity Commission, Genetic Information Discrimination. https://www.eeoc.gov/genetic-information-discrimination.

U.S. Food & Drug Administration. *Approved cellular and gene therapy products*. https://www.fda.gov/vaccines-blood-biologics/cellular-gene-therapy-products/approved-cellular-and-gene-therapy-products.

4

Healthcare Laws and Compliance

CHAPTER OBJECTIVES

1. List federal and state agencies that oversee and resolve matters that require disciplinary action.
2. Discuss the Emergency Medical Treatment and Active Labor Act and Clinical Laboratory Improvement Act of 1988.
3. Discuss the Patient's Bill of Rights.
4. Discuss compliance plans and the role of the compliance officer.
5. Identify the purpose of disciplinary actions and list examples of ethical and illegal actions that would warrant disciplinary actions.
6. Describe key types of compliance violations.
7. Discuss fraud and abuse in healthcare and the relevant laws.

KEY TERMS

Abuse Improper practices, outside the acceptable standards of practice.

Anti-Kickback Statute A federal law that prohibits the exchange or offer to exchange anything of value in an effort to induce or reward the referral of business.

Bias A preference of one thing over another, usually unfairly favoring one over another.

Centers for Medicare and Medicaid Services (CMS) The federal agency that oversees most of the regulations related to the healthcare system and provides government-subsidized medical coverage, such as Medicare, Medicaid, and State Children's Health Insurance Program (SCHIP).

Clinical Laboratory Improvement Act of 1988 (CLIA) Regulates all laboratory facilities for safety and handling of specimens to ensure accuracy and timeliness of testing regardless of where the test is performed.

Compliance Adherence to guidelines and regulations set forth by an organization and/or a governing body.

Compliance officer An individual in an organization or practice who is designated to maintain and inspect the adherence to all areas of regulations and guidelines.

Compliance plan Policies and procedures used to ensure that guidelines and regulations are obeyed, including auditing, monitoring, and protocol for taking action when infractions are discovered.

Emergency Medical Treatment and Active Labor Act (EMTALA) of 1986 Federal law that any hospital emergency room that receives payments from federal healthcare programs to provide medical screening and treat and stabilize any patient regardless of insurance status.

False Claims Act Federal law that prevents an individual or organization from knowingly creating a false record or submitting a false claim to any federal government payer.

Fraud Deliberate, intentional act to mislead for financial gain.

Health Information Technology for Economic and Clinical Health (HITECH) Act An Act that provides the authority to establish programs to improve healthcare quality, safety, and efficiency through the promotion of health information technology.

Office for Civil Rights (OCR) Federal agency that enforces federal civil rights laws, conscience and religious freedom laws and a number of other laws and regulations.

Medical practice acts Laws defined by each of the states that regulate the licensing and medical laws for that state and define the scope of practice for licensed and unlicensed individuals in the healthcare field.

Office of Inspector General (OIG) Independent agency that functions under the Department of Justice to investigate and protect the integrity of the Department of Health and Human Services (HHS) and their recipients, as well as all federal healthcare programs.

Office of the National Coordinator for Health IT (ONCHIT) The principal federal entity charged with coordination of nationwide efforts to implement health information technology and facilitating the exchange of electronic health information

Patient's Bill of Rights Basic rules of conduct between patients and medical caregivers.

Qui tam In Latin meaning "who as well"; a type of lawsuit where a private citizen exposes fraud upon the government and files a lawsuit on the government's behalf.

Sanctions Penalties to serve as punishment or enforcement of rules and regulations.

Stark law A set of federal laws designed to maintain the integrity of the medical field; includes antitrust and antikickback laws to prevent physicians from gaining financially from solicitation of services or monopolization of services.

Whistleblower An individual, usually an employee, who turns in his or her employer for potential fraud and abuse.

INTRODUCTION

Since health care deals with the lives and health of people, it is understandably one of the most regulated industries in the United States. There are many laws and regulations to protect that set privacy and usage standards for patient information, ensure quality patient care, prevent fraud, and protect healthcare staff. Healthcare regulations and standards are necessary to ensure compliance and to provide safe health care to every individual who accesses the system. The healthcare regulatory agencies, in turn, monitor practitioners and facilities, provide information about industry changes, promote safety, and ensure legal compliance and quality services.

In addition, healthcare organizations and healthcare professionals are subject to inspection, review, reporting requirements, and enforcement actions by a variety of state and federal agencies, and they must follow myriad local, state, and federal regulations. This chapter will provide an overview of some of the major laws, acts, and regulations that healthcare organizations need to stay in compliance and to protect patients.

REGULATING AGENCIES

Employers and professional agencies, such as certification boards, licensing boards, and other state and federal agencies, all work together to oversee the healthcare industry to ensure that the rights of patients and the general public are safeguarded. Regulating and accrediting agencies must also oversee **compliance** to ensure that all healthcare professionals and organizations adhere to guidelines and regulations set forth by an organization and/or a governing body. It is the duty of all healthcare professionals to monitor themselves and uphold the ethical standards of the profession. If a healthcare professional commits an illegal or unethical act, it is ultimately the responsibility of the employer or governing body to impose **sanctions** that would be appropriate for the violations that occurred.

The various regulatory bodies protect the public from a number of health risks and provide numerous programs for public health and welfare. Together, these regulatory agencies protect and regulate public health at every level by providing quality control and monitoring safety, ethics, and legal patency of healthcare organizations.

Healthcare regulations are developed and implemented not only by all levels of government—federal, state, and local—but by private organizations as well. Federal, state, and local regulatory agencies often establish rules and regulations for the healthcare industry, and their oversight is mandatory. Some other agencies, such as those for accreditation, require voluntary participation but are still important because they provide rankings or certification of quality and serve as additional oversight, ensuring that healthcare organizations promote and provide quality care.

As a federal regulating agency, the U.S. Department of Health and Human Services (HHS) has eleven operating divisions, including eight agencies in the U.S. Public Health Service and three human services agencies. These divisions administer a wide variety of health and human services and conduct life-saving research for the nation, protecting and serving all Americans. Four federal agencies account for administering more than 600 regulatory requirements that healthcare systems and healthcare providers must comply with, many of them related to medical records and health information technology. Healthcare providers and professionals are subject to additional regulation and oversight from many other sources.

The **Centers for Medicare and Medicaid Services (CMS)** oversee most of the regulations related directly to the healthcare system, including the funding for healthcare services (Fig. 4.1). CMS provides government-subsidized medical coverage to more than 100 million people through several programs:

- Medicare for the elderly and disabled
- Medicaid for lower-income individuals and families
- Children's Health Insurance Program (CHIP) for health insurance coverage for children under 19.

Medicare is the government's health insurance program for people aged 65 or older. Some people under age 65 may qualify for Medicare with disabilities, permanent kidney failure, or other chronic diseases.

Although much of its funding is federal, Medicaid is administered at the state level. Medicaid provides coverage for some low-income people, families and children, pregnant women, the elderly, and people with disabilities. In some states, Medicaid has been expanded to cover all adults below a certain income level. Medicaid programs must follow federal guidelines, but coverage and costs may be different from state to state.

In all states, CHIP, formerly known as State Children's Health Insurance Program (SCHIP), provides low-cost health coverage to children in families that earn too much money to qualify for Medicaid. In some states, CHIP covers pregnant women. The program has an extensive history of providing insurance to underprivileged children and receives funding from respective states and the federal government. Today, the Affordable Care Act (ACA) makes this service accessible to the largest number of low-income children in the country's history (Box 4.1).

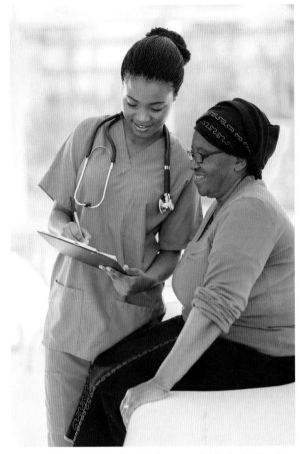

Fig. 4.1 The Centers for Medicare and Medicaid Services (CMS) provides government-subsidized medical coverage to more than 100 million people through several programs, such as Medicare and Medicaid. (iStock.com/Michaeljung.)

BOX 4.1 Provisions of the Affordable Care Act

In March 2010, the Affordable Care Act (ACA) was enacted. Provisions included:

- expand access to insurance coverage
- increase consumer insurance protections
- emphasize prevention and wellness
- improve health quality and system performance
- promote health workforce development
- curb rising health costs

CMS is also responsible for ensuring compliance to the Health Insurance Portability and Accountability Act (HIPAA). HIPAA, which works to reduce costs while protecting patients and providing better medical care, is a major piece of healthcare regulation and was instituted to improve the efficiency and effectiveness of the healthcare system. HIPAA will be further discussed in the chapter on medical records.

Another agency is HHS's **Office for Civil Rights (OCR)**, which enforces federal civil rights laws, conscience and religious freedom laws, HIPAA, and a number of other laws and regulations. OCR works closely with both doctors and patients to ensure that every patient knows their rights and privacies concerning personal health information and medical treatment options. As a government agency, the OCR also investigates health information privacy and patient safety confidentiality complaints to decide if a discriminatory act or a violation of law has occurred and takes action to correct those problems. Under HIPAA, the OCR can levy significant fines to healthcare providers and their business associates if personal health information is lost or stolen.

The **Office of the National Coordinator for Health IT (ONCHIT)** is the principal federal entity under HHS charged with coordination of nationwide efforts to implement health information technology and facilitating the exchange of electronic health information. ONCHIT is also charged with the promotion, assistance, and governance of the health information exchange (HIE) process as it pertains to protected health information. It is ONCHIT's duty to coordinate and oversee the nationwide adoption of electronic medical records while providing guidance for the electronic exchange of health information.

The ONCHIT is authorized by the **Health Information Technology for Economic and Clinical Health (HITECH) Act**. The HITECH Act established ONCHIT in law and provides the HHS with the authority to establish programs to improve healthcare quality, safety, and efficiency through the promotion of health information technology, including electronic health records (EHRs) and private and secure electronic health information exchange.

Office of the Inspector General (OIG) is the governmental wing responsible for protecting patient privacy, ensuring quality care, and combating fraud by ensuring healthcare organizations are compliant with federal healthcare laws and HHS programs. The OIG is an independent agency that functions under the Department of Justice to investigate and protect the integrity of the HHS and its many branches and programs, such as the Medicare and Medicaid programs. There are more than 70 OIG offices throughout the United States that help to monitor and combat fraud, waste, and abuse. For example, the OIG has made efforts to target hospitals and healthcare systems to enforce the Stark law, which prohibits physician self-referral, and the Anti-Kickback Statute, which prohibits illegal remuneration involving any federal healthcare programs, such as Medicare or Medicaid.

MEDICAL PRACTICE ACT

The practice of medicine is governed by each state's medical board. State medical boards are the agencies that license medical doctors, investigate complaints, discipline physicians who violate the medical practice act, and refer physicians for evaluation and rehabilitation when appropriate. The overriding mission of medical boards is to serve the public by protecting it from incompetent, unprofessional, and improperly trained physicians. Medical boards accomplish this by striving to ensure that only qualified physicians are licensed to practice medicine and that those physicians provide their patients with a high standard of care.

Each state has laws and regulations that govern the practice of medicine and specify the responsibilities of the medical board in regulating that practice. As part of their enforcement of healthcare professionals, individual states may enact their own **medical practice act**, which establish laws that govern healthcare professionals' scope of practice and licensing requirements. In all 50 states, medical practice acts have been established by statute to govern the practice of medicine. States' medical practice acts are laws and provide important safety measures to ensure that patients and the general public are protected against unlicensed and unqualified physicians and fraudulent and unsafe medical practices.

State medical boards establish the standards for the profession through their interpretation and enforcement of this act. Depending on the state and applicable laws, these agencies can apply sanctions that include loss or suspension of license, limitations and restrictions of licensing, loss of membership in the organization, censure, mandatory remediation, or treatment for violations involving substance abuse or psychological impairments and required continuing education. These sanctions would be imposed in addition to any applicable criminal charges, fines, and sentences.

OTHER QUALITY STANDARDS AND REGULATIONS

Emergency Medical Treatment and Active Labor Act

The Emergency Medical Treatment and Active Labor Act (EMTALA) of 1986 requires any hospital emergency department that receives payments from federal healthcare programs, such as Medicare and Medicaid, to provide an appropriate medical screening to any patient seeking treatment. This was enacted to eliminate "patient dumping" where a facility would transfer a patient based on a potentially high-cost diagnosis or refuse to treat a patient based on his or her ability to pay.

This legislation requires the emergency department to determine whether a condition is emergent or not and to provide stabilizing treatment in the case of an emergency medical condition. It does not require that treatment be given for nonemergency conditions. Furthermore, outpatient clinics are not medically equipped to handle emergencies and therefore are not bound by the EMTALA.

Clinical Laboratory Improvement Act

The Clinical Laboratory Improvement Act (CLIA) of 1988 is a group of laws that regulate all laboratory facilities for safety and handling of specimens. The objective of CLIA is to regulate accuracy and timeliness of testing regardless of where the test is performed. The Food and Drug Administration (FDA) is the federal agency that authorizes and implements the CLIA laws and determines the test complexity categories.

All laboratory testing sites—medical offices, hospitals, and laboratories—are given a CLIA number and are required to maintain certain standards of operation. The CLIA number certifies the complexity of the laboratory tests that can be performed in that particular laboratory. Without a CLIA certification, a site is not able to legally perform laboratory tests in the United States. Violation of CLIA regulations is punishable by fines and exclusion from federal health plans.

Each laboratory test is categorized by level of complexity. For moderate to highly complex tests, these are referred to as "nonwaived" tests, and laboratories or sites that perform these tests need to have a CLIA certificate, be inspected, and meet the CLIA quality standards based on the FDA requirements. Conversely, CLIA-waived tests are simple tests with a minimal risk for an incorrect result. These tests are cleared by the FDA for home use, and tests approved for waiver by the FDA using the CLIA criteria.

Sites performing only waived testing must have a CLIA certificate and follow the manufacturer's instructions; other CLIA requirements do not apply to these sites. A complete list of CLIA-waived tests may be found at https://www.accessdata.fda.gov/scripts/cdrh/cfdocs/cfClia/analyteswaived.cfm.

The Joint Commission (TJC)

To ensure quality health care, many hospitals seek accreditation. The Joint Commission (TJC), formerly called the Joint Commission on the Accreditation of healthcare Organizations (JCAHO), is a private, nonprofit organization that establishes the standards and guidelines for medical care. TJC accredits more than 4000 facilities throughout the United States, which accounts for approximately 78% of hospitals. Being accredited allows hospitals to receive payment from federally funded programs, such as Medicare and Medicaid.

PATIENT'S BILL OF RIGHTS

The Patient's Bill of Rights, also known as the U.S. Advisory Commission on Consumer Protection and Quality in the Health Care Industry, was passed to provide guidelines and policies to ensure the protection and safety of patients. Most medical practices, hospitals, insurance companies, and even governments have adopted some form of the Patient's Bill of Rights. In fact, many hospitals and medical offices have the Patient's Bill of Rights is usually posted throughout the facility, as well as distributed along with the practice's privacy release of information policies.

The Patient's Bill of Rights outlines basic rules of conduct and interaction between patients and healthcare professionals to ensure the delivery of safe and effective patient care. The objectives of the Patient's Bill of Rights are:

1. to help patients feel more confident in the U.S. healthcare system by ensuring that it is fair and works to meet patients' needs, gives patients a way to address any problems they may have, and encourages patients to take an active role in getting or staying healthy
2. to stress the importance of a strong relationship between patients and their healthcare providers

BOX 4.2 Patient's Bill of Rights

1. You have the right to be treated fairly and respectfully.
2. You have the right to get information you can understand about your diagnosis, treatment, and prognosis from your healthcare provider.
3. You have the right to discuss and ask for information about specific procedures and treatments, their risks, and the time you will spend recovering. You also have the right to discuss other care options.
4. You have the right to know the identities of all your healthcare providers, including students, residents, and other trainees.
5. You have the right to know how much care may cost at the time of treatment and long term.
6. You have the right to make decisions about your care before and during treatment and the right to refuse care. The hospital must inform you of the medical consequences of refusing treatment. You also have the right to other treatments provided by the hospital and the right to transfer to another hospital.
7. You have the right to have an advance directive, such as a living will or a power of attorney for healthcare. A hospital has the right to ask for your advance directive, put it in your file, and honor its intent.
8. You have the right to privacy in medical exams, case discussions, consultations, and treatments.
9. You have the right to expect that your communication and records are treated as confidential by the hospital, except as the law permits and requires in cases of suspected abuse or public health hazards. If the hospital releases your information to another medical facility, you have the right to expect the hospital to ask the medical facility to keep your records confidential.
10. You have the right to review your medical records and to have them explained or interpreted, except when restricted by law.
11. You have the right to expect that a hospital will respond reasonably to your requests for care and services or transfer you to another facility that has accepted a transfer request. You should also expect information and explanation about the risks, benefits, and alternatives to a transfer.
12. You have the right to ask and be informed of any business relationships between the hospital and educational institutions, other healthcare providers, or payers that may influence your care and treatment.
13. You have the right to consent to or decline to participate in research studies and to have the studies fully explained before you give your consent. If you decide not to participate in research, you are still entitled to the most effective care that the hospital can provide.
14. You have the right to expect reasonable continuity of care and to be informed of other care options when hospital care is no longer appropriate.
15. You have the right to be informed of hospital policies and practices related to patient care, treatment, and responsibilities.
16. You also have the right to know who you can contact to resolve disputes, grievances, and conflicts. And you have the right to know what the hospital will charge for services and their payment methods.

3. to stress the key role patients play in staying healthy by laying out rights and responsibilities for all patients and healthcare providers

The Patient's Bill of Rights is not a law but a guideline of what a patient should be guaranteed when seeking healthcare services. Some of these guarantees include the following:

- The right to respectful care
- The right to receive current, relevant, and understandable information
- The right to know the identity of everyone involved in his or her care
- The right to make decisions about the plan of care before undergoing treatment
- The right to privacy

It also requires that patients and healthcare professionals collaborate and participate in a patient's care. To this end, the Patient's Bill of Rights recommends that patients must provide information about their medical history and ask for clarification when they do not understand information or instructions being given to them. Patients must follow the hospital rules and be respectful toward other patients and medical staff and other hospital employees (Box 4.2).

COMPLIANCE PLAN

To ensure compliance with all healthcare laws and regulation, almost all healthcare organizations create a **compliance plan**. A compliance plan is a written set of policies and procedures that describe how an organization will operate and conduct itself in an ethical and compliant manner. It also includes guidelines and regulations and protocols for addressing infractions when discovered.

The OIG offers guidelines on how to create and implement a compliance program for individual and small group physician practices, as well as larger healthcare organizations. The goal of the OIG's compliance program is to detect erroneous claims or prevent the engagement of unlawful conduct, especially involving any federal healthcare programs, such as Medicare and Medicaid. The OIG's compliance program includes seven key components:

- Conduct internal monitoring and auditing.
- Develop written standards and procedures, such as a compliance plan.
- Designate a compliance officer.
- Conduct appropriate training and education.
- Respond to detected offenses and develop a corrective action plan.
- Develop open lines of communication.
- Enforce disciplinary standards.

The OIG recommends the focus of a compliance plan, including coding and billing; reasonable and necessary services; documentation; and improper inducements, kickbacks, and self-referrals. When creating a compliance plan, a physician group can add specific policies and procedures for any other risk areas that are specific to its practice.

An important component of a compliance program and plan is the designation or hire of a specific individual to act as a **compliance officer** to ensure that these policies and procedures are being followed and that any violations are being appropriately addressed. The position of the compliance officer may be a dedicated full-time position, or it may be included in the duties of an existing supervisor or manager in any given area or department. The role of the compliance officer is to ensure that the compliance plan is followed by all employees and to provide training on the policy and procedures.

Ongoing monitoring is crucial to determine whether a compliance plan is working and to keep up with ever-changing standards and rules. Education and training should be tailored to a specific practice specialty. For additional information on the OIG's compliance programs, visit the OIG website at: https://oig.hhs.gov/compliance/101/index.asp.

ENFORCEMENT AND DISCIPLINARY ACTIONS

There are a number of different disciplinary actions that a healthcare professional may receive from one of the regulating agencies, including sanctions, monetary fines, and even imprisonment. State and federal regulations focus on violations in the areas of fraud, substance abuse, illegal activities, practicing without a license or practicing outside the scope of practice, and malpractice.

Illegal and unethical acts can be penalized by law, licensing and/or ethics boards, certification boards, and employers, with consequences varying depending on the severity of the act or lack of action. In the case of a minor infraction, the consequences may include a performance improvement plan or corrective action plan by an employer or a temporary loss of license or small fine/penalty to an accrediting agency. In the case of a more serious infraction or violation, the healthcare professional may incur permanent loss of license, heavy fines and penalties, and imprisonment. For example, if a physician is found to be guilty of illegal billing practices, the state licensing board may revoke the physician's license and ability to practice medicine.

In the healthcare field, violations can range from the unethical treatment or negligence of care of a patient to a violation of privacy, fraud, or other illegal actions (Box 4.3). In addition to the legal consequences of breaking a law, employers and agencies may also impose sanctions that extend beyond these. Although committing an illegal act may lead to fines and possible imprisonment, professional and workplace sanctions depend on professional codes of conduct and may include corrective actions, termination of employment, or loss of license (Box 4.4).

BOX 4.3 Examples of Healthcare-Related Offenses That May Warrant Disciplinary Action

- Violation of patients' rights (e.g., HIPAA or confidentiality breach)
- Working outside of the employee's scope of practice
- Failure to perform at the accepted standard of care
- Fraud/abuse
- Abandonment of patient(s)
- Falsifying documentation
- Lack of documentation
- Negligence
- Violation of Stark law

BOX 4.4 Examples of Work-Related Violations That May Warrant Disciplinary Action

- Violation of time-off policy or sick-time policy
- Violation of dress code policy
- Violation of the code of ethics
- Violation of duties—either failing to perform the job or working outside of the job description
- Violation of the integrity of the institution, such as embezzlement or slander against the institution
- Abandonment of responsibility or position
- Noncompliance with continuing education or annual in-service requirements
- Physical or emotional impairment on the job
- Sexual harassment
- Assault
- Battery
- Violation of employment protection acts
- Violation of consumer protection acts

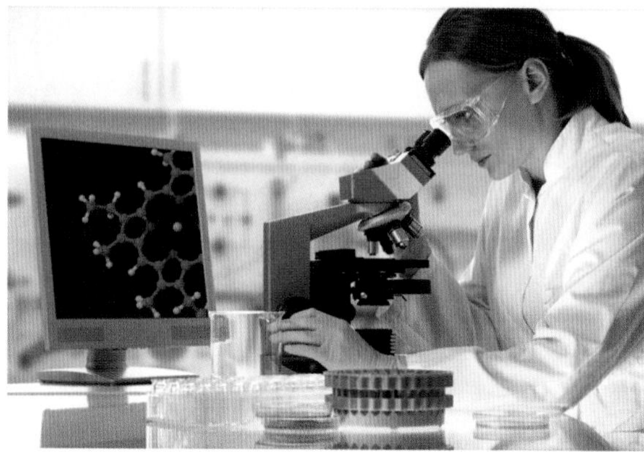

Fig. 4.2 Examples of fraud include billing for services not provided, up-coding services for larger reimbursement, or down-coding (under coding) for services provided. (AlexRaths/iStock/Thinkstock.com.)

FRAUD AND ABUSE LAWS

Fraud and abuse in healthcare are a national problem that costs consumers, insurance companies, and governments billions of dollars a year. Fraud is the intentional act to misrepresent facts or mislead for financial gain. Fraud in health care is an intentional misrepresentation, deception, or act of deceit for the purpose of receiving greater reimbursement. It is a criminal offense that can lead to, for example, healthcare professionals and medical billing and coding personnel incurring fines, loss of license, and even imprisonment. Examples of fraud include billing for services not provided or up-coding services to gain larger reimbursement for services provided (Fig. 4.2). It is important to note that it is the attempt at deceit that is fraud, regardless of whether it is successful. Abuse in health care is a reckless disregard or conduct that goes against acceptable business and/or medical practices resulting in greater reimbursement.

Fraud and abuse can bring big financial penalties to a physician or medical practice. According to the Department of Justice, there were more than $4.7 billion in settlements and judgments involving fraud and false claims against the government in 2016. More than half of the penalties were given to pharmaceutical companies, medical device companies, hospitals, nursing homes, laboratories, and physicians. These convictions included inadequate or unnecessary medical procedures and treatments, kickbacks to healthcare professionals, and overcharging for Medicare and Medicaid programs.

As an employee in any healthcare organization, it is important to understand that the penalties outlined earlier in the text are levied not just on the physician but may also be levied on the employer. Coding and billing personnel can also be subject to fines and imprisonment if they take part in a fraudulent activity, even if they were only following the physician's or employer's direction.

As a result, a number of laws and guidelines, especially by the federal government, are in place to prevent, identify, and penalize acts of fraud and abuse in health care. Federal healthcare fraud statute prohibits "knowingly and willfully executing, or attempting to execute, a scheme or artifice in connection with the delivery of or payment for healthcare benefits, items, or services to either:

- Defraud any healthcare benefit program
- Obtain (by means of false or fraudulent pretenses, representations, or promises) any of the money or property owned by, or under the control of, any healthcare benefit program."

Violations of key federal fraud and abuse laws can be either civil or criminal offenses.

DISCUSSION

On July 13, 2017, Attorney General Jeff Sessions and Department of Health and Human Services Secretary Tom Price, MD, announced the largest ever healthcare fraud enforcement action by the Medicare Fraud Strike Force. This action involved charging more than 412 people, which included 115 physicians, nurses, and other licensed medical professionals, for their alleged participation in healthcare fraud involving approximately $1.3 billion in false billings. "Healthcare fraud is not only a criminal act that costs billions of taxpayer dollars—it is an affront to all Americans who rely on our national healthcare programs for access to critical healthcare services and a violation of trust," said Secretary Price.

1. What kind of penalties should these healthcare professionals receive as a result of their actions?
2. What safeguards can a medical clinic or healthcare organization put in place to prevent fraud from medical billing?

Civil Laws in Fraud and Abuse

The two most common fraud and abuse violations of civil law are the False Claims Act and the Stark law. If found in violation, there are no criminal penalties or prison time, but financial penalties may be severe.

False Claims Act

Under the **False Claims Act (FCA)**, it is a federal crime for an individual or organization to knowingly create a false record or submit a false claim to any federal government payer. Many states have adopted similar regulations. Some examples of violations of the FCA would be altering a medical record to support a higher level of service or submitting claims to Medicare for services that were not provided.

An important component of the FCA includes protection for whistleblowers. A **whistleblower** is someone who turns in his or her employer for potential fraud and abuse. The employee is protected from discrimination, retaliation, harassment, suspension, or termination as a result of his or her participation in an investigation. If an employee reports fraud and is then discriminated against because of it, he or she may be entitled to reinstatement without loss of seniority and compensation to cover any damages incurred.

A specific type of violation of the FCA is a ***qui tam*** lawsuit, which is Latin meaning "who as well," in which the whistleblower files a lawsuit on behalf of the government. A *qui tam* lawsuit may help the government prevent fraud and recover millions of dollars that have been stolen from the U.S. Treasury and taxpayers. For example, if a physician is fraudulently billing and receiving payment for services that he or she did not perform, an employee or a patient may file a suit on behalf of the government. In this *qui tam* case, the "whistleblower" or plaintiff may be entitled to a percentage of the recovered money. The individual, or *qui tam* relator, can receive up to 15%–25% of the total amount recovered if the government prosecutes and 25%–30% if litigated by the *qui tam* plaintiff.

Besides Medicare and Medicaid fraud, other common violations of the FCA involve prescription drug fraud. The U.S. FDA approves all prescription drugs for specific indications and medical use. If a physician decides to prescribe a drug for a different indication than its approved use, this practice is known as "off-label" use prescribing and does not violate any law. However, if the drug manufacturer promotes the drug for an "off-label" use, or a different indication than its approved use, this would be a violation of the FCA.

Under the FCA, civil penalties can reach $20,000 per false claim plus triple damages. Administrative sanctions can reach $20,000 per line item on a false claim and bring exclusion from participation in Medicare and other state healthcare programs. A guilty verdict can also bring criminal fines up to $100,000 and up to 10 years' imprisonment.

Physician Self-Referral Law (Stark Law)

The Physician Self-Referral Law, or **Stark law**, is a collection of federal laws designed to maintain the integrity of the medical field and includes antitrust and antikickback laws that prevent physicians from gaining financially from solicitation or monopolization of services. For example, suppose a physician encourages her patients to seek physical and massage therapy at a particular clinic because she is part owner in that clinic—a fact she fails to share with her patients. Another example of a Stark law violation would be if a physician refers all of his patients to a radiology center that is owned by his immediate family. A person who violates the Stark law may face various civil sanctions including fines of up to $15,000 per claim.

Criminal Laws in Fraud and Abuse

In addition to civil penalties, the federal government may also bring a criminal case against an individual or a healthcare institution for violating fraud and abuse statutes. In general, these statutes require some level of intent, with a conviction being a felony and resulting in financial penalties and prison time. The most common criminal fraud and abuse statutes are the Anti-Kickback Statute and the Criminal Health Care Fraud Statute.

Anti-Kickback Statute

The Anti-Kickback Statute (AKS) is a federal law that prohibits the exchange or the offer to exchange anything of value in an effort to induce or reward the referral of business in a federal program.

Suppose a physician strongly encourages his patient on Medicare to take a particular medication because he receives a financial incentive from the drug manufacturer. Or a local hospital provides special events tickets to physicians who send their patients to the facility's ancillary departments.

The AKS is in place to prevent kickbacks because these actions are not in the best interest of the patient. Kickbacks create a bias toward promoting certain specialists, treatments, drugs, and other services or products because the promotion results in personal financial gain for the physician.

Penalties for violating the AKS include up to $25,000 in penalties, as well as a felony conviction punishable by up to 5 years in prison. Violators also face exclusion from participation in federal programs.

Criminal Healthcare Fraud Statute

The Criminal Health Care Fraud Statute prohibits "knowingly and willfully executing, or attempting to execute, a scheme or artifice in connection with the delivery of or payment for healthcare benefits, items, or services to either:

- Defraud any healthcare benefit program
- Obtain (by means of false or fraudulent pretenses, representations, or promises) any of the money or property owned by, or under the control of, any healthcare benefit program."

An example of a violation of this statute is a coordinated scheme among several physicians and medical clinics to defraud the Medicare Program by submitting claims for power wheelchairs that were not medically necessary. Fines, imprisonment, or both may be imposed for violating the Criminal Health Care Fraud Statute.

Exclusions Authorities

The OIG can exclude individuals and organizations who commit healthcare fraud and abuse from participating in federal and state healthcare programs, such as Medicare and Medicaid. In fact, the OIG maintains a database of individuals and entities that are excluded from participating in federal healthcare programs called the *List of Excluded Individuals/Entities.* Violations of any of the following laws may be cause to be placed on the exclusion list and include the following:

- Patient abuse and neglect
- Felony violations for non–healthcare-related offenses such as fraud, theft, or financial misconduct
- Felony or misdemeanor violations for the manufacture or distribution of narcotics
- Misdemeanors related to healthcare fraud and abuse
- Suspension of license as a result of incompetence, poor performance, and breaches of financial integrity
- Provision of unnecessary or substandard care
- Defaulting on healthcare education loans

Under the Exclusion statute, there are two forms of exclusion: *Mandatory Exclusions* and *Permissive Exclusions.* The OIG enforces mandatory exclusions. Individuals or organizations may be placed on the Mandatory Exclusions list if they commit violations that include healthcare fraud; illegal manufacturing, distributing, prescribing, or dispensing of controlled substances; and abuse and neglect involving Medicare or Medicaid patients. The OIG also has the discretion to enforce Permissive Exclusions. An individual or organization may be placed on the Permissive Exclusions list if convicted of fraud, committing a controlled substance–related misdemeanor, or obstructing an audit or investigation.

An excluded individual or organization may be found civilly liable under the FCA for knowingly submitting false claims and may face fines of up to $10,000 per item on that claim and up to three times the total damages. Furthermore, not only will an individual placed on the Exclusions list not receive payment from any federal or state programs, but also an organization may not receive payment for services provided by the excluded individual in its employ.

APPLY THIS

Using the following scenarios, determine whether disciplinary action should or should not be taken and, if so, what sanctions would be implemented.

1. A nurse is writing a prescription for a patient and signing the physician's name.
2. An employee meets a patient in the supermarket and discusses the patient's office visit earlier that day.
3. An employee is in the break room and is relating a joke that is of a sexual nature and a coworker overhearing the joke is embarrassed and offended.
4. A billing department employee discusses with a patient over the phone the possible payment plan options for the bill.
5. A physician has already treated a patient when she realizes that the insurance policy will not be in effect for another week. The physician tells the front desk staff to change the date of treatment so that it will fall within the dates of coverage.

CONCLUSION

In the healthcare field, there must be laws and guidelines in place to protect not only the employer and employee, but also the public. Maintaining clear and concise policies and procedures is essential to upholding effective standards of practice and providing quality healthcare for patients. Organizations function best when employees know and understand the laws and guidelines of what is expected of them.

CHAPTER REVIEW QUESTIONS

1. Which of the following provides basic rules of conduct between patients and healthcare professionals?
   A. Patient's Bill of Rights
   B. EMTALA
   C. Compliance plan
   D. CLIA
2. An employee discovers that her clinic has been billing for medical services that it never provided to patients. She reports it, which makes her a/an
   A. compliance officer.
   B. inspector general.
   C. whistleblower.
   D. excluded individual.
3. The OIG stands for
   A. Office of Investigation for the Government.
   B. Office of Inspector General.
   C. Occupational Investigative Group.
   D. Office of Internal Governing.
4. The deliberate act of misrepresentation to gain financially is
   A. abuse.
   B. fraud.
   C. sanctioning.
   D. All the above
5. Which of the following may result in an employee being sanctioned?
   A. Reporting an employer's illegal activities
   B. Committing fraud
   C. Following the state's medical practice act
   D. Assisting in the screening of a patient arriving at the emergency department
6. The medical practice act is written and regulated by
   A. the federal government.
   B. the Centers for Medicare and Medicaid.
   C. the state's medical board.
   D. the Office of Inspector General.
7. The federal agency that oversees program-sponsored health coverage is
   A. CLIA.
   B. OIG.
   C. CMS.
   D. ACA.
8. The Act that regulates hospitals and the way they screen patients to ensure their condition is an emergency or is stable is the
   A. ACA.
   B. EMTALA.
   C. CLIA.
   D. OIG.

9. The objectives of the Patient's Bill of Rights include all the following except

A. ensures that every American has insurance coverage.

B. stresses the role of patients in their health.

C. stresses the importance of the relationship between the patient and the healthcare provider.

D. Helps patients feel more confident in the healthcare system and give them a way to address problems in their health.

10. A conflict of interest would fall under which law or regulation?

A. Anti-Kickback Statute.

B. Exclusion Rule.

C. Clinical Laboratory Improvement Act.

D. Stark Law.

SELF-REFLECTION QUESTIONS

1. You are asked to appoint a compliance officer. What qualities would you look for?
2. Consider your future career. What areas of fraud and abuse can occur?
3. What steps could be put into place to prevent cases of fraud and abuse in a medical office?

INTERNET ACTIVITIES

1. Look up *qui tam* under the guidelines of Medicare at https://www.cms.gov.
2. Using the following links, review and complete a compliance self-assessment form for a place you have worked or for a work setting in which you hope to be employed. Reflect on what this experience has shown you about expectations in your field:
   - http://www.cms.gov/Medicare/Compliance-and-Audits/Part-C-and-Part-D-Compliance-and-Audits/Downloads/Compliance-Program-Effectiveness-Self-Assessment-Questionnaire.pdf
   - http://www.opm.gov/policy-data-oversight/work-life/reference-materials/workplaceviolence.pdf
3. Investigate one or more of the following laws and write an assessment of how it relates to your chosen field of healthcare:
   - Emergency Medical Treatment and Active Labor Act (EMTALA)
   - Medicare Access and CHIP Reauthorization Act of 2015 (MACRA)
   - Clinical Laboratory Improvement Act of 1988 (CLIA)
   - Health Information Technology for Economic and Clinical Health Act (HITECH)
   - Health Insurance Portability and Accountability Act (HIPAA)
   - Stark law
4. Research some professional organizations in your field and determine if there are any specific laws that will regulate you in the future.

ADDITIONAL RESOURCES

Manatt, P., & Phillips, L. L. P. (September 2015). Major settlements for healthcare providers under the Stark Law and False Claims Act. Available from: https://www.lexology.com/library/detail.aspx?g=a5682620-4a75-4705-a803-2fab586464ce.

Office of Inspector General, U.S. Department of Health and Human Services. A roadmap for new physicians: fraud & abuse laws. Available from: https://oig.hhs.gov/compliance/physician-education/01laws.asp.

Office of Inspector General, U.S. Department of Health and Human Services. State False Claims Act Reviews. Available from: https://oig.hhs.gov/fraud/state-false-claims-act-reviews/index.asp.

https://www.ncsbn.org

https://www.ama-assn.org/ama/pub/physician-resources/medical-ethics/code-medical-ethics/frequently-asked-questions.page

http://www.ama-assn.org/delivering-care/frequently-asked-questions-ethics

https://www.cms.gov

https://www.oig.hhs.gov/oei/reports/oei-01-89-00560.pdf

https://www.ocr.gov

https://www.cms.gov/Outreach-and-Education/Medicare-Learning-Network-MLN/MLNProducts/downloads/fraud_and_abuse.pdf

https://www.ncsl.org/research/health/the-affordable-care-act-brief-summary.aspx

5

Torts in Health Care

CHAPTER OBJECTIVES

1. Discuss what is the basis of torts and how it relates to malpractice.
2. Describe the different types of torts.
3. List and describe the different types of intentional torts.
4. Explain the importance of consent and the different types of consent.
5. List and describe specific types of quasi-intentional torts.

KEY TERMS

Assault Placing someone in immediate fear or apprehension of harmful or unpleasant touching without the person's consent.

Battery Harmful or offensive touching of another person without consent or without a legally justifiable reason.

Breach of confidentiality The public revelation of confidential or privileged information without an individual's consent.

Consent The acknowledgment of a person (usually the patient) regarding the risks and alternatives involved in a treatment and the permission for the treatment to be performed. This can be in some cases a verbal consent but in the medical field is usually a written document.

Defamation Any intentional false communication, either written or spoken, that harms a person's reputation; decreases the respect, regard, or confidence in which a person is held; or induces disparaging, hostile, or disagreeable opinions or feelings against a person.

Explicit consent Also known as express or direct consent, it means that an individual is clearly presented with an option to agree or disagree or to express a preference or choice, often verbally or in writing.

False imprisonment Restraint of a person so as to impede his or her liberty without justification or consent.

Implied consent Consent that is not expressly granted by a person, but rather inferred from a person's actions and the facts and circumstances in a specific situation.

Intent The willful decision to bring about a prohibited consequence.

Intentional infliction of emotional distress Type of conduct that deliberately causes severe emotional trauma to the victim.

Intentional tort A category of torts that describes a civil wrong resulting from an intentional act on the part of another person or entity.

Invasion of privacy The wrongful intrusion into private affairs with which the perpetrator or the public has no concern.

Liability Obligations under law arising from civil actions or torts.

Libel Written, printed, or other visual communication that harms another person's reputation.

Quasi-intentional Tort A voluntary act that directly causes damage to a person's privacy or emotional well-being, but without the intent to injure or to cause distress.

Slander Spoken or verbal communication in which one person discusses another in terms that harm the person's reputation.

Strict liability A person places another person in danger, even in the absence of negligence, simply because he or she is in possession of a dangerous product, animal, or weapon.

Trespass An unlawful intrusion that interferes with one's person, property, or land.

INTRODUCTION

In the previous chapters, negligence and malpractice were discussed and the importance of healthcare professionals to take the necessary legal and ethical steps to protect themselves against liability. In addition, healthcare professionals must be aware of other potential areas of liability that may cause harm or injury to a patient or another person.

TORTS

A **tort** is a wrongful act that results in injury to another's person, property, reputation, or the like, and for which the injured party is entitled to compensation. A tort is a violation of civil law but does not include a breach of contract or trust. A tort occurs when there is an act of negligence caused by carelessness, for example, and not intentionally. When a tort or a negligence occurs in health care, it is often referred to as *malpractice* or a professional negligence (Fig. 5.1). There are many reasons that result in a tort in health care with the most common being: an improper or misdiagnosis; a procedure that was performed and unnecessarily or incorrectly; or complications from a procedure or treatment that resulted in harm to the patient.

The basis of tort law is that people are liable for the consequences of their actions. Courts impose liability for torts to compensate an injured party for an act or an omission that causes harm. Under most tort laws, the injury or harm suffered does not have to be physical.

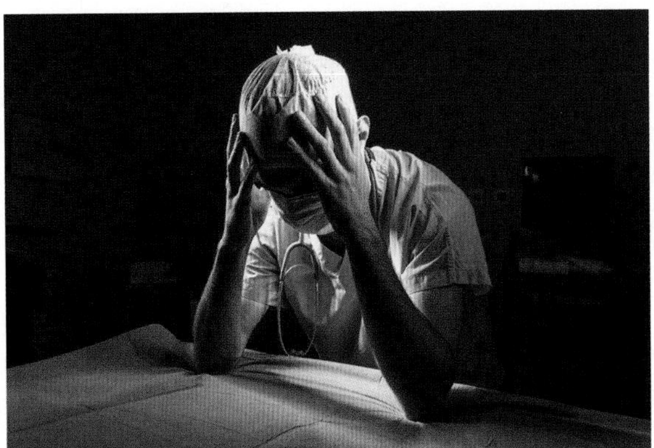

Fig. 5.1 A tort in health care is often called malpractice and may be due to a misdiagnosis or an incorrect procedure or treatment. (iStock.com/Devseren.)

Torts may include emotional distress or a violation of personal rights, such as a loss of the right to privacy. The person who commits the tort, called the *tortfeasor*, is not considered "guilty," as that is a term used in criminal law and not civil law. Instead, the tortfeasor is "liable," rather than guilty. Tort liability is meant to monetarily reimburse the tort victim for the harm caused by the tortfeasor.

APPLY THIS

Paula has been a registered nurse for more than 15 years in the hospital's intensive care unit (ICU). On a particular day, she was hoping to end her shift early and do her round of patients faster than they usually do it. This includes properly monitoring patients and their vital signs and charting in their medical records any changes in their progress. On her next shift at work, she was asked to report to the hospital's risk management department. Paula was informed that one of her patients had a complication overnight. The patient's blood pressure dropped, and the night shift nurses could not confirm that the patient's medication was administered, since it was not charted in his medical records by Paula.

1. What error(s) did Paula make in this situation?
2. What kind of punishment is possible in this situation?
3. What are the circumstances that define this as a possible violation of civil vs. criminal law?

TYPES OF TORTS

There are many different types of torts, but the three main types are: negligence, strict liability, and intentional torts or wrongs (Box 5.1).

BOX 5.1 Different Types of Torts

- Assault
- Battery
- Defamation
- Intentional infliction of emotional distress
- Invasion of privacy
- Malpractice
- Negligence
- Nuisance
- Product liability
- Trespass

NEGLIGENCE

As discussed in Chapter 1, negligence is a breach of established standards of care. It is a failure to take reasonable care or steps to prevent loss or injury to another person. In health care, negligence occurs when a healthcare professional fails to take reasonable care or steps to prevent loss or injury to a client.

It is not a deliberate act but results in a harm to another person. For an act of negligence to occur, it must violate the following basic elements: duty of care, dereliction of duty, result in direct cause of harm, and that it caused damage or injury. Negligent torts occurred when the tortfeasor's actions were unreasonably unsafe.

STRICT LIABILITY

Strict liability is the relationship to or ownership of the thing that caused harm. Strict liability exists when a person places another person in danger, even in the absence of negligence, simply because that person is in possession of a dangerous product, animal, or weapon. Most cases of strict liability are regarding defective products. For example, if a flu vaccine was not prepared or packaged appropriately and people get sick, this may be a case of a strict liability tort.

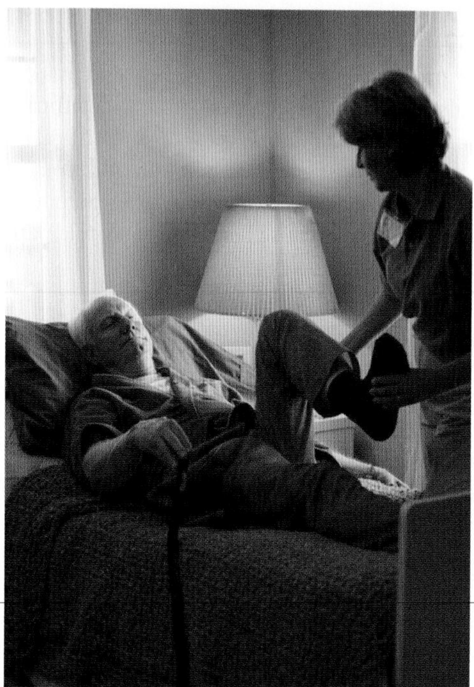

Fig. 5.2 To determine intent, we do not necessarily have to establish that the accused individual had a desire to cause harm or injury to a person. (Copyright © Photodisc/Photodisc/Thinkstock.com.)

INTENTIONAL TORTS

An **intentional tort** occurs when a person intends to perform an action that causes harm to another. For an intentional tort to be proven, it is not required for the person causing the harm to intentionally cause the injury; the person must only intend to perform the act. In general, intentional torts require that there be an intentional interference, or an intent, with an individual's person, reputation, or property.

Intent is generally the willful decision to bring about a prohibited consequence. In both civil and criminal laws, intent plays a key role in determining liability and responsibility. However, for an intentional tort to occur, it does not necessarily have to be established that the accused individual had a desire to bring about harm or injury to another person (Fig. 5.2). Instead, it is enough to be able to demonstrate that any reasonable person would or should be substantially certain that specific results will follow from his or her actions. The willful decision to bring about a prohibited consequence. For example, a surgical technician is late for work and needs to prepare the surgical tools and supplies before the morning's surgery. Because she is running late, she does not double check that the surgical tools have been properly sterilized. As a result, the surgical tools used on the patient were not sterile, and the patient developed an infection after surgery. Although the surgical technician did not intend to cause harm to the patient, any reasonable person would conclude that the surgical technician's action would have these results.

Intent may also be transferred. For example, suppose you intend to shoot person A, but you miss and shoot person B instead. Even though you have no intent to harm person B, the law deems that you had the intent to harm person B. Thus, in transferred intent, it is a rule of law that "intent follows the bullet."

APPLY THIS

Transferred intent does not often occur in the healthcare setting. Describe an example of transferred intent. Would this be a violation of civil law, criminal law, or both?

TYPES OF INTENTIONAL TORTS

The primary types of intentional torts are assault, battery, false imprisonment, intentional infliction of emotional distress, and trespass. Each type of intentional tort requires the presence of specific elements to be met for the tort to have been committed.

Assault

The first type of intentional tort is **assault**, which is placing someone in immediate fear or apprehension of harmful or unpleasant touching without the person's consent. To commit an assault, the person must be aware, or fearful, that the other person is about to make unwanted physical contact with another person. For example, a patient is in bed crying and becomes increasingly distraught and agitated. A home health aide caring for the patient tries to calm the patient without success and becomes frustrated. The home health aide raises her hand over her head and threatens to strike the patient if she does not stop crying. The home health aide does not have to say anything to the patient or even make contact for this to be an act of assault. If the patient sees the home health aide raising her hand and believes she may be hit, then the patient is put in imminent fear of assault. If, on the other hand, the patient is crying into her pillow and does not see the home health aide raising her hand to strike, the patient was not aware of the threat and, thus, assault was not committed.

In most cases, assault cannot be committed by mere words or a threat. Words, without an act, cannot constitute an assault. For example, if a person is pointing a gun at you but does not say anything, this is a case of assault because the intent to harm is real and apparent even without the expressed verbal threat. In addition, a person threatens to shoot you and points a gun at you. Later, you discover that there are no bullets in the gun; this is still a case of assault. However, if the person verbally threatens to shoot you but no gun is visible, there is no assault.

Battery

In many cases, assault and battery are grouped together. However, they are two separate intentional torts, with the assault often preceding the battery. A **battery** is harmful or offensive touching of another person without consent or without a legally justifiable reason. Without the consent of the patient, or an absence of an emergency, any touching of a patient may be considered battery. For battery to occur, the following elements must be met:

- There was an intent to cause contact.
- Contact occurs.
- Contact is harmful.
- No consent was given.

Committing battery does not mean you try to maliciously hurt or strike a person. Although hitting, spitting at, kicking, or slapping a patient are all forms of battery, it can be subtler than that. Any touching or contact, such as inserting an intravenous device or performing an injection, may be battery if done without the consent of the person or without authorization by the healthcare provider overseeing the patient's care.

In some cases, an individual does not need even to make contact with another person to commit battery. Instead, if the individual just touches something near the person without his or her consent, then battery may have been committed. For example, a patient wants to leave the hospital against medical advice. If you grabbed the patient's purse or suitcase from his hand, even if it is just to get him to listen to you, this may be a case of battery even though your intent was to help the patient.

In addition to being a civil or intentional tort, battery may also be considered a crime, depending on the type of intent. A criminal battery requires the presence of an intent to do wrong or to cause harmful or offensive contact. A defendant found guilty of the crime of battery may also be sued in civil court for damages for the same offense or incident.

APPLY THIS

A patient arrives in the emergency department suffering from psychosis. He becomes violent and starts attacking other patients and the medical staff. In attempts to restrain him, his arm gets broken. The patient's family sues the hospital for his injury.

1. What kind of tort can the hospital be sued for? Do they have grounds for suing the hospital?
2. Should the hospital be liable for the injury?

Types of Consent

For battery to occur, the touching must be done without permission or **consent**, unless it is an emergency. There are many distinct types of consent, but the two primarily related to health care are *general consent* and *informed consent*.

General consent. General consent is an individual's permission to be touched. General consent can be *explicit* or *implied*. Explicit consent, also known as express or direct consent, means that an individual is clearly presented with an option to agree or disagree or to express a preference or choice, often verbally or in writing. Explicit consent is usually required when clear, documentable consent is required, and the purpose for which it is being provided for is sensitive, such as the collection, use, or disclosure of personal information. For example, all patients admitted to a hospital are required to sign a general consent form, which grants permission for employees of the hospital to "touch" the patient in order to provide medical care and treatment.

Conversely, implied consent is not expressly granted by a person, but rather inferred from a person's actions and the facts and circumstances of a particular situation. There are many situations when healthcare professionals routinely obtain implied consent when treating a patient. For example, a medical assistant may ask a patient to roll his sleeve up while she is holding a syringe. If the patient rolls his sleeve up, this is implied consent for him to receive the shot (Fig. 5.3).

Implied consent may also be given in emergency situations. The situation must be life threatening or pose a risk of significant physical injury to the patient if the procedures are not performed. Only those procedures that are absolutely necessary are authorized, and explicit consent should be obtained as soon as possible. Furthermore, only a healthcare provider, such as a physician, can make the determination that a true emergency exists that necessitates proceeding without explicit or informed consent, which will be discussed next.

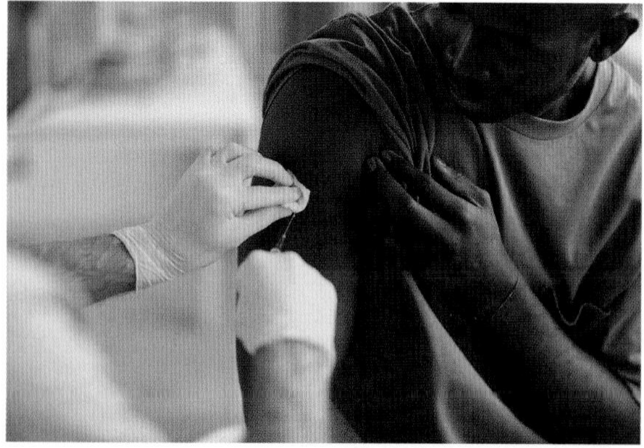

Fig. 5.3 Implied consent is based on inference and from the patient's action, such as rolling up the sleeve in anticipation of an injection. (iStock.com/SeventyFour.)

All states have statutes that specify when consent is implied. Thus, healthcare professionals must be aware of their individual state laws and ensure they are following them in order to protect patients' rights and to prevent any occurrence of negligence.

RELATE TO PRACTICE

An individual was watching other people stand in line to receive a vaccination. He spoke very little English and did not ask people why they were standing in line but decided to stand in line anyway. When he got closer to the front of the line, he held up his arm to the physician, who proceeded with the injection. When he realized what had happened, he filed a lawsuit against the healthcare provider and clinic alleging battery.

1. Was this a case of battery? Why or why not?
2. What kind of consent was given?
3. Should the court dismiss the battery claim? Why or why not?

Informed consent. General consent often gets confused with informed consent. **Informed consent** is the process by which the treating healthcare provider discloses appropriate information to a competent patient so that the patient may make a voluntary choice to accept or refuse treatment. The healthcare provider must detail all possible risks and potential prognoses for having a treatment or procedure performed and the available alternatives. Failure to obtain informed consent may lead to a case of medical negligence; however, the failure to obtain general consent or permission to touch the patient may lead to a case of battery.

To prevent allegations of battery, always have the patient's written consent to perform a procedure. Perform only the procedure authorized, and do not exceed the scope of the patient's consent. Unless it is an emergency, healthcare professionals should not proceed with any procedure without the consent of the patient. Obtaining consent is fundamental to the practice of medicine.

However, there are some situations when general consent by itself may not be enough to avoid the risk of battery. A medical *battery* can be committed in specific situations in which there was consent to perform one particular procedure, but a different procedure was performed instead. For example, in the case of *Pizzaloto v. Wilson,* the patient gave consent for the surgeon to perform excisions to remove adhesions and small cysts caused by ovarian endometriosis. During the surgery, the surgeon noted that the patient's reproductive organs had sustained severe damage and determined that the patient was, as a result, sterile. The surgeon proceeded to perform a hysterectomy, removing the patient's uterus and both of her ovaries. When the patient woke up from surgery, she was angry with the actions taken by the surgeon and filed a lawsuit. The court ruled that the patient (plaintiff) was entitled to recover damages and awarded her $10,000 because there was no emergency present and thus the surgeon committed battery because no consent had been given for this specific procedure.

APPLY THIS

A patient needs to receive a barium swallow but refuses to swallow the contrast medium. The nurse in charge of the patient takes the cup and forces the patient to drink it. You are an employee, and you observe this incident.

1. What offense(s) is the nurse committing?
2. What are your legal and ethical responsibilities as an employee?
3. What kind of rights does the patient have?

False Imprisonment

False imprisonment is the unlawful detention of a person, in which that person is deprived of personal liberty of movement against his or her will. To be falsely imprisoned, the confinement itself must be within a specific area by means of physical barriers and/or by physical force or threat of physical force, and the person must be aware of the confinement. Thus, any person who intentionally restricts another's freedom of movement without his or her consent (and without legal justification) may be liable for a charge of false imprisonment, which is both a crime and a civil violation. False imprisonment can occur in a room, on the streets, or even in a moving vehicle, just as long as the subject is unable to move freely, against the person's will.

All states have false imprisonment laws to protect against unlawful confinement. To prove a false imprisonment, the following elements must be present:

- There must have been a willful detention.
- The detention must have been without consent.
- The detention was unlawful.

In health care, false imprisonment generally arises in three circumstances: in the psychiatric setting with involuntary commitments; with the use of restraints, either physical or chemical; and in situations in which a patient attempts to leave the hospital against medical advice. However, in most situations, patients do have the right to refuse treatment and can leave against medical advice. But there are limited and defined situations in which patients may be legally detained.

Involuntary Commitment

In the psychiatric setting, a patient may be detained or involuntarily admitted if all the following legal requirements are met:

1. The statutory provisions for the reason for involuntary commitment, such as danger to self or others, exist.
2. All statutory requirements for physician examination have been met in a timely manner.
3. All appropriate documentation exists in the chart to support the action of involuntary admission.
4. All the patient's rights have been preserved.
5. All statutory time limits have been met, but not exceeded, for holding an individual against his or her will.

All healthcare professionals must use great caution when deciding to admit and confine a patient involuntarily and must ensure that all the previously mentioned legal requirements are met. For example, in the case *Brand v. University Hospital*, the plaintiff was out of town when she became ill. As she was driving to the local hospital, she experienced a seizure, became unconscious, and was involved in an accident. She was transported from the scene of the accident to the local hospital. In the emergency department, the treating physician gave her the option of either being admitted for a neurological workup or of being discharged to follow up with her own neurologist. The patient chose the latter and called friends to drive her home. One of her friends, a former drug addict, assumed the patient's behavior was due to a drug problem and then transported the patient to the behavioral treatment unit of University Hospital. The patient was so groggy that she was unaware until the next morning that she was in a locked psychiatric ward. She asked to be transferred to the medical ward of the hospital and insisted that the psychiatrist call the other hospital and her neurologist. Neither the psychiatrist nor the hospital staff at the treatment unit listened to the patient for more than 36 h. The patient sued University Hospital. The trial court originally dismissed the plaintiff's claim, but the appeals court overturned that decision, and the plaintiff was allowed to proceed against the hospital staff and physician.

In this case, the legal requirements for an involuntary admission were not met. There was no documentation that the patient was a danger to herself or others and there was insufficient physician examination. Thus, the staff of the behavioral unit had no right to detain the patient involuntarily.

Physical or Chemical Restraints

In many hospitals and nursing homes, some patients may have to be restrained to prevent injury to themselves or to others. If there is a need to use restraints, it must be documented in the patient's medical records. Otherwise, it may be a case of false imprisonment. Use of any other type of restraint, such as sheets to hold patients in wheelchairs, Posey belts, or any other form of physical restraint, should be implemented only as a last resort and must be used only as approved by hospital policy and the healthcare provider. Obtain written consent for the use of any type of restraint whenever possible.

With limited exceptions, healthcare professionals and organizations should operate under the assumption that they can never hold a patient against his or her will. However, there have been cases in which involuntary admission was necessary. In the case of *Mawhirt v. Ahmed*, a patient brought a lawsuit against the healthcare professionals and hospital for false imprisonment secondary to an involuntary admission and the use of both physical and chemical restraints. The plaintiff was suffering from paranoid delusions and that the CIA and Mafia were trying to harm him. Two physicians determined he was a danger to himself and others and proceeded with the appropriate procedures for the involuntary admission. The nursing staff documented the psychotic, delusional behavior of the plaintiff, as well as behavior that suggested that the plaintiff could harm himself or threaten other patients. They followed the institution's guidelines for the administration of chemical restraints and the procedures established for the use of physical restraints. As such, the court dismissed the plaintiff's claims.

Against Medical Advice

Another situation that raises possible issues of false imprisonment involves patients wishing to leave the hospital against medical advice (AMA). Although healthcare professionals have a duty to provide patient care, they cannot prevent a competent patient from refusing treatment or leaving the care of a healthcare provider or hospital. This means the patient cannot be barred from exiting or leaving. In addition, no healthcare professional or hospital employee can prevent the patient from collecting clothes and other personal belongings. In fact, no attempt can be made to prevent the patient from leaving, including touching the patient or his or her belongings in an effort to make the patient stay.

For example, a 67-year-old man's nephew admitted him to a nursing home. The man attempted to remove himself but was physically prevented from leaving the nursing home for 51 days. After several attempts to leave, he was placed in a restraint chair and denied use of the phone or even access to his own clothes. As the man was competent, he could not be detained against his will. The court found that the actions of the nursing staff were in disregard of the man's rights and were willful, reckless, and malicious in detaining him.

In addition, a hospital cannot detain or stop a patient from leaving, even for financial reasons. When the physician has written a discharge order, the hospital cannot keep the patient even if he or she has not made payments for the services rendered. Even though the patient obviously has the obligation to pay for these services, the hospital can hold the patient only until the patient indicates how he or she will pay for services.

In the case of a minor, the hospital can attempt to obtain a court order to require the family to keep the child in the hospital. But any attempt to physically restrain the child or the parent in the absence of a court order exposes the hospital to liability (Fig. 5.4).

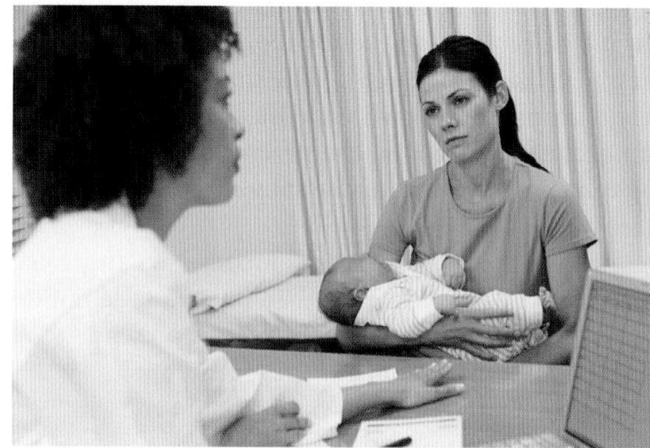

Fig. 5.4 In the case of a minor, the hospital can attempt to get a court order to require the family to keep the child in the hospital, but any attempt to physically restrain the child or the parent in the absence of a court order exposes the hospital to liability. (Copyright © Monkey Business Images/Monkey Business/Thinkstock.com.)

Intentional Infliction of Emotional Distress

A tort of intentional infliction of emotional distress involves conduct that is so terrible that it causes severe emotional trauma in the victim. To establish such a tort, the plaintiff must show that the defendant's conduct is outrageous and beyond the bounds of common decency. Insulting behavior is not enough; the actions must be egregious.

In the case of *Williams v. Payne* et al., the police suspected that the plaintiff had ingested crack cocaine. The plaintiff was brought to Pontiac Osteopathic Hospital, where the sheriff asked the physician to pump the plaintiff's stomach. The physician was aware that the sheriff did not have a warrant for the search. After placing the plaintiff in four-point restraints, the physician forcefully and, over the objections of the plaintiff, performed a gastric lavage. Afterward, the plaintiff was involuntarily catheterized. The court refused to dismiss the claim and allowed the claim to continue to the jury.

Trespass to Land

The tort of trespass occurs when a person, without the consent of the owner, enters on another's land or causes anyone or anything to enter the land. Harm to the land is not required; but, without harm to the land, courts usually award only nominal damages.

Cases of trespass in health care most often occur when healthcare professionals are guests in their patients' homes. Although healthcare professionals are there to perform necessary medical procedures, they are still guests in the patients' homes and may be there only with the approval and consent of the patient. At any time that a patient instructs a healthcare professional to leave his or her home, that person must leave. If that person does not leave, trespassing has been committed. In fact, the patient is authorized to use reasonable force to remove a trespasser from his or her home. Even if a healthcare professional's motives are noble in refusing to leave the property, such as wanting to perform necessary wound care for the patient's benefit, it is not a defense against the tort of trespass. Other potential claims for trespass to land include those against a patient who refuses to leave a facility after being discharged and against visitors in a facility who refuse to leave after visiting hours.

QUASI-INTENTIONAL TORTS

Quasi-intentional torts are voluntary acts that directly cause damage to a person's privacy or emotional wellbeing, but without the intent to injure or to cause distress. Quasi means "resembling" because these types of torts resemble intentional torts, but are different because they are based on speech. Quasi-intentional torts include defamation, invasion of privacy, and breach of confidentiality.

Defamation

Defamation is a false statement that wrongfully damages the reputation of another person. There are two types of defamation: libel and slander. Libel refers to written, printed, or visual defamatory statements, and slander refers to spoken defamatory statements.

To be liable for defamation, you must make a defamatory statement that is published or broadcasted to third parties; you cannot defame someone by telling only that person. In addition, the speaker must know or should know that the statement is false.

In defining a defamatory statement, the courts have looked to whether the statement exposed the plaintiff to public hatred, contempt, ridicule, or degradation. There also must be proof that there was actual harm to the person's reputation.

However, there are defamatory statements called *defamatory statements* per se for which no proof is needed because the statement is so damaging and presumed harmful. An example would be an allegation of sexual misconduct or criminal behavior or that an individual is afflicted with a disease that is stigmatized, such as syphilis, gonorrhea, leprosy, or human immunodeficiency virus (HIV) and acquired immunodeficiency syndrome (AIDS). In the case of *defamatory statements* per se, the plaintiff does not need to prove actual damage to reputation.

There may be qualified privileges that protect a person from a defamation suit. One of the most common examples of qualified privilege is the reporting of elder or child abuse. As long as the report is made in good faith, the healthcare professional or anyone reporting the abuse is protected from liability.

Invasion of Privacy

Invasion of privacy is the quasi-intentional tort of unjustifiably intruding upon another's right of privacy by any of the following actions:

- Appropriating his or her name or likeness
- Placing a person in a false light
- Publishing private facts
- Unreasonably interfering with his or her seclusion

Whereas defamation is the result of making false statements, in most instances of invasion of privacy, the information is true, but that person wants the information to be kept private. In addition, although defamation causes injury to reputation, invasion of privacy causes injury to feelings.

Appropriating Likeness and Placing a Person in a False Light

In the healthcare setting, the most common example of *appropriating likeness* is the use of photographs or video images of the patient without consent or exceeding the scope of the consent. For example, in the case of *Vassiliades v. Garfinckel* et al., a plastic surgeon used before-and-after pictures of a patient in a public demonstration without the patient's consent.

If a patient gives consent to the use of his or her likeness for teaching or treatment purposes, the scope of the consent cannot be exceeded. If the patient does not give consent, then no likeness can be used at all for any reason.

DISCUSSION

A local politician had extensive cosmetic dental work and plastic surgery performed in the clinic where you work. You tell a family member who works with the local politician. The local politician (patient) learns of this and believes her privacy has been breached. What are the legal and ethical ramifications?

Breach of Confidentiality

A **breach of confidentiality** is the public revelation of confidential or privileged information without an individual's consent. As health care becomes more dependent on technology, this has created more occurrences of breaches of confidentiality. Although allowing easier access to patient records and information to be shared among other healthcare providers, electronic health records still need to be maintained and secured to prevent unauthorized access.

In the case of *Ruocco v. Emory Hospital*, the plaintiff filed a lawsuit alleging invasion of privacy, negligent maintenance of records, negligent supervision, intentional infliction of emotional distress, and defamation. The plaintiff was a nurse, employed by the hospital, and was taking part in a hepatitis study. She received injections as part of the study. When she missed several weeks of work, one of the physicians in the study accessed her electronic medical record without the plaintiff's permission. Although he was not the plaintiff's treating physician, he accessed her records by claiming he was. In addition, he did not tell the plaintiff he accessed the records, and, in fact, in his deposition, he stated that he never intended to tell her. The plaintiff learned of the unauthorized access when she accessed her own records and saw that someone had accessed her records without her consent.

As a result of increases of breaches in confidentiality over electronic access to medical records, in 1996 Congress enacted the *Health Insurance Portability and Accountability Act of 1996* (HIPAA), calling for regulations to establish criteria for a federal standard in authorizing the release of medical information. In February 2000, the U.S. Department of Health and Human Services published the final rules to establish the federal criteria. (HIPAA will be discussed in further detail in the medical records chapter.)

Whether a healthcare professional has access to written medical records or to electronic computerized records, the responsibility to keep information confidential does not change (Fig. 5.5). Any information that a healthcare professional learns while caring for a patient is confidential, even if it does not relate directly to the treatment of the patient.

APPLY THIS

An adult patient is a member of a religious group that does not believe in receiving blood transfusions. The patient undergoes a surgical procedure and begins to hemorrhage. He is unable to voice his objections or express his wishes. You are aware of this patient's religious beliefs and that he does not want to receive blood. On the admission sheet, the area for religion is blank. He has no family. To prevent him from dying, the surgeon wants to give him a blood transfusion.

1. What should you do?
2. What are the ethical dilemmas and legal implications if he receives blood?
3. What are the legal and ethical implications if the patient is a minor and the parents refuse a blood transfusion?

Publicizing Private Facts

The most basic right of patients is the expectation that their personal and medical information will be kept confidential by the healthcare professional and organization. Every state mandates that the patient's

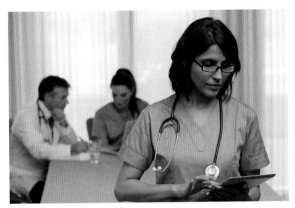

Fig. 5.5 Whether a healthcare provider has access to the traditional written medical record or to computerized records, the responsibility to keep information confidential does not change. (Copyright © Wavebreakmedia Ltd./Wavebreak Media/Thinkstock.com.)

confidentiality be maintained and outlines only limited situations in which a healthcare professional or organization may release information concerning a patient without his or her consent.

Being a healthcare professional and working in a medical facility does not give one the right to unlimited access to all patients' medical records. The law allows a healthcare professional and hospital staff to view and use only the medical records of the patients they are treating and to access and use only the information necessary to provide care. For example, in the case of *Estate of Behringer v. Princeton Medical Center*, a successful ear, nose, and throat surgeon was admitted for tests and was diagnosed with AIDS at the same hospital where he practices. No special steps were taken to protect the medical record or the patient's privacy. In fact, the physicians and nurses who cared for the surgeon spoke openly about his condition to individuals who were not involved in his care. By the time the physician was discharged from the hospital, numerous people in the community knew of his condition and his practice was negatively affected. The court upheld that there was an invasion of the surgeon's privacy.

CONCLUSION

The act of providing patient care and treatment may give rise to potential liability for torts and acts of malpractice. To prevent these types of liabilities, healthcare professionals must always have the patient's consent to perform specific procedures and not exceed that consent. Always maintain the patient's confidentiality and speak about the patient's condition only to those individuals who are actively involved in the patient's care. Understand that the patient has an absolute right to refuse treatment. In addition, the patient cannot be physically restrained or confined even when the patient is leaving the treatment facility against medical advice.

Very few patients ever become plaintiffs. However, a patient can quickly become one if the healthcare professional does not exercise good medical judgment or does not have respect for the patient's rights, privacy, and freedom.

CHAPTER REVIEW QUESTIONS

1. Publishing private but true facts about someone is defined as
   A. libel.
   B. slander.
   C. invasion of privacy.
   D. negligence.
2. If a patient has given consent for a procedure and a different or separate procedure is performed, the physician can be held liable for
   A. defamation.
   B. battery.
   C. assault.
   D. invasion of privacy.
3. Knowingly printing or publishing false information about someone is known as
   A. invasion of privacy.
   B. slander.
   C. breach of confidentiality.
   D. libel.
4. If you raise your hand or fist in such a manner that another person becomes fearful that you are going to strike him or her, you have committed
   A. assault.
   B. battery.
   C. defamation.
   D. libel.

5. A patient is scheduled to have a procedure performed, but states that he or she does not want the procedure. If the healthcare professional disregards the patient's wishes and performs the procedure anyway, the provider has just committed
   A. assault.
   B. invasion of privacy.
   C. breach of confidentiality.
   D. battery.
6. Which of the following is *not* an example of a tort?
   A. A phlebotomist forcibly grabs a patient, who is resisting getting her blood drawn.
   B. A surgeon operates on the wrong patient because he did not verify the patient's identity.
   C. A patient is prescribed penicillin and has an allergic reaction to it. The medical office did not ask the patient about any allergies to the drug.
   D. A physician misdiagnoses a patient's tumor as being cancerous when it is not.
7. A medical assistant administers a shot to a patient but forgets to properly dispose of the needle. The next patient comes into the patient room and accidently gets pricked by the open needle. What kind of tort is this?
   A. Assault.
   B. Intentional tort.
   C. Negligence.
   D. Strict liability.
8. A nurse put on her stethoscope and tells the patient she is going to listen to the patient's lungs. The patient starts to unbutton his shirt. This is an example of which kind of consent?
   A. Explicit consent.
   B. Implied consent.
   C. General consent.
   D. Informed consent.
9. A voluntary act that damages a person's privacy or well-being is a
   A. breach of confidentiality.
   B. intentional tort.
   C. quasi-intentional tort.
   D. intentional infliction of emotional distress.
10. A person's computer was hacked, and her information was released on the internet. This is an example of
    A. invasion of privacy.
    B. slander.
    C. breach of confidentiality.
    D. libel.

SELF-REFLECTION QUESTIONS

1. What role does *intent* play in an intentional tort?
2. How does *consent* play a role in the defense of an intentional tort?
3. How can charting and medical records help prevent a successful lawsuit based on false imprisonment?
4. Is there ever an instance when a patient's consent may not be necessary besides in an emergency? When the patient is not competent? When it is the only way to save the patient's life?

INTERNET ACTIVITIES

1. Using legal websites and search engines, find a case based on a lack of informed consent in your current or future profession.
2. Perform a web search for informed consent. What information must be disclosed during informed consent, and who is responsible for obtaining the informed consent?

ADDITIONAL RESOURCES

https://www.ama-assn.org
https://www.apa.org
https://www.ast.org
https://www.aama-ntl.org
https://www.loc.gov

BIBLIOGRAPHY

Aiken, T. (Ed.). (2004). *Legal, ethical, and political issues in nursing* (2nd ed.). Philadelphia: F.A. Davis.

Big Town Nursing Home, Inc. v. New, 461 S.W.2d 195 (Tex. 1970).

Blackman for Blackman v. Rifkin, 759 P.2d 54 (Colo. 1988).

Brand v. Univ. Hosp., 525 S.E.2d 374 (Ga. 1999).

Davis v. St. Jude Med. Ctr., 645 So. 2d 771 (La. App. 5th Cir. 1994).

DiLeo v. Nugent, 592 A.2d 1126 (Md. 1991).

Doe v. Methodist Hosp., 639 N.E.2d 683 (Ind. 1994, rev'd, 690 N.E.2d 681) (Ind. 1997).

Estate of Behringer v. Princeton Med. Ctr., 592 A.2d 1251 (N.J. 1991).

Id. at 1273.

Feeney v. Young, 191 A.D. 501, 181 N.Y. Supp. 481 (N.Y. 1920).

Guin v. Sison, 552 So. 2d 60 (La. 1989).

Ironside v. Simi Valley Hosp., No. 95–6336, slip op. (6th Cir. 1996).

Mawhirt v. Ahmed, 86 F.Supp.2d 81 (E.D. N.Y. 2000).

Montgomery v. Bazaz-Shegal, 742 A.2d 1125 (Pa. 1999).

Novak v. Cobb County Kennestone Hosp. Auth., No. 94–8403, slip op. (11th Cir. 1996).

O'Brien v. Cunard S.S. Co., 28 N.E. 266 (1881).

Phipps v. Clark Oil and Ref. Corp., 408 N.W. 2d 569, 573 (Minn. 1987).

Pizzaloto v. Wilson, 437 So. 2d 859 (La. 1983).

Roberson v. Provident House, 576 So. 2d 992 (La. 1991).

Ruocco v. Emory Hosp., No. 97-VS0132401.

Saur v. Probes, 476 N.W.2d 496 (Mich. 1991).

Schlesser v. Keck, 271 P.2d 588 (Calif. 1954).

Schloendorff v. Soc'y of N.Y. Hosp., 105 N.E. 92 (1914).

Simpkins v. District of Columbia et al., No. 94-5243, slip op. (D.C. Cir. 1997).

Smith v. St. Paul Fire and Marine Ins. Co., 353 N.W.2d 130 (Minn. 1984).

St. Paul Fire and Marine Ins. Co. v. Asbury, 720 P.3d 540 (Ariz. 1986).

St. Paul Fire and Marine Ins. Co. v. Shernow, 610 A.2d 1281 (Conn. 1992).

Vassiliades v. Garfinckel's, Brooks Bros., 492 A.2d 580 (D.C. 1985).

Williams v. Payne et al., 73 F. Supp. 2d 785 (E.D. Mich. 1999).

6

Medical Malpractice and Liability

CHAPTER OBJECTIVES

1. Define and explain malpractice.
2. List the four legal conditions that determine negligence in the healthcare setting.
3. Recognize the concept of "*respondeat superior*" and its role in malpractice cases.
4. Identify and explain the three categories of dereliction of duty (breach).
5. Outline the three categories of damages that are required in malpractice cases.
6. Describe the process of establishing a case of malpractice or negligence.
7. Define and explain defenses in malpractice cases.
8. Discuss the issues of malpractice and negligence as they relate to emergency care.
9. Define liability prevention strategies for both individual employees and managers in the healthcare setting.

KEY TERMS

Affirmative defense A defense strategy that allows the defendant (usually provider or facility) to present the argument that the patient's condition was the result of factors other than negligence on the defendant's part.

Alternative dispute resolution (ADR) The procedure for settling disputes by means other than litigation.

Arbitration The process of resolving a dispute outside the courts with a person or persons assigned by the court to mediate in a civil suit and then decide the outcome of the dispute.

Assumption of risk A legal defense that asserts that the plaintiff was aware of risks and accepted the risks associated with the activity involved.

Claims-made policy Insurance policy in which coverage is triggered on the date that the insured first becomes aware of the possibility of a claim and notifies the insurer.

Comparative negligence A legal defence that proves the plaintiff's own actions, or lack of action, contributed to the damages done.

Compensatory damages The amount awarded to the plaintiff in a court case to reimburse the plaintiff for loss of income or pain and suffering.

Contributory negligence A defense strategy that allows the defendant to present the argument that the patient's condition was the result of factors other than negligence on the defendant's part.

Damages The actual injury or loss suffered by a defendant in a suit; usually given a monetary award by the court based on the extent of the loss or injury.

Defensive medicine The practice of ordering unnecessary tests, treatments, and other procedures to protect against medical malpractice.

Denial Legal assertion of innocence; made only if all four elements of negligence are false.

Dereliction (of duty) A neglect or negligence of one's duty.

Direct cause In a negligence case, the correspondence between the dereliction of duty and the actual damage sustained by the plaintiff.

Discovery rule Law or statute that states the statute of limitations does not begin until the discovery of the diagnosis or injury.

Duty In a malpractice suit, the proof of responsibility of the parties involved.

Emergency Medical Treatment and Active Labor Act (EMTALA) A federal law that requires anyone coming to an emergency department be stabilized and treated, regardless of his or her insurance status or ability to pay.

Good Samaritan Law Law providing immunity for those who render health care in an emergency or disaster without reimbursement.

Liable Having legal responsibility for one's own actions.

Litigious Highly inclined or prone to engage in lawsuits to settle disputes.

Malfeasance The performance of an illegal act.

Malpractice The failure of a professional to meet the standard of conduct that a reasonable and prudent member of the same profession would exercise in similar circumstances and that results in harm.

Mediation The process by which a neutral third party who is trained in mediation techniques facilitates and assists in resolving a dispute.

Misfeasance Poor performance of a duty or action, causing damage.

Nominal damages A small payment or award given by the court.

Nonfeasance A failure to perform an action when needed.

Occurrence-basis policy An insurance policy that covers claims taking place during the policy period, regardless of when claims are made.

Patient abandonment A legal claim that occurs when a healthcare provider terminates the professional relationship with a patient without reasonable notice and when continued care is medically necessary.

Premium The amount of money an insurer charges to provide the coverage described in the policy.

Punitive damages An award granted by the courts to punish the defendant for the damages done based on a malicious or intentional act.

Release of tortfeasor Law that asserts that once the person causing damage (the tortfeasor) is released from further liability in a previous suit's settlement, he or she cannot be held liable in a subsequent suit.

Res ipsa loquitur Clear evidence of negligence and that there was no other possible way that the plaintiff could have effected a different outcome or contributed to the damages or injury.

Res judicata Law that forbids suing a subsequent time for the same damages once a case has already been resolved.

Respondeat superior Legal doctrine stating that, in many circumstances, an employer is responsible for the actions of employees performed within the course of their employment.

Risk management The process of identifying threats that could harm the organization, its patients, staff, or anyone else within the organization.

Settlement Legal agreement that is reached between two parties in a civil matter.

Statute of limitations Defense against a tort action; requires that a claim be filed within a specific amount of time of discovering that a wrong has been committed.

Vicarious liability The liability of an employer for the actions of its designated agents.

INTRODUCTION

Every profession and industry have some risk of liability to their clients or to the public. Consider a truck driver and the kind of damage he could cause if he was under the influence of drugs or alcohol while driving an 80,000-ton truck and for an accident occurred. Similarly, in the healthcare setting, people's lives are dependent on all healthcare professionals upholding a standard of care and conducting themselves in a professional and ethical way to prevent any injury to patients.

Even with the best intentions and many safeguards in place, accidents can happen, and mistakes can occur. In our legal system, when a party has been injured or harmed, the party responsible for the action or inaction that resulted in the injury needs to be held responsible. This is when negligence and medical malpractice laws protect those individuals who suffer damages or injury.

As a healthcare professional, it is critical to have a thorough understanding of the duties and responsibilities when practicing your profession to avoid causing such damage and injury to your patients. This chapter will discuss what constitutes malpractice and how is it determined and how healthcare professionals may protect themselves against such liability and negligence.

MALPRACTICE AND NEGLIGENCE

As we discussed in previous chapters, one of the most common types of violation against civil law is a tort. A *tort* is a civil wrong that results in injury to another's person, property, reputation, safety, or the like, and for which the injured party is entitled to compensation. A specific type of tort is *negligence*, which is a failure to use care or act in a certain way that a reasonably prudent and careful person would under similar circumstances. It is an act of omission or failure to do what a person of ordinary prudence would have done under similar circumstances. For example, a driver is texting while driving and causes an accident that harms another driver. This would be considered a case of negligence because a reasonable and careful person would not text while driving.

In the healthcare setting, malpractice may occur. **Malpractice** is a type of negligence in which a party (or parties) responsible for the care or treatment of an individual either acts or fails to act, resulting in damages, injuries, and/or direct losses to the individual. Medical malpractice occurs when the bond of trust between a healthcare professional and patient has in some form been breached, treatment was not provided, and/or the standard of care not been met, resulting in injury or even death to the patient. When determining if a case of malpractice has occurred, one must understand negligence and the four legal conditions that determine it: *duty*, *dereliction of duty (breach)*, *direct cause*, and *damages*.

Duty

The first legal condition that must be met in a negligence case is **duty**. This is the existence of a legal responsibility on the part of the physician or healthcare provider to provide care or treatment to the patient. Duty is often the easiest to establish because it is created whenever a healthcare provider undertakes the care of a patient. A duty does not exist where no relationship is established between the healthcare provider and patient, such as providing emergency care to an accident victim by the roadside.

To establish that a healthcare provider has a duty, the patient should ask the following questions:

1. Who are the responsible parties involved?
2. Was there a professional relationship established between the patient and healthcare provider?

Part of identifying the responsible party or parties involves a concept referred to as ***respondeat superior***, which in Latin means "*let the master answer*." In other words, an employer is responsible for the actions of employees performed within the course of their employment. Often, it is the individual with the highest license or training or the highest authority of an organization who is the one ultimately responsible for the actions of his or her employees or subordinate workers (Fig. 6.1). However, this does not exclude any healthcare professional from responsibility. But it legally requires that the person most responsible provides training, education, and supervision to his or her subordinate staff to ensure adherence to policies, procedures, and scope of practice. For example, if a respiratory care therapist is sued for actions that harmed a patient, his employer—the hospital—can be sued for negligence. As a result, the hospital can be sued under **vicarious liability**, which is based on the legal concept of *respondeat superior*. The hospital can be sued on the basis both that it had control, or should have had control, over the actions of the respiratory care therapist, and that he or she was working in the course and scope of his or her employment with the hospital.

There are times when an employer may not agree with the employee's view of that incident, which may result in a conflict over liability. For example, the employer

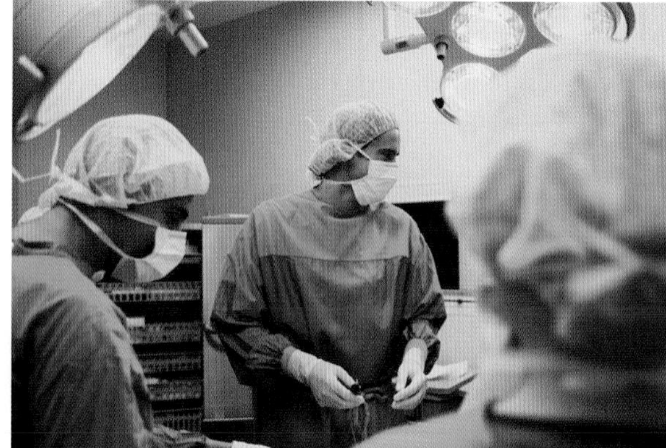

Fig. 6.1 In *respondeat superior*, the individual with the highest license or training and/or the owner or highest authority of an organization is ultimately the individual responsible for actions of their subordinate workers. (Copyright © Jochen Sand/DigitalVision/Thinkstock.com.)

may take the position that the employee was not acting within the scope of the employee's duties. If the employer proves this is true, the employee will be liable, and the employer's insurer has no duty to assist in the employee's defense if a lawsuit was to occur.

APPLY THIS

Bob works as a patient care technician at Green Hills Medical Center. One evening, as Bob is entering the hospital, he hears squealing brakes. Bob looks around the corner of the building but does not see anything except the taillights of a fast-moving car as it turns onto a side street. Bob shrugs his shoulders and goes into the hospital to start his shift.

The following day, Bob reads in the newspaper that a young man died last night after being dumped outside Green Hills Medical Center. The family of the young man is threatening to sue the hospital and anyone else who was there who did not help their family member. Bob realizes that he might have witnessed this situation and is worried that he might be involved in this lawsuit.

1. What should Bob do?
2. Could the family sue Bob for malpractice? Could they sue the hospital for malpractice?

Dereliction of Duty (Breach)

A dereliction of duty, or breach, occurs when one party or parties has a duty of care toward another party or parties but fails to live up to that reasonable care or standard. After establishing whether there was a duty, a dereliction of duty must be determined. Did that person breach his or her duty by failing to act with the same reasonable care an ordinary person would use in the same circumstances? Although this standard may vary by state and jurisdiction, in medical malpractice, the standard is usually determined by the standard of care (discussed in Chapter 2).

In a medical malpractice case, the question is not whether a healthcare provider acted as a reasonable individual off the street, but whether the provider acted in a way that a reasonable medical professional with the same training and knowledge would have acted. For example, an examination performed by any dermatologist in a specific should be able to identify a suspicious mole and recommend a biopsy as confirmation. Or a nurse would verify the expiration date on a medication before administering it. These are examples of standards of care and what a patient should expect from a healthcare professional.

Categories of Derelictions or Breaches

There are generally three types of derelictions of duty (or *feasance*):

- Malfeasance—an intentional action or performance of an illegal or wrongful act. An example might be a physician working outside his or her scope of practice, such as a family physician performing an invasive surgical procedure that a surgeon should be performing instead.
- Nonfeasance—a failure to perform an action that should have been taken. An example would be a nurse who did not ask about known allergies, resulting in the patient having a severe allergic reaction from a treatment.
- Misfeasance—the poor performance of an action that results in damage. An example would be a surgical technician failing to properly sterilize surgical equipment, causing a bacterial infection in a patient.

Direct Cause

If it has been established that the healthcare provider is responsible (has a duty in this situation) and that there was a dereliction in this duty, the patient will next need to prove direct cause. Using a previous example, if the patient had an allergic reaction to a medication that was administered and the nurse had not verified the patient's allergies, this would be a direct cause of the patient's injuries. A direct relationship must be proven between the alleged misconduct and the subsequent injury. In this case, the patient's allergic reaction was directly from the treatment, and it could not be from anything else.

Damages

Once negligence has been established and that the damages or losses incurred by the patient were directly related to that negligent act, the court must determine the damage that was caused by the negligence. This often means a calculation of monetary damages that can be awarded to the injured party. This may include recovery for any permanent disability, loss of employment or wages, pain and suffering, medical or hospital expenses, permanent mental disability, future loss of earnings if unable to return to employment, and loss of enjoyment attributable to the injuries and/or disabilities suffered.

In a medical malpractice case, most damages are designed to compensate a patient for harm caused by a healthcare provider's mistake. Damages generally fall into the following categories:

- Compensatory damages—Compensation for the actual injury and harm that the patient has suffered.

Compensatory damages aim to make the plaintiff "whole." Compensatory damages may be either for *economic losses,* such as loss of income, medical and hospital bills, physical therapy, and medical equipment, or for *noneconomic losses,* such as pain and suffering, mental anguish, loss of quality of life, or loss of the ability to work. If there were no actual damages, the patient may receive **nominal damages**, which are small awards given when no major damages were suffered but the patient is still entitled to some type of compensation.

- **Punitive damages**—Awards based on an intentional or wrongful act that was performed. Punitive damages are often awarded as a punishment for the wrongful act. In measuring punitive damages, the question is asked, "Should the healthcare provider be punished for what happened?" Often, to be awarded punitive damages, the negligent act must be intentional and/or particularly reckless in nature. For example, punitive damages may be awarded if a hospital knowingly allowed a surgeon who has a suspended medical license to perform surgery that resulted in harm to a patient.

APPLY THIS

As a certified nursing assistant, you are assigned to a different unit to work with the nursing staff. You discover one of the nurses is your sister's best friend. During your time working with her, she is often missing from the unit, and you cannot find her to report on your patients.

During one of your rounds, you find that the blood pressure of one of the patients is very high and that she complains of a headache. You let the nurse know and ask her to confirm your reading. Instead of checking on the patient, however, she leaves to make a personal phone call. Several hours later, you walk into the same patient's room, and she is now drooling and cannot move the left side of her body. When it is reported to your supervisors, the nurse implores you not to tell the nurse manager because she is already on probation.

1. Who is responsible in this situation?
2. Are the four elements of negligence present in this scenario? What are they?
3. Are there issues that can affect the licenses of both the nurse and the certified nursing assistant?

Patient Abandonment

Patient abandonment is a legal claim that occurs when a healthcare provider, usually a physician, terminates the professional relationship with a patient without reasonable notice and when continued care is medically necessary. Patient abandonment is a type of medical malpractice due to a breach in duty of care. When a patient is seen by a healthcare provider for a diagnosis or treatment, a professional relationship begins. This professional relationship continues until either the healthcare provider or the patient terminates the relationship. The healthcare provider–patient relationship is both an ethical relationship governed by the state medical boards and a legal relationship defined by the courts or by state law. For patient abandonment to occur, the following conditions must be met:

- A professional relationship was established and clearly existed
- Medical care for the patient was still necessary
- Medical care abruptly ceased with no time for the patient to seek new care and treatment from another provider
- Injury or damage to the patient resulted directly from the abandonment

Box 6.1 provides common examples of patient abandonment.

To legally terminate the healthcare provider–patient relationship, the healthcare provider must give the patient proper notice that the healthcare provider is terminating the relationship and give the patient sufficient time to find another provider before finally refusing to treat the patient any further. Giving proper notice to a

BOX 6.1 Examples of Patient Abandonment

- Taking a vacation without providing coverage from another healthcare provider and in the same specialty
- Failing to follow up with a patient after prescribing medication
- Failing to respond to patient communications, such as phone calls and emails
- Prematurely discharging a patient from the hospital or without proper instructions
- Failing to provide adequate staffing to appropriately care for a patient
- Appointment being scheduled out too far to provide effective care

BOX 6.2 Common Reasons to Terminate a Healthcare Provider–Patient Relationship

- The patient fails to pay the medical bills.
- The patient is rude, disruptive, uses improper language, exhibits violent behavior, or threatens the safety of the office staff or other patients.
- The patient requires more highly specialized services than the healthcare provider can provide.
- The patient continually cancels or misses appointments.
- The patient does not adhere or refuses to comply with the treatment plan.
- The office staff is uncomfortable working with or communicating with the patient.
- The patient did not provide an honest medical history or was misleading in the information provided, thereby compromising the efficacy of treatment.

patient usually includes telling the patient, either on the phone or face to face, that the relationship is being terminated and writing the patient a letter confirming the termination. The letter should be sent by certified mail, return receipt requested. Place a copy of the letter and the postal receipt in the patient's medical record. Proper notice might also include assistance in helping the patient find a new provider or even recommendations for new providers. The healthcare provider should tell the patient the reasons why the provider is terminating the relationship (Box 6.2).

Healthcare providers must provide sufficient time for the patient to find another provider and the amount of time depends on the nature of the patient's condition and location. For example, for a minor injury or condition, such as a needing treatment for a urinary tract infection, 1- or 2-weeks' notice might be sufficient time. For a more serious condition, such as a patient with uncontrolled hypertension or diabetes, 1 or 2 months may be necessary. If the patient lives in a rural area where there are very few healthcare providers, even more time will be required. During this time, the healthcare provider must continue providing the same level of care.

ESTABLISHING A CASE OF NEGLIGENCE

In a negligence case, the plaintiff (patient) must prove the four legal conditions occurred with a "preponderance of evidence" and that the healthcare provider acted below the accepted standard of care. In other words, the responsibility rests on the plaintiff to prove the case, as opposed to the defendant. However, often there are no witnesses to the negligent act or there is insufficient evidence or documentation, such as the patient's medical records.

In these situations, some states allow plaintiffs to use the legal concept of *res ipsa loquitur*, which was discussed in Chapter 1. *Res ipsa loquitur* means that there is clear evidence of negligence and that there was no other possible way that the patient (plaintiff) could have suffered the damages or injury except as a result of the negligence. For example, a surgeon performs an operation to amputate a patient's right arm but instead amputates the left arm. Clearly, the surgeon performed a negligent act, and the patient had nothing to do with the surgeon's action. To establish negligence under *res ipsa loquitur,* one or more of the following must be true:

- Evidence regarding the actual negligent act and cause of injury is unobtainable.
- The healthcare provider has superior knowledge or means of obtaining evidence about the cause of the injury.
- The type of injury does not ordinarily occur in the absence of negligence.
- The patient was not responsible for the injury.
- The healthcare provider was responsible for the patient's welfare at the time of the injury.
- The healthcare provider had exclusive control over the circumstances that led to the injury.

Although this may vary with individual states, under *res ipsa loquitur* negligence cases, the presumption is that the defendant is negligent and the burden of proof falls on the defendant to prove there was no negligence.

The Trial Process

Lawsuits alleging medical malpractice are generally filed in a state trial court. Such trial courts are said to have jurisdiction over medical malpractice cases, which is the legal authority to hear and decide the case. Some towns may be located in two judicial districts, giving the injured patient an option to file suit in more than one trial court.

Under limited circumstances, a medical malpractice case may be filed or moved to a federal court. This can occur if the underlying case invokes a federal question or federal constitutional issue or if the parties live in different states.

In the United States, the right to a jury trial is regarded as a fundamental constitutional right. A jury trial is a legal proceeding where a group of individuals chosen from the public is asked to consider the evidence presented during the case and make a decision. The choice of jurors is guided by court rules and with the participation of lawyers from both sides. Demographic information about the jurors is known to both parties, each of whom can usually strike a limited number of jurors to assure impartiality of the jury panel. In contrast to a jury trial, a bench trial is one in which a judge or a panel of judges makes the ultimate decision. In the United States, a physician can expect a jury trial in nearly all cases of medical malpractice, assuming the case is not resolved prior to trial.

It should be noted that most medical malpractice cases do not go to trial court and are often resolved out of court through a settlement. A **settlement** is a legal agreement that is reached between two parties—the plaintiff and the defendant—in a civil matter. Through a settlement, the patient (plaintiff) agrees to give up the right to pursue any further legal action in connection with the accident or injury, in exchange for an agreed-on sum of money from the defendant (healthcare provider, hospital, or an insurance company). Most states have passed laws that limit the amount of compensation a plaintiff can receive from a medical malpractice lawsuit. Most of these compensation caps for damages apply to *noneconomic* losses, such as for the patient's pain and suffering.

DEFENSES AGAINST MALPRACTICE

According to a survey by the American Medical Association, more than 60% of physicians older than the age of 55 have been sued for malpractice at least once. Although most of those lawsuits are dropped or dismissed, all healthcare professionals, not just physicians, must be aware of the potential risk from a growing **litigious** society, or one that is more highly inclined or prone to engage in lawsuits. As a result, more and more healthcare providers are practicing **defensive medicine**, which is the practice of ordering unnecessary tests, treatments, and other procedures to protect against medical malpractice.

If the allegations are entirely false or the lawsuit is baseless, the defendant may assert his or her innocence. The **denial** defense can be used only if *all* aspects of the complaint are false, or all four elements of negligence have not been established.

Before a case goes to court, both parties may agree to try an **alternative dispute resolution (ADR)**, which is usually less formal, less expensive, and less time consuming than a trial. Although there are many types of ADR for civil cases, the most common are mediation and arbitration. In **mediation**, an impartial person, called a "mediator," helps the parties try to reach a mutually acceptable resolution of the dispute. The mediator does not decide the dispute but helps the parties communicate so they can try to settle the dispute themselves. Mediation leaves control of the outcome with the parties.

In contrast, **arbitration** appoints a neutral person, called an "arbitrator," to hear arguments and evidence from each side and then decide the outcome of the dispute. Arbitration may be either "binding" or "nonbinding." Binding arbitration means that the parties waive their right to a trial and agree to accept the arbitrator's decision as final. Generally, there is no right to appeal an arbitrator's decision. However, nonbinding arbitration means that the parties are free to request a trial if they do not accept the arbitrator's decision.

APPLY THIS

A patient is admitted to the emergency department due to several days of severe abdominal pain. The patient is diagnosed with gallstones that have perforated the gallbladder and have become gangrenous. The patient also suffers from poorly controlled type 2 diabetes. The patient undergoes surgery, and the gallbladder is removed, but the patient suffers from jaundice postsurgery. After follow-up testing, it is determined that the bile duct from the gallbladder was damaged during the emergency surgery and the patient needs another surgical procedure to repair the damage.

1. Would the conditions of negligence be met in this case?
2. Are there any other mitigating factors involved?
3. Would the patient receive any kind of damages? Which kind of damages?

Statute of Limitations

Some technical defenses can prevent a case from ever going to trial. For example, most states have a statute of limitations on lawsuits, including medical malpractice, which means that the plaintiff has a limited number of years after the injury or discovery of the injury to file a lawsuit. Depending on the state and the type of lawsuit, the statute of limitations may be 2 years or as long as 10 years, with most medical malpractice cases usually having a statute of limitations of 6 years. If the lawsuit is not filed within the timeframe, the plaintiff has lost the right to file a lawsuit against the defendant.

The statute of limitations starts at the time of the accident or injury; however, it is not always clear when an injury occurred, especially in a medical malpractice case. As a result, many states have a discovery rule, which is a law that states that the statute of limitations does not begin until the discovery of the injury. For example, if a physician amputates a right arm when he or she should have removed the left, the date of the malpractice and the start of the statute of limitation are clearly the date the surgery occurred and when the patient realized the wrong arm had been removed. However, in the case of mesothelioma from exposure to asbestos, evidence of potential injury can take years or even decades to discover. The statute of limitation may not begin until the diagnosis was made or, in some cases, even afterward, for example, when a person investigates the cause of the cancer.

Another technical defense is the *res judicata*, in which the patient cannot sue a second time for the same damages once a case has already been resolved. Similarly, the release of tortfeasor asserts that, if the person causing damage (the tortfeasor) is released from further liability in a previous suit's settlement, he or she cannot be held liable in a subsequent suit.

Affirmative Defense

Another type of defense against a malpractice lawsuit is an affirmative defense, which is created for the defendant to argue against the plaintiff's claim in a lawsuit. An affirmative defense strategy allows the defendant to present the argument that the patient's condition was the reason for the injury and not the result of the defendant's negligence. In most cases, an affirmative defense is taken to limit damages and not to admit to negligence or any level of culpability. The most common examples of affirmative defenses are *contributory negligence* and *comparative negligence.*

Contributory Negligence

In contributory negligence, a party who negligently harms another party is not deemed responsible if the injured party is himself or herself negligent in action to any extent. For example, a patient suffers from complications from a surgical procedure, but the patient also did not follow the physician's discharge instructions. Based on contributory negligence, the physician can prove that the patient is partially responsible for his or her injury, making the physician not legally liable to the plaintiff.

Comparative Negligence

In comparative negligence, the defendant still seeks to show that the action or inaction of the plaintiff was a contributing factor in the damages that he or she incurred. However, instead of proving no liability to the injury, the defendant seeks to reduce the compensation to the injured party. In both instances, the plaintiff's negligence must be proved by the defendant.

Assumption of Risk

Another defense against malpractice is the assumption of risk defense, which asserts that the plaintiff was aware of the risks and accepted the risk associated with the activity involved. For an assumption of risk, the patient must first give consent, or acknowledge the risks and alternatives involved in a treatment usually given verbally or by a written document. Thus, before undergoing any medical treatment or procedure, healthcare providers, medical clinics, and hospitals must require patients to sign a *consent to treat* form, as well as a form that explains the risks of the procedure.

The assumption of risk defense relies on accurate documentation. For example, before any procedure, a patient is required to sign an informed consent form, which lists and details all possible risks involved in a treatment or procedure, and possible outcomes or complications. The informed consent form also details the possible ramifications or consequences of not having the procedure. However, regardless of what the patient consents to or signs, this defense does not exempt a healthcare professional from liability if his or her actions were reckless or intentional and resulted in harm to the patient.

APPLY THIS

A patient is seen by a gastroenterologist, and it is recommended that the patient undergo a colonoscopy procedure for diagnostic purposes. The physician reviews the risks of having the procedure performed and the consequences of not having the procedure performed with the patient. The patient signs an informed consent form. Before the procedure, the medical assistant reviews the preparation instructions with the patient. In the instructions, it is clearly noted that the patient should stop taking any medication that may cause bleeding problems, such as aspirin, at least 7 days before the surgery. However, the patient continues to take a single 81-mg dose of aspirin each evening.

On the day of the procedure, both the medical assistant and the gastroenterologist review the preparation instructions with the patient, with the patient confirming that he followed all of them. Several days later, the patient complains of bleeding and must be hospitalized. The patient files a lawsuit against the gastroenterologist.

1. Who is responsible in this case?
2. What kind of defense(s) could the gastroenterologist use against this lawsuit?

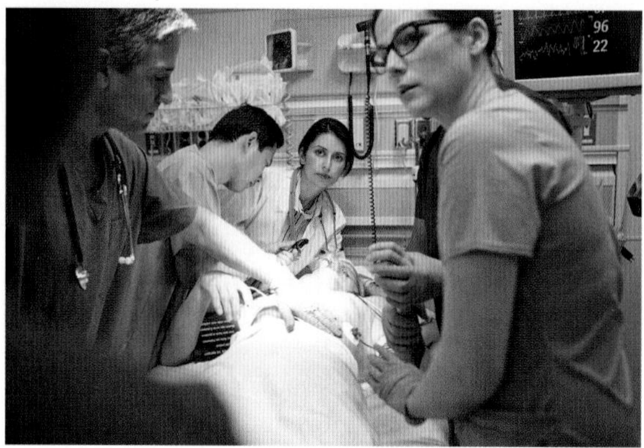

Fig. 6.2 EMTALA, sometimes referred to as the "anti-dumping law," was designed to prevent hospitals with emergency departments from transferring uninsured or patients with Medicaid without screening, treating, and stabilizing the injured or ill person. (iStock.com/Monkeybusinessimages.)

EMERGENCY CARE

One of the highest-risk areas for medical malpractice is in emergency medicine, often because decisions on patient care must be made immediately and consent may not always be given. Because of this, most states provide some protection from lawsuits for emergency medical services personnel, such as firefighters, first responders, and emergency medical technicians (EMTs). Depending on the state and, as long as the emergency personnel does not act intentionally or in a reckless manner, he or she would not be liable for malpractice. In fact, even if liability was found with the emergency personnel, it would be his or her employer who would be deemed liable and financially responsible.

However, this protection from malpractice does not extend to the physicians, nurses, and other healthcare professionals working in the emergency department at a hospital where the medical malpractice standards and standard of care apply. All hospitals with emergency departments that receive federal reimbursements, such as Medicare and Medicaid funding, are subject to the **Emergency Medical Treatment and Active Labor Act (EMTALA)**. EMTALA, sometimes referred to as the "anti-dumping law," was designed to prevent hospitals with emergency departments from transferring uninsured or patients with Medicaid without, at a minimum, providing medical screening and treat and stabilize the injured or ill person to the extent possible (Fig. 6.2). In almost all cases, the hospital is liable for the actions of the healthcare providers working in its emergency department, even if the provider is not an employee of the hospital but an independent contractor. It is presumed that the patient was visiting the hospital's emergency department and not there to see a specific healthcare provider. Penalties for violating EMTALA may result in the hospital or physician's ability to receive Medicare payments, fines, and the hospital may be sued for personal injury in civil court under a "private cause action."

Good Samaritan Laws

What happens if you witness a car accident, and you stop to help? Will you be sued if you accidently injured someone while trying to help in this situation? Would it be worse if it was discovered that you are a healthcare professional?

In general, no one is obligated to provide assistance during an emergency situation. Fortunately, many people do. To protect these people from liability, there are laws to provide basic legal protection for those who assist a person who is injured or in danger called the Good Samaritan laws. Although it may vary, every state has some form of Good Samaritan law. The Good Samaritan laws provide protection to any individual who provides assistance in an emergency situation, as long as the actions are not reckless and do not needlessly endanger the person the individual is trying to assist.

In addition, in the United States, healthcare professionals are not legally required to provide medical assistance to injured persons if they have not established a relationship, or duty, to them. If a healthcare professional responds in good faith in an emergency or accident, he or she may also be protected under the Good Samaritan laws. The Good Samaritan laws will apply to healthcare providers and other allied health professionals as long as they are providing assistance near the accident or emergency when they are off duty and no physician–patient relationship or any other kind of professional duty exists. In these circumstances, these healthcare professionals are covered under the Good Samaritan laws and cannot be sued for malpractice (Fig. 6.3).

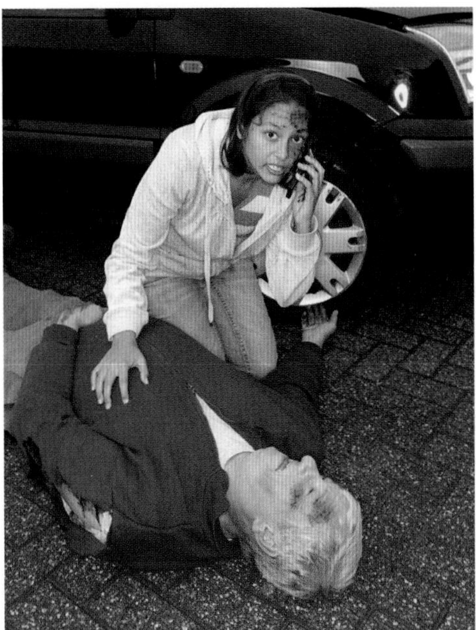

Fig. 6.3 A *Good Samaritan law*, active in most states, provides immunity to medical professionals who provide health care in an emergency without reimbursement or without proper facilities available. (Copyright © Studio-Annika/iStock/Thinkstock.com.)

However, a healthcare provider who voluntarily aids an individual in an emergency owes that individual the same duty of care and treatment as that of a reasonably competent provider under the same or similar circumstances. For example, a family physician cannot be held to the same standards of care as a surgeon during an emergency. The family physician may be liable if he or she volunteers to perform a procedure that he or she has not been properly trained to perform.

APPLY THIS

A middle-aged male present at the emergency department of a local hospital with symptoms suggestive of a stroke. After a thorough examination, a vascular surgeon is assigned to operate on the patient. After a brief postsurgical hospital stay, the surgeon releases the patient with a prescription for Coumadin and orders a follow-up appointment in 7 days to monitor the effects of the drug. The patient fails to comply and does not follow up on any of his appointments.

Over the next 12 months, the patient has prescriptions for Coumadin refilled. Also, during this time, the patient has the prescription transferred at least twice to different pharmacies. The last pharmacy incorrectly refills the prescription and gives the patient twice the dosage originally prescribed. As a result, the patient dies of internal bleeding caused by long-term Coumadin use. The executor of the patient's estate brings a lawsuit against the surgeon and the pharmacy.

1. Who was negligent—the surgeon, the pharmacy, or both?
2. Was the patient guilty of any negligence? If so, what kind?

PREVENTION OF LIABILITY AND MALPRACTICE

Unlike other professions, healthcare professionals are dealing every day with the well-being and lives of their patients. Thus, it is critical that healthcare professionals always remind themselves of their duty and responsibility to their patients. Mistakes in judgment and errors will occur, but the following are some best practices to help prevent malpractice:

- Always work within your scope of practice.
- Never promise a cure to a patient.

- Carefully identify and confirm identification of a patient before treatment.
- Always verify a patient's allergies.
- Document every patient encounter.
- Stay current in your respective profession and field.
- Treat all patients with dignity and respect.
- Work only within your job description and knowing the policies and procedures of the employer.

Risk Management

Because of the high risk, severe penalties, and costs of medical malpractice, many clinics and almost every hospital have risk management. **Risk management** in health care is the process of identifying threats that could harm the organization, its patients, staff, or anyone else within the organization.

Risk management focuses on *loss reduction* and *loss prevention*. Loss reduction involves the steps taken after an event or incident occurs and it is aimed at minimizing the adverse impact. Loss prevention is a planned, systemic, and proactive process to identify activities, issues, and situations that may result in potential liability. Loss prevention is the preferred method since the cost of prevention is often much less than the cost of the damage. It often includes education and training programs for staff, such as providing new employee orientation, an employee handbook, continuing education, and other activities to reduce specific risks.

Many healthcare organizations with risk management will employ a supervisor or manager, whose role is to prevent incidents and to minimize the damages after an event to reduce liability. The risk management managers may be a physician, nurse manager, an attorney, or a healthcare administrator. The risk management manager's duties would include monitoring the safety of staff and patients and preventing any incidences of negligence and malpractice (Fig. 6.4).

Duties of a Risk Management Manager

The primary role and duties of the risk management manager is mainly in the areas of safety of staff and patients, communication, and documentation.

Safety of Staff and Patients

- Implementing a quality improvement (QI) plan to keep all practice activities compliant and well aligned with all standards and regulations

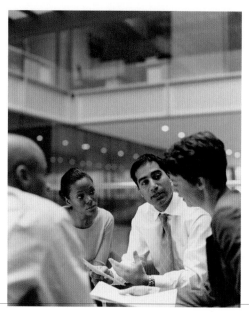

Fig. 6.4 The duties of the risk management supervisor would include monitoring the safety of staff and patients and preventing any incidences of negligence and malpractice. (Copyright © Digital Vision/DigitalVision/Thinkstock.com.)

- Training of staff and regularly assessing skill competencies, credentialing, and continuing education, including appropriate training in operation of equipment
- Maintaining appropriate safety standards of the premises and physical environment
- Monitoring safe handling of drugs, as well as hazardous materials on site
- Enforcing Occupational Safety and Health Administration guidelines and other federal and state regulations and credentialing
- Ensuring that appropriate liability insurance is acquired and maintained
- Overseeing sterilization of materials and equipment
- Maintaining safety standards of equipment
- Regularly reviewing the facility's disaster plan

Communication

- Ensuring that all staff members are current on the policies and procedures that pertain to their roles and job duties in the practice
- Ensuring that all patient health information and confidentiality is safeguarded in both electronic and physical areas of the practice

- Communicating with patients to ensure that the practice is running well, and that patients' needs are being met—patient phone calls are being responded to in a timely manner, the staff are polite and respectful when communicating with patients, and the staff is adhering to high standards of professionalism
- Overseeing that all written communications for the patients are current and readily available, such as patient education materials, preoperative instructions, and informed consent forms

Documentation

- Establishing and implementing all forms required for patient encounters
- Providing a means for staff to ensure that all communication with a patient—including verbal and via phone and text—is appropriately documented
- Keeping records of cancellations and no-shows, as well as recording appropriate follow-up and patient compliance incidents
- Confirming all charges and verifying all monies collected to avoid errors in the patients' balances and in the billing to the insurance carriers
- Scheduling regular audits of billing and coding to correct any problems quickly and efficiently

The risk management manager should ensure the medical practice has in place a compliance plan and policies and procedures that must be followed to ensure that both clinical and administrative sides of the practice are compliant. Every practice must have documented policies, a current compliance plan, enforced job descriptions specific for each employee, up-to-date education and in-services, and an effective system of checks and balances to protect all areas of the practice from litigation and liability. The risk management manager should provide in-services and training for all staff so that everyone is up to date on any new rules and regulations and advances in technology. Regardless of the type of healthcare organization, the role of the risk management manager is paramount to the operations of the practice and the safety and care of the patients.

Professional Liability

Professional liability insurance, sometimes known as medical malpractice insurance in healthcare, is one type of insurance that protects physicians and other licensed healthcare professionals from liability associated with presumed wrongful practices resulting in bodily injury, medical expenses, and property damage, as well as the cost of defending lawsuits related to such claims. Professional liability insurance usually covers malpractice for the healthcare professionals and the employees of the facility, as long as they are working within their scope of practice and are on duty.

Professional liability insurance operates in a similar fashion as health insurance. The overall purpose of insurance is to spread the risk of financial loss among members of a group who have a commonly shared risk; for professional liability insurance, it is usually shared based on profession or business. A small fee, or **premium**, is paid by each insured member and put into a fund by the insurer. The insurer then uses this fund to pay for claims against any of the members. This avoids potentially devastating financial costs associated with defending a member against a lawsuit or claim. Regardless of whether the lawsuit is frivolous and lacks merit, the healthcare professional will still need legal protection, which may be very costly without some type of liability insurance. For example, medical liability insurers were found to have paid $274,887 on average on liability claims.

Types of Professional Liability Policies

There are generally two basic types of professional liability or malpractice insurance: *occurrence-basis policy* and *claims-made policy*. Some liability insurers may offer only claims-made policies while others offer both but may limit access to occurrence-basis coverage to a few medical specialties. There are several important differences between claims-made and occurrence-basis coverage, the most important being the time at which the claim is filed.

Occurrence-Basis Policy

An **occurrence-basis policy** provides lifetime coverage for incidents that occurred while the policy was in effect, regardless of when the claim is filed. For example, you purchased an occurrence-basis policy with coverage from March 1, 2016, through March 1, 2017, but then decide not to renew the policy. If a claim is made on July 4, 2016, based on an incident that occurred during the policy period, coverage applies. You would not, however, have coverage for any incident that occurred before the beginning effective date of the policy unless you purchased *prior acts coverage*, which will be discussed later in this chapter.

Occurrence-basis coverage offers the safest protection because a healthcare professional may never know when a claim will be submitted. Most healthcare facilities usually obtain occurrence-basis policies. Even if the employee is no longer working for the facility, the facility will still be protected and have coverage for an incident that occurred while that employee was employed. Although occurrence-basis policies were the most common types of liability insurance, more insurers are increasingly omitting occurrence policies in favor of claims-made policies.

Claims-Made Policy

The predominant form of coverage offered by medical liability insurers is a claims-made policy. A **claims-made policy** is a type of coverage provided for any claim made while the policy is in effect and provides coverage only for claims when both the incident and the resulting claim happen during the period the policy is effective. Claims-made policies provide coverage so long as the insured continues to pay premiums for the initial policy and any subsequent renewals. Each succeeding year the policy is continuously renewed, the "coverage period" is extended. Once premiums stop, the coverage stops. Claims made to the insurance company after the coverage period ends will not be covered, even if the alleged incident occurred while the policy was in force.

For example, you purchase a claims-made policy with coverage from March 1, 2017, through March 1, 2018. But at the end of that term, you decide not to renew because you are no longer employed as a healthcare professional. If a claim is made against you on March 10, 2017, coverage applies. However, if the incident occurred on March 10, 2017, but the claim was not made against you until June 1, 2018, you are not covered under this policy.

There are some claims-made policies that do provide coverage if the insurer is notified before the expiration of the policy of an incident that could evolve into a claim. Also, some policies provide, at no extra charge, a 60-day extension after expiration of the policy during which the liability insurer will defend a claim filed during the extended coverage. If neither of these two modifications for coverage exists, then the healthcare professional should consider purchasing tail coverage, which will be discussed in the next section.

RELATE TO PRACTICE

A patient was treated as an outpatient at a medical clinic and prescribed a sulfa drug. The patient is allergic to sulfa drugs, which was documented in the patient's medical record. However, the medical scribe did not transcribe the allergy note into the computerized patient record. On discharge from the facility, the nurse failed to check the patient's written medical record. In addition, the pharmacist who dispensed the drug did not note the allergy.

After taking one dose of the sulfa drug, the patient had a severe allergic reaction that ultimately led to her death. The patient's family sued the pharmacist and the medical clinic for the negligence of the nurse and the medical scribe.

1. Who should be liable in this situation? Who has the *duty*?
2. If the claim against the medical scribe was made after she left the clinic's employ, did the clinic's occurrence-basis liability insurance provide coverage to defend her?

DISCUSSION

The role of medical malpractice lawsuits contributes to the large costs of the U.S. healthcare system is a subject of an intense national debate. As a result, many states have adopted a variety of administrative and legislative actions, collectively referred to as "tort reform" measures. These measures include actions such as ending lawsuits in which one defendant can be responsible for paying all the damages if other defendants lack the resources to pay; reducing the monetary damage awarded if the injured party has workers' compensation and health insurance; limiting the fees that a lawyer can claim; and limiting the length of time after an injury that a lawsuit may be brought to trial.

1. What kind of tort reform do you think should be enacted, if any?
2. What role do you think the government should have in limiting malpractice lawsuits?
3. Do you think there are too many malpractice lawsuits? Or do patients need a way to protect themselves against negligent healthcare providers?

CONCLUSION

Healthcare professionals will always be at risk for malpractice because of the nature of their work. As a result, healthcare professionals must be keenly aware of their duty in their profession, keep within their scope of practice, and take steps to ensure that patients receive the best quality of care. In addition, having a thorough understanding of existing laws and standards in regard to negligence will help protect against malpractice lawsuits.

CHAPTER REVIEW QUESTIONS

1. In negligence, a healthcare provider who cares for a patient but fails to provide a reasonable standard of care is an example of
   A. duty.
   B. damages.
   C. dereliction of duty.
   D. direct cause.
2. An example of a high-risk area for malpractice in the healthcare setting would be in
   A. the emergency department.
   B. administration.
   C. laboratory facilities.
   D. the radiology department.
3. Which of the following would be an important element in a malpractice case?
   A. What the physician thinks is right
   B. What the hospital thinks happened
   C. What the patient feels is fair
   D. What the documentation reflects happened
4. Who can be named in a malpractice case?
   A. Only a physician
   B. Only a hospital
   C. Only the person who allegedly directly injured the patient
   D. All parties who were involved in the case where the alleged injury occurred
5. The discovery rule applies to
   A. the patient's ability to work.
   B. the first time an injury occurs in a facility.
   C. the discovery of a new treatment for an illness.
   D. the statute of limitations for suing for an injury or illness.
6. Which of the following type of damages in malpractice awards a patient for "pain and suffering"?
   A. Economic loss
   B. Noneconomic loss
   C. Nominal damages
   D. Punitive damages
7. Which legal theory is similar to the concept of *respondeat superior*?
   A. Quasi-intentional tort
   B. Occurance-basis policy
   C. Vicarious liability
   D. Negligence
8. A patient sues a physician for negligence. However, the physician wants to reduce the compensation because the patient failed to schedule follow-up medical visits to monitor his disease. This is an example of
   A. comparative negligence.
   B. contributory negligence.
   C. compensatory negligence.
   D. assumption of risk.
9. At which point of a malpractice lawsuit would an alternative dispute resolution occur?
   A. Before an incident of negligence occurs
   B. Before the trial.
   C. During the trial.
   D. After a trial.
10. Which of the following is true of lawsuits?
    A. Most lawsuits may be filed or heard in a federal court.
    B. Most lawsuits are filed in a state trial court.
    C. Most lawsuits are heard by a trial court by a jury trial.
    D. Most lawsuits rarely get resolved and fail to reach a settlement.

SELF-REFLECTION QUESTIONS

1. How would you protect yourself from negligence in your current or future healthcare profession?
2. Knowing of the Good Samaritan laws, how willing would you be to stop to help in an emergency?
3. Although, in the United States, healthcare professionals are not required to assist in the event of a medical emergency, many other countries, such as Australia and many in Europe, do impose a legal obligation to assist. Do you think the federal government should enact a Good Samaritan law? Should there be a requirement for healthcare professionals?

INTERNET ACTIVITIES

1. Access the following article regarding new legislation on malpractice and write a summary of the article: http://articles.courant.com/2013-03-29/health/hc-er-malpractice-bill-20130329_1_malpractice-suits-public-health-committee-change-malpractice-law.
2. Research the scope of practice for your profession in your state to ensure you know the individual state guidelines for your field.
   Research the Good Samaritan law in your state.
3. Search the Internet or discuss a case and the disciplinary actions that have been taken against healthcare professionals in your current or future profession.

ADDITIONAL RESOURCES

http://www.imri.com
http://www.naplia.com
http://www.eckenrode-law.com/resources/defending_med_malpractice.pdf
https://www.ncbi.nlm.nih.gov/pmc/articles/PMC3792272/
http://www.abpla.org/what-is-malpractice
https://www.thedoctors.com
https://www.medicalmalpracticehelp.com
https://www.cms.gov
https://www.ama-assn.org
https://www.findlaw.com

BIBLIOGRAPHY

Bal, B. S. (2009). An introduction to medical malpractice in the United States. *Clinical Orthopaedics and Related Research*, *467*(2), 339–347. https://doi.org/10.1007/s11999-008-0636-2.

Dobbyn, J. F. (1989). *Insurance law* (pp. 152–160). St Paul, Minn: West Publishing.

Glannon, J. W. (1995). *The law of torts* (pp. 375–378). Boston: Little, Brown.

Harris County Hosp. Dist. v. Estrada, 872 S.W.2d 729 (Tex. 1993).

Kim, T. F. *Most doctors sued sometime in career*. Available from http://www.insurancejournal.com/news/national/2011/08/19/211634.htm.

Prosser, W. (1975). *Handbook of the law of torts* (pp. 468–475). St Paul, MN: West Publishing.

Smith, J. W. (1998). *Hospital liability, § 5.01(3), § 5.01(6), § 5.01(7), § 5.02(3)*. New York: Law Journal Seminars-Press.

7

Healthcare Business and Operations

CHAPTER OBJECTIVES

1. Describe types of healthcare providers and professionals.
2. Explain the role of credentialing, licensing, and registration in health care.
3. List and describe types of practice structures.
4. Identify and describe different types of health insurance plans and related patient costs.
5. Discuss the different types of managed care organizations.
6. Discuss the different types of government healthcare programs and who are eligible.

KEY TERMS

Allied health professional A large and varied group of health care–related professions and personnel whose functions include assisting, facilitating, or complementing the work of physicians and other healthcare providers in the healthcare system.

Associate practice A legal agreement in which physicians share staff and overhead expenses of operation but do not share in the legal responsibility or in the profits of the business.

Certification A process that verifies the qualifications of professionals and assesses their background and their ability to legally and/or competently work in their field.

Credentialing The process of verifying an individual's professional qualifications.

CHAMPVA Acronym denoting Civilian Health and Medical Program of the Department of Veterans Affairs. Coverage designed specifically for disabled veterans and their dependents. Also known as *Veterans Health Administration*.

Coinsurance The percentage of payment that is agreed on by the insured as their portion of any claims; cost-sharing.

Copay A fixed amount determined by the health insurance policy that is paid for services to offset premiums paid by the insured.

Deductible An amount of money that is paid by the insured before the insurance company pays for services. Usually a fixed amount paid annually.

Gatekeeper A person, such as the primary care physician, or an organization that is appointed by a managed care carrier to maintain and approve services to reduce costs and unnecessary spending.

Group practice A medical practice with three or more physicians of the same or similar specialty, who share the same overhead and staff and practice medicine together.

Health Maintenance Organization (HMO) A type of managed care company that serves participating patients by offering services at a fixed rate within the group of participating providers and facilities.

Incident to billing A method of billing outpatient services provided by a nonphysician provider when working under the direct supervision of a physician.

Indemnity plans Fee-for-service plans that allow the patient to direct his or her health care. Typically require the patient to pay deductible and a percentage (cost-share) of the allowed charge. Allows both in-network and out-of-network coverage.

Licensing An official permission to perform certain duties.

Limited Liability Company (LLC) A legally structured company in which the members of the company cannot be held personally liable for the debts or actions of the company or another party in the company.

Managed Care Organization (MCO) Provides healthcare plans that balance healthcare delivery while controlling costs by limiting the providers who can be seen by the patient and discounting payments to those providers.

Medicaid Federal program administered by each individual state that provides healthcare coverage for indigent and/or medically needy patients.

Medicare Federal program that provides medical insurance coverage to members older than age 65 or to those who are deemed permanently disabled.

Nonphysician providers Also called *mid-level providers,* providers who are educated and skilled to perform medical services and procedures similar to those of physicians.

Point of Service Plan (POS) Insurance plan that combines some elements of HMO and PPO plans, and allows members to choose a primary care provider who will directly refer to in-network providers when needed.

Preferred Provider Organization (PPO) A type of managed care organization that allow members to see any in-network provider without first obtaining a referral from the patient's primary care provider.

Primary care physician (PCP) A designated provider who oversees the care and manages the healthcare services for an individual.

Professional corporation (PC) A specific legal company structure that is designed for provision of professional services for their clients, such as lawyers, physicians, or architects.

Registration A professional organization in a specific healthcare field administers examinations and/or maintains a list of qualified individuals.

Sole proprietorship A single professional-owned business in which an individual employs other professional in the same field. In medical practice, a single physician-owned practice that employs other physicians to work for the practice.

Solo practice Single owner/operator of the company or business. In the medical field, this would represent a single-physician practice.

Specialist In the medical field, an individual who has undergone further specific training in a certain discipline and practices medicine in that discipline, such as dermatology or endocrinology.

Third-party payers Usually refers to an insurance company but can be any other person or organization that is responsible for the medical care coverage of a patient.

TRICARE Government medical program for active-duty military and their dependents, as well as coverage for military retirees (after 20 or more years of service).

INTRODUCTION

Many people do not view the practice of medicine as a business; however, it is a business that has customers (patients), and it must generate revenue to keep in operation. Not every medical practice or healthcare organization uses the same type of business structure or model, and there are many factors that influence the type of business structure a practice may choose.

Some of these factors include the types of patients who are served, the specialty and the types of medical services provided by the healthcare provider, changes in reimbursement and billing procedures for healthcare providers, and legal strategies that offer protection against personal financial liabilities. This chapter will discuss the different type of business structures in health care, the various types of healthcare professionals and business providers, and insurance and government coverage plans.

TYPES OF HEALTHCARE PROFESSIONALS

As a result of healthcare reform and increasing demand for health service, there has been incredible growth in healthcare professionals, particularly the different types and specialties. Healthcare professionals range from physicians and specialists to mid-level providers to allied health professionals. All these healthcare professionals provide patient care but have different functions and roles in various healthcare organizations, as well as training and education.

Medical Doctors

Medical doctors, also commonly called *physicians*, are licensed by their state medical boards to treat patients. All licensed physicians have undergone a minimum of undergraduate education and completed medical school and residency requirements. Fully licensed physicians may be either medical doctors (MDs) or doctors of osteopathic medicine (DO). Both credentials are equivalent in the practice of medicine, although one may find more DOs practicing primary care than MDs.

The major difference between the two is the type of medical school that was attended by the physician. An MD, or allopathic physician, receives more traditional training, whereas a DO is trained in an osteopathic philosophy that treats the mind, body, and spirit. An osteopathic physician's training includes musculoskeletal manipulation treatment to treat a wide variety of disorders.

Specialists

Medical specialists are fully licensed MDs or DOs who have completed additional advanced training in a specific area of medicine (Fig. 7.1). After completing the training and passing the appropriate board examination, these physicians will have the credentials of either "board certified" or "fellowship" in those specialties. The different specialties are governed by a variety of different associations and organizations, such as the following:

- AMA—American Medical Association
- American College of Surgeons
- American College of Physicians
- Board specialty organizations in each specialty area

Box 7.1 lists some of the different medical specialties.

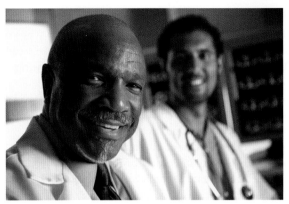

Fig. 7.1 Specialists are fully licensed medical doctors who have undergone further schooling and training in a specific area of medicine. (Copyright © Medioimages/Photodisc/Thinkstock.com.)

BOX 7.1 Examples of Medical Specialties

- Allergy and immunology
- Anesthesiology
- Cardiology
- Dermatology
- Emergency medicine
- Geriatric medicine
- Hematology
- Infection control
- Nephrology
- Neurology
- Nuclear medicine
- Obstetrics and gynecology
- Oncology
- Otorhinolaryngology
- Pathology
- Pediatrics
- Physiatry—Physical medicine and rehab
- Preventive medicine
- Psychiatry
- Radiology
- Rheumatology

Surgical specialties include the following:

- General surgery
- Neurosurgery
- Plastic surgery
- Oral surgery
- Orthopedic surgery
- Thoracic surgery

Other Types of Doctors

In addition to MDs and DOs, there are other types of doctors who provide more focused and specialized care to patients. Some other doctors include the following:

- DC—Doctor of Chiropractic
- DMD—Doctor of Dental Medicine
- DDS—Doctor of Dental Surgery
- OD—Doctor of Optometry
- PharmD—Doctor of Pharmacy
- DPM—Doctor of Podiatric Medicine

Their requirements for licensure to practice vary and depend on their specialty.

Nonphysician Providers

Another group of healthcare professionals are the **nonphysician providers (NPPs)**, also called *mid-level providers* or *practitioners*. They are not physicians but may perform some of the same highly skilled services and procedures, such as minor surgery and writing prescriptions, and they are usually able to bill insurance companies for their services (Fig. 7.2). Examples of nonphysician providers are the following:

- NP—Nurse Practitioner
- PA—Physician Assistant
- CRNA—Certified Registered Nurse Anesthetist
- LSW—Licensed Social Worker
- PT—Physical Therapist
- OT—Occupational Therapist
- CNM—Certified Nurse Midwife

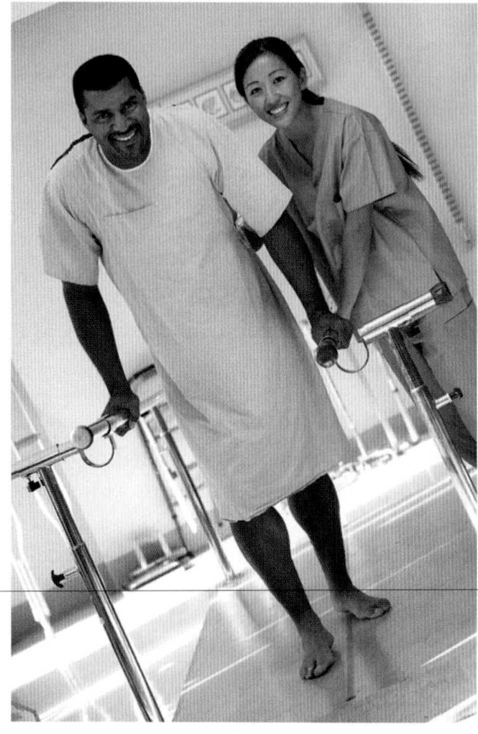

Fig. 7.2 Nonphysician or mid-level providers are not physicians, but they may perform similar services such as writing prescriptions, and they usually bill insurance companies for their services. Examples of nonphysician providers are nurse practitioners, physician assistants, and physical therapists. (Copyright © BananaStock/BananaStock/Thinkstock.com.)

Allied Health Professionals

Allied health professionals are proving to be essential members of the healthcare team. Instead of billing separately to insurance companies for their services, however, they operate as paid employees, or sometimes as outside contractors paid by the employer or facility. There are an estimated 80 different allied health professions with different education and licensure requirements (Box 7.2).

With so many different healthcare professions, patients may sometimes confuse them. It is important, however, for each healthcare professional to identify him- or herself to patients. In fact, in most medical clinics and hospitals, all healthcare professionals are required to wear identification badges or name tags that indicate their specialty and credentials. Students also need to be sure to identify themselves as such.

BOX 7.2 Examples of Allied Health Professionals

- RN—Registered Nurse
- CMA/RMA—Certified or Registered Medical Assistant
- CMT—Certified Medical Transcriptionist
- CNA—Certified Nursing Assistant
- CPC—Certified Professional Coder
- Dental Assistant or Hygienist
- EMT—Emergency Medical Technician
- Laboratory or Medical Technologist
- LPN—Licensed Practical Nurse
- Pharmacy Technician
- Phlebotomist
- RHIT—Registered Health Information Technologist
- RT—Respiratory Therapist
- X-Ray Technician
- Sonographer

Credentialing and Registration

For almost every healthcare profession, credentialing is an important process of verifying an individual's professional qualifications. Almost all healthcare professionals will have some type of certification, which verifies the qualifications of professionals and assesses their background and their ability to legally and/or competently work in their field. Almost every member on a healthcare team will need to be credentialed in one form or another, especially if the team member is providing direct patient care. Similarly, registration is when the professional organization in a specific healthcare field administers examinations and/or maintains a list of qualified individuals. Box 7.3 summarizes some of the healthcare professions and their credentials and the agencies that oversee the profession.

Licensing

In addition to credentialing, several healthcare professions may need to be licensed in their field, which require a higher standard of requirements and qualifications to work in their profession. Licensing is an official permission to perform certain duties. The difference is that licenses are legal requirements, while certifications are desired but not required for employment. However, some employers may require certification. For example, physicians and nurses must be licensed by the state in which they are employed. Medical billers, however, do not require a license, but may have a form of certification in their field.

Most states also have a medical practice act that governs the practice of medicine in the state. There are

BOX 7.3 Examples of Credential and Provider Agency of Healthcare Professionals

Professional	Credential	Provider Agency
Physicians		
Medical Doctor	MD	Federation of State Medical Boards (FSMB) and the National Board of Medical Examiners® (NBME®)
Doctor of Osteopathy	DO	National Board of Osteopathic Medical Examiners (NBOME)
Physician Assistant	PA	National Commission on Certification of Physician Assistants (NCCPA)
Nurses		
Advanced Practice Registered Nurse	APRN	State Board of Nursing, National Council of State Boards of Nursing (NCSBN)
Registered Nurse	RN	State Board of Nursing, National Council of State Boards of Nursing (NCSBN)
Licensed Practical Nurse/Licensed Vocational Nurse	LPN or LVN	State Board of Nursing, National Council of State Boards of Nursing (NCSBN)
Medical Assistants	CMA	American Association of Medical Assistant (AAMA)
	RMA	American Medical Technologist (AMT)
	CCMA	National Healthcareer Association (NHA)
	NCMA	National Center for Competency Testing (NCCT)
	NRCMA	National Association for Health Professionals (NAHP)
Medical Biller/Coders	CCS, CPC, CPB	American Health Information Management Association (AHIMA)
	CPC	American Association of Professional Coders (AAPC)
	CPB	American Association of Professional Coders (AAPC)
Pharmacists	Pharm. B.S. or Pharm. D.	American Council on Pharmaceutical Education (ACPE)
Pharmacy Technicians	CPhT	Pharmacy Technician Certification Board (PTCB)
Surgical Technicians	CST	National Board of Surgical Technology and Surgical Assisting (NBSTSA)
Emergency Medical Technicians and Paramedics	NRP	National Registry of Emergency Medical Technicians (NREMT)

medical practice acts for many healthcare professions, including physicians, nurses, physical and occupational therapists, and dentists. These acts often specify the requirements for medical licensing and credentialing in the state, such as education requirements, renewal, continuing medical education, licensure fees, and training.

TYPES OF MEDICAL PRACTICE STRUCTURES

There are many different types of corporate structures for medical practices and even many different variations within those structures. The following is a summary of the most commonly available types of medical practice settings.

Solo Practice

In a solo practice, a single physician is the only provider within that practice and does not share patients with any other physicians. In this type of business arrangement, a "covering physician" is necessary when the physician either is on vacation or unable to see patients. Most physicians in solo practice are specialists and are often structured as a professional corporation (PC). A professional corporation is an organization of professionals in the same field or trade, such as physicians. One of the advantages of this structure is the ability to run the practice based on the way one wants and without question from a partner or associate. The financial risk is higher, however, as overhead costs are not being shared by other physicians.

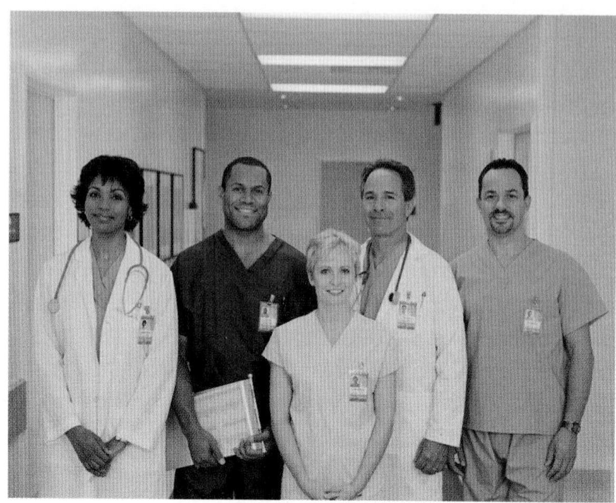

Fig. 7.3 In a sole proprietorship, the provider has legal agreements to hire other physicians or nonphysician providers to work. (Copyright © Ryan McVay/DigitalVision/Thinkstock.com.)

Sole Proprietorship

A sole proprietorship is similar to a solo practice except that the physician has legal agreements to hire other physicians or nonphysician providers to work for him or her (Fig. 7.3). The physician owner still owns and operates the practice but can employ other providers to work on an hourly or daily basis. In turn, the other providers do not usually share in corporate profits.

Associate Practice

An associate practice is a common structure in which two or more providers, usually in the same or similar specialty, share the overhead expenses. However, they do not share in the profits, losses, or liabilities of the other physician's practice. This corporate structure can be organized as individual professional corporations or could be established as limited liability companies (LLCs).

An LLC is essentially a hybrid entity that combines the characteristics of a corporation and a partnership or sole proprietorship. Members of an LLC cannot be held personally liable for the company's or another physician's debts or liabilities.

Group Practice

Group practices are a corporate structure that assigns designated officers to manage the group's business operations. Although group practices vary in size, compensation structure, and profit sharing, they share in the same benefits and profits. Group practices enable the individual providers to be covered when they are unable to see patients. In addition, they allow the providers to share overhead and staffing costs, and they offer the providers protection from liability. Many group practices purchase and own their own buildings, which affords them the ability to control their own costs and, in some cases, even collect rent from other physicians or practices who rent space from them.

The group practice structure usually provides profit sharing and incentives for physicians working together and offers benefits to each provider depending on the level of provider and the length of time associated with the group. This has become one of the most common medical practice structures because it both benefits and protects individual physicians or providers.

Other Structures

Some physicians or healthcare professionals prefer to simply be directly hired by a hospital or medical practice. If hired by the hospital, the healthcare professionals are employees and receive a salary or wage and any other benefits, such as liability insurance; however, they do not benefit from any profit sharing. Many hospitals are structured this way for hiring of staff physicians and other ancillary specialties, such as emergency department physicians, radiologists, and anesthesiologists. Although healthcare professionals may lose some autonomy, they may find that they have a consistent salary and thus less risk than if they started or joined a private practice. Furthermore, declining reimbursement and the increasing costs involved in meeting quality measurements have resulted in many physicians looking at hospital employment as a good alternative to solo or group practice. Many physicians may choose to relinquish the business responsibilities associated with being in private practice in order to focus on practicing medicine.

Another common medical practice structure is the Health Maintenance Organization (HMO), which provides an integrated structure where many types of providers and facilities join to create a network. When first introduced, most providers in an HMO model were direct employees of the HMO. Now, however, HMOs have adopted more of a group practice model where they contract with independent practices as opposed to employing their own physicians and healthcare professionals. HMOs will be discussed in further detail in the next section.

TYPES OF HEALTH INSURANCE COVERAGE

The various types of health insurance coverage for patients can be confusing. Health insurance plans vary widely regarding the patient's liability or the patient's responsibility for payment.

Traditional Indemnity Plans

Indemnity plans, or fee-for-service plans, allow patients to direct their health care and visits to almost any physician, healthcare professional, or hospital they like. The insurance company then pays a set portion of the total charges. Although providers and facilities can choose to contract with the insurance company, indemnity plans offer both in-network and out-of-network benefits. No primary care provider is required, and patients are able to contact specialists directly without a referral.

Indemnity plans are attractive to some employers because the employees are paying part or all of the monthly premiums for their employees. Indemnity plans also typically require the employee to pay a deductible before the insurance carrier will cover any of the claims. Under the Affordable Care Act, many patients found themselves in high-deductible health plans (HDHPs) for indemnity or managed care plans. In HDHPs, deductibles were sometimes more than $10,000 per year for a family, although monthly premiums for coverage were usually much lower. This works well for patients who are rarely sick or do not often seek medical care, take few medications, and mainly need health insurance to cover them in emergency situations or in cases of catastrophic illness.

Some employers may also offer a health savings account (HSA) or something similar to help offset the high deductible. HSAs allow employees and employers to contribute pretax funds to meet the deductible costs. If the funds are not used in a given year, they carry over, tax-free, until they are needed. Although these funds can be used only for healthcare expenses before retirement, the employee can withdraw the money and use it for nonmedical withdrawals after age 59 1/2.

After a patient's deductible is met, there is typically a coinsurance in which the insurance carrier pays a percentage, and the patient pays the remainder of the bill. For example, if a patient has an 80/20 plan, this means that the insurance carrier is paying 80% of the allowable fees and the patient will be responsible for the remaining 20%. The providers contract with the insurance company, agreeing to accept an adjusted fee scale. Thus, under the terms of the agreement, fees are based on what the insurance company allows for the service, not on what is billed by the provider. If the provider does not contract with, or "participate," with the insurance carrier, the provider is considered "out-of-network" and will usually be paid by the insurance carrier at a lower percentage, for example, 70/30 or 60/40.

Managed Care Organizations

Managed Care Organizations (MCOs) were first introduced in the 1970s as a way of balancing healthcare delivery while controlling costs. Under an MCO, an insurer-controlled costs by limiting the providers who can be seen by the patient and discounting payments to those providers. People had to enroll in an MCO's plan, who were called *members,* and they had to agree to restrictions on the providers they could see for treatment. In return, they would receive comprehensive medical coverage at a lower rate. Traditionally, MCOs focused on preventative care and, thus, had a more extensive network of primary care providers than specialists. The two most common types of MCOs are HMOs and Preferred Provider Organizations (PPOs).

Health Maintenance Organizations

In an HMO, healthcare services are offered by a network of providers who agree to supply medical services to its patients, or members. Members enrolled in the HMO are covered only if they visit participating providers in that plan. Members also had to select a **primary care physician (PCP)**, who would manage the member's health and give referrals for any specialists needed for consultation. In this way, the PCP serves as a **gatekeeper**, who is a person in the HMO who maintains and approves services to reduce costs and unnecessary spending (cost containment).

Gatekeepers authorize the patient's referrals, hospitalizations, and laboratory studies and prevent unnecessary and costly tests and visits to specialists. This centralized approach also helps to improve the level of communication between multiple providers to prevent unnecessary tests and overtreatment, which will lead to improved health outcomes.

HMO plans typically have lower premiums and lower cost-sharing than other types of MCOs. If the patient has an HMO plan, there is no **coinsurance** amount due but a flat **copay** for the services provided. For example, the member may have a $5, $10, $20, or higher copay depending on the plan and type of services rendered, such as prescriptions or hospital services, but it will be a set amount due at the time of service.

When first introduced, there were, however, several issues with HMOs. First, HMOs were unpopular with many providers because they financially penalized them if there were too many referrals. This was at odds with a physician's duty. It is important for all healthcare professionals always to keep the patient's needs as the priority. Thus, if the physician deems it medically necessary, the physician is ethically bound to treat or refer the patient regardless of the potential costs. As a result, the policy of financially penalizing HMO providers was discontinued.

A second issue for HMO plans was that some areas lacked participating providers, thereby limiting physician access for members. Also, if a patient wanted to see a physician who was not in the network, the patient would have to pay for those services completely on his or her own. In 1970, the number of HMOs declined to fewer than 40. But, as a result of the enactment of the Health Maintenance Organization Act of 1973, HMOs began to grow rapidly.

APPLY THIS

Megan sees Dr. Penden for a medical visit. Dr. Penden's fee is $120 for an office visit but charges only Megan $80 based on her insurance plan.

1. Megan's policy has a coinsurance of 80/20. How much would Megan have to pay? How much would her insurance carrier have to pay?
2. Megan's policy also requires a copay of $20. How much would she have to pay now along with her coinsurance of 80/20?
3. How much would Megan have to pay if she did not have insurance?

Preferred Provider Organizations

Preferred provider organizations (PPOs), sometimes referred to as a *participating provider organization* or *preferred provider option,* are some of the most popular types of MCOs. PPOs allow patients to see any in-network provider without first obtaining a referral from the patient's primary care provider, or gatekeeper. PPOs typically allow out-of-network benefits but pay a lower percentage of the cost than in-network. Similar to an indemnity plan, patients usually have a deductible, copays, and coinsurance.

Under these plans, if a member sees a provider who is in-network, the member pays the flat copay amount. If the member chooses to see a provider who does not participate with the plan, the member must pay up front and then be reimbursed based on his or her out-of-network benefits. These types of plans are very popular, especially with large employers, as they allow members more flexibility in choosing their providers but also help control costs.

Point of Service Plans

Point of service plans (POSs) combine some elements of HMO and PPO plans. They usually require that a member choose a primary care provider to direct referrals to in-network providers when needed. Most in-network services are not subject to a deductible. Out-of-network services are allowed but will be subject to both a deductible and coinsurance.

Other Commercial Payers

Other types of commercial plans include self-insured models. One type is the employer-sponsored Employee Welfare Benefit Plan under the Employment Retirement Income Security Act (ERISA) of 1974, which establishes a savings account for employees and provides funds to that account to cover employees' claims instead of paying premiums for health insurance. There are pros and cons to this type of policy for the employer. Health claims are not prepaid through premiums. If an employee does not have many medical claims, the amount of money paid by the employer is low. However, one major hospitalization by an employee could deplete the account. For this reason, an employer will often have a combination of the self-insured model up to a set amount and then an insurance carrier to cover anything beyond that amount.

Government Health Care Programs

In addition to private insurance, the federal government spends more than $1.6 trillion a year on healthcare expenditures that cover about one-third of Americans. There are six major government healthcare programs: Medicare, Medicaid, the State Children's Health Insurance Program (SCHIP), the Department of Defense TRICARE and TRICARE for Life programs (DOD TRICARE), the Veterans Health Administration (VHA) program, and the Indian Health Service (IHS) program. Many of these government healthcare programs are discussed in more detail in the Healthcare Standards and Compliance chapter, and only a few of the major government healthcare plans will be discussed in this section.

Medicaid

Medicaid is a federal program that is governed and managed by each individual state to provide aid to the indigent or medically needy patient. As a joint federal and state program, Medicaid is the largest source of funding for medical and health-related services for more than 74 million people with low income and/or disability in the United States.

Local departments of social services will usually manage who is eligible for coverage and any other benefits that might be awarded to an individual, called a *beneficiary*. Although an individual may not meet the financial criteria for need, he or she may be considered medically needy because of a catastrophic illness or injury. Also, in many states, special programs are in place for needy children and pregnant women to ensure that they are covered by Medicaid programs. Most Medicaid programs do not require any contributions from the beneficiary, but the child coverage in most states has a minimal premium that the parent(s) must contribute.

Although these are federally funded programs, each individual state regulates the programs so the conditions, eligibility requirements, and benefits vary by states. In addition, on the state distribution level, these programs usually use local managed care carriers to administer and manage the beneficiaries. Furthermore, beneficiaries can choose from a selection of these managed care plans, giving the Medicaid beneficiaries more choices when looking for providers.

Medicare

Medicare is a federal insurance program that provides healthcare coverage for eligible recipients aged 65 or older. Medicare is funded by a payroll tax, premiums and surtaxes from beneficiaries, and general revenue. Unlike Medicaid, Medicare is administered solely by the federal government, although there are currently 30–50 private insurance companies contracted by the federal government to provide medical services to beneficiaries.

Medicare also provides health insurance to younger people with disability status as determined by the Social Security Administration, including specific diseases. A permanently disabled person may apply for Medicare coverage if he or she is unable to work for more than 24 months. The 24-month waiting period may be reduced to 2 months, for example, in cases of end-stage renal disease (ESRD). Medicare coverage is also available to permanently disabled children.

There are three parts to Medicare:

- Medicare part A: Covers hospital claims
- Medicare part B: Covers all outpatient services
- Medicare part D: Covers the prescription drug plan

Medicare has a deductible for each part and covers 80% of the allowable charges, leaving the beneficiary to cover the remaining 20% as out-of-pocket costs. In many cases, Medicare beneficiaries carry a secondary insurance plan to help cover those coinsurance amounts. A beneficiary may have Medicare and Medicaid if he or she is medically and/or financially eligible, often referred to as a "Medi–Medi" plan.

Medicare Part C is for the eligible Medicare beneficiary who opts to be covered by a managed care Medicare plan. As with a managed care plan, these plans use local participating physicians and require the beneficiaries to pay a flat copay amount instead of the 80/20 coverage in other Medicare plans. In addition, Medicare Part C provides coverage for hospital and outpatient services, with other plans also offering drug and vision coverage.

Tricare

TRICARE, formerly known as the Civilian Health and Medical Program of the Uniformed Services (CHAMPUS), provides insurance coverage for active military beneficiaries and their dependents, as well as for retired military personnel who have served for 20 years or more. Military personnel who serve only a few years and do not meet eligibility for TRICARE may be eligible for other veterans' benefits.

For those not eligible for TRICARE, the Civilian Health and Medical Program of the Department of Veterans Affairs, or Veterans Health Administration (CHAMPVA), is coverage designed specifically for disabled veterans and their dependents. CHAMPVA covers veterans' families not eligible for TRICARE who are:

- Dependents of veterans who have a 100% permanent disability received while on active duty
- Dependents of veterans who died from a disability received while on active duty

Civilian healthcare professionals can register with TRICARE and CHAMPVA to be approved providers to these beneficiaries. Most of these plans require the beneficiary to pay some out-of-pocket cost-share amount, similar to a commercial health insurance plan.

SHIFTS IN MEDICAL PRACTICES

In the 1800s, it was common for physicians to open a medical office attached to their home and have a private or solo practice. However, with changing demographics and increased costs and liabilities, the number of physicians working in solo practices has significantly diminished and are joining group practices. In a group practice, multiple physicians share ownership of the practice and it allows them to share costs, overhead expenses, and other expenses and risks to remain profitable.

Cost Sharing

Consider the cost to open a new medical practice. There is the cost of the building, utilities, staff, benefits, insurance, equipment, computers, office and medical supplies, and advertising. Now, consider the number of patients a physician would need to see every day just to meet all the overhead expenses.

With reimbursement payments from Medicare and other payers being reduced as much as 5% and the costs of running a practice having increased up to 50% since 1990, according to the Medical Group Management Association, cost sharing provides a significant benefit in reducing the financial risk and pressure on individual physicians. For example, with overhead expenses ranging around 60% of a practice's revenues, two physicians or a large group practice can share the overhead costs of staff salaries, supplies, and building and occupancy costs.

Expanded Scope of Nonphysician Providers

In addition to adopting a more corporate structure, more medical clinics and healthcare organizations are employing nonphysician providers (NPPs), such as physician assistants and nurse practitioners, who can assist in seeing a majority of patients that higher cost physicians would. As a result, employment of these NPPs has greatly expanded in recent years. Originally, these NPPs worked under the direct supervision of a physician. Guidelines specified that the physician had to be in the office while the NPP was seeing patients in case there were issues or questions. In addition, they were utilized only for seeing overflow patients and routine follow-up care without any complicating factors.

In addition, NPPs and their services were billed to the insurance company or third-party payers as if the physician had seen the patient. This is called "incident to billing" and is a method of billing outpatient services provided by an NPP. However, in the last several years, NPPs, particularly nurse practitioners (NP), physician assistants (PA), and clinical nurse specialists (CNS), have been given their own benefit category and may provide services without direct physician supervision. They can bill directly for services if they are licensed by their state to perform these services. In fact, in several states, nurse practitioners are able to practice independently and open their own practices, although a majority of insurance carriers do reduce the amount of reimbursement for services provided by an NPP instead of a physician.

CONCLUSION

Over the last several decades, the changes in the healthcare field have been dramatic, especially regarding how medical services are paid for and delivered. The types of providers of care, the types of services rendered, and the insurance carriers available to cover these services have changed as well.

In addition, changes in healthcare reform have continued to bring new insurance coverage options. As our healthcare needs continue to change and advance, our healthcare delivery system must be ready to adapt to meet the demands and needs of patients and the healthcare professionals.

CHAPTER REVIEW QUESTIONS

1. What type of practice structure would include a physician who hires other physicians?
   A. Solo practice
   B. Group practice
   C. Sole proprietorship
   D. All the above
2. What type of insurance covers patients who are indigent?
   A. Medicare
   B. Medicaid
   C. TRICARE
   D. HMO
3. What type of provider would have the initials DC after his or her name?
   A. Podiatrist
   B. Pharmacist
   C. Chiropractor
   D. None of the above
4. An example of a gatekeeper is
   A. an employer.
   B. a PCP.
   C. a mid-level provider.
   D. None of the above
5. All the following are considered physicians or medical doctors, *except*
   A. surgeon.
   B. DO.
   C. psychiatrist.
   D. NP.
6. Healthcare professionals that meet legal requirements to practice in their field are
   A. certified.
   B. licensed.
   C. registered.
   D. credentialed.
7. Which of the following statements is false about physicians in solo practices?
   A. Physicians in solo practice are often structured as a professional corporation.
   B. It is a type of medical practice that a single physician is the provider and owner.
   C. The physician does not share patients with other physicians.
   D. The financial risk and liability are less in solo practices compared to others.
8. Which of the following types of medical practices have the advantage of shared risk and liability?
   A. Group practice
   B. Sole practice
   C. Associate practice
   D. Professional corporation
9. The health insurance plan that allows the most flexibility for patients is the
   A. preferred provider organization (PPO).
   B. health maintenance organization (HMO).
   C. managed care organization (CMO).
   D. Indemnity plan.
10. Which of the following is not a government-sponsored program?
    A. Health Maintenance Organization
    B. TRICARE
    C. Medicare
    D. Medicaid

SELF-REFLECTION QUESTIONS

1. What are the education requirements for nurse practitioners? Should they be paid the same or less than a physician when performing the same procedures?
2. Do you think the government has a responsibility to provide health care to its citizens?
3. In what type of practice structure would it be most beneficial for you to work?
4. How do the different types of insurance coverage affect a patient's treatment?

INTERNET ACTIVITIES

1. Investigate these and other sites to find out details and facts about the Affordable Care Act and the push to repeal it and replace it with a different plan:
   https://obamacarefacts.com/affordablecareact-summary/
   https://obamacarefacts.com/the-difference-between-obamacare-and-trumpcare/
2. Find out the details of who is eligible for Medicaid in your state and the eligibility requirements. See https://www.cms.gov.
3. Research the different credentialing agencies and which one governs your profession.

ADDITIONAL RESOURCES

http://econofact.org/evidence-on-the-value-of-medicaid
https://www.excellusbcbs.com
https://www.cms.gov
https://www.ama-assn.org
https://www.americanbar.org
http://www.bioethics.net
https://www.tricare.mil
https://www.verywell.com/hmo-ppo-epo-pos-whats-the-difference-1738615

BIBLIOGRAPHY

Gottlieb, J., & Shepard, M. (July 2, 2017). *Evidence on the value of medicaid*. Available from: https://www.kff.org/other/state-indicator/number-of-hmos/?currentTimeframe=0&selectedRows=%7B%22wrapups%22:%7B%22united-states%22:%7B%7D%7D%7D&sortModel=%7B%22colId%22:%22Location%22,%22sort%22:%22asc%22%7D.

8

Workplace Issues and Employment Laws

CHAPTER OBJECTIVES

1. Describe the importance of professionalism and emotional intelligence for healthcare professionals.
2. List the different components in an employee handbook.
3. Discuss the different federal agencies that enact and enforce employment protection laws.
4. List groups considered protected classes by the federal government.
5. Define and describe types of harassment and workplace discrimination.
6. Define the different laws to protect patients and consumers in fair collections process.

KEY TERMS

Americans with Disabilities Act of 1990 (ADA) Laws enacted in 1990 to protect citizens with disabilities from discrimination with regard to employment, education, and public accommodation.

Civil Rights Act of 1964 Law that made it illegal to discriminate against someone for his or her color, sex, race, religion, or national origin with regard to voting and public access.

Consumer Credit Protection Act Law that requires providers to be up front about fees and finance charges when offering credit.

Contract An agreement between individuals or parties creating mutual obligations and enforceable by law.

Discrimination Treatment of a person or thing, either in opposition of or in favor of, based on bias or prejudice.

Due process Procedures or actions followed to safeguard individual rights. In the workplace, the process to safeguard an employee if he or she feels his or her rights are in jeopardy.

Emotional intelligence (EI) An individual's skill to perceive, understand, reason with, and manage his or her emotions and the emotions and behaviors of others.

Emotional quotient (EQ) A measurement of emotional intelligence.

Employment-at-will The employment contract that allows either the employer or the employee to terminate employment without cause.

Equal Employment Opportunity Act of 1972 Act that prohibits employment discrimination based on race, color, national origin, sex, religion, age, disability, political beliefs, and marital or familial status.

Equal Pay Act of 1963 Act that prohibited wage differentials based on sex.

Fair Credit Billing Act Law that requires businesses to provide prompt written response to billing complaints and investigation of possible billing errors.

Fair Credit Reporting Act Law that protects patients from inaccurate information on their credit reports.

Fair Debt Collection Practices Act Law that prohibits debt collectors, including physician office staff, from using deceptive or abusive practices in the collection of consumer debts.

Family Medical Leave Act (1993) Law that requires employers with 50 or more employees to allow eligible employees to take unpaid leave to help care for a family member's illness or to stay at home after the birth or adoption of a child.

Occupational Safety and Health Act of 1970 Act that defines and enforces safety regulations for the health and protection of employees in the workplace.

Occupational Safety and Health Administration (OSHA) Federal agency within the Department of Labor that designs, regulates, and monitors standards for employee safety.

Professionalism An individual's conduct in the workplace.

Sexual harassment Use of power or intimidation over an individual for sexual favors; unwanted or unwelcomed sexual advances and actions or behaviors with sexual implications or innuendoes leading another individual to feel uncomfortable or offended.

Workers' compensation A form of mandated insurance program that covers medical costs and wage replacement for employees injured on the job.

Workplace violence Any act or threat of physical violence, harassment, intimidation, or other disruptive behavior that causes fear for personal safety in the workplace.

INTRODUCTION

One of the most important relationships a professional has is the employer–employee relationship. In the healthcare setting, having a strong relationship often results in job satisfaction, motivation, productivity, and transparency. As a result, it is important to clearly describe that relationship with well-defined policies and procedures, so that the expectations are clearly understood by the employee and easily enforced by the employer. Many of these policies and procedures for the workplace have been developed by the federal government to provide protection to both the employer and the employee through every phase of his or her employment, from hiring to termination.

Healthcare professionals are particularly vulnerable because of their workplace setting and their daily interactions with patients, who present with various physical and mental illnesses. Thus, employers need to take necessary steps to understand the various employment laws to provide a safe work environment. Employees need to uphold the standards established by the employer and in the employment laws and perform their duties as defined by their job description with efficiency and productiveness.

PROFESSIONALISM

No matter how skilled or well-trained an individual may be, he or she must also be professional. In fact, a lack of professionalism may prevent an individual from being interviewed for a job, offered employment opportunities, or promoted, and it may even lead to termination. **Professionalism** is generally how one conducts oneself at work. It encompasses what are often referred to as *soft* or *interpersonal skills* and helps an individual successfully interact with others in the workplace. Professionalism may be difficult to define because it is not just one quality or skill. In fact, it is a blending or integration of a series of qualities, which include the following:

- Respectfulness
- Competence
- Dependability
- Trustworthiness
- Commitment
- Approachability
- Accountability

Professionalism is often based on one's values and understanding of his or her professional role, and it is evidenced in one's behavior and conduct (Fig. 8.1). An individual's attitude, communication style, and the

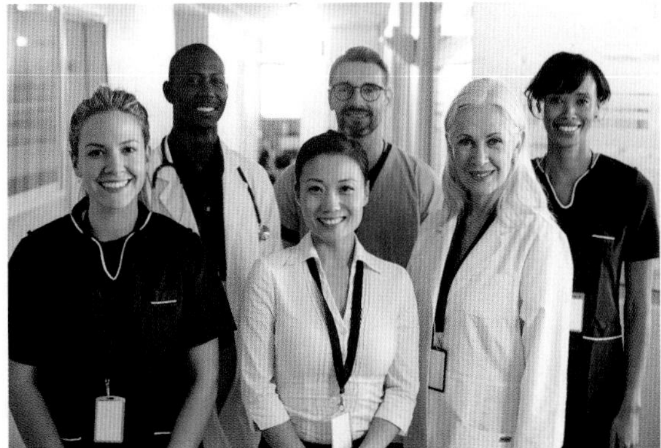

Fig. 8.1 Professionalism is essential to healthcare professionals and is often based on one's values and understanding of one's role at work. (iStock.com/Monkeybusinessimages.)

way he or she approaches conflict all speak toward professionalism.

Regardless of the profession or industry, professionalism is critical to success. Employers need employees who can conduct themselves professionally and appropriately in all circumstances. In fact, high levels of professionalism are essential in the healthcare field. Anyone can be trained to take a blood pressure reading or perform an injection, for example, but it is not always as easy to train an employee to provide patient care with respect and empathy, to be dependable and reliable, or to get along with coworkers. To be professional, healthcare professionals must leave personal problems out of the work environment and maintain a high level of integrity. They must not react to situations with emotion but with thoughtful assessment and appropriate response. They must communicate clearly and not divulge confidential patient information.

APPLY THIS

A coworker has been coming into work repeatedly late and seems very preoccupied with issues she is having outside of work. Her work performance has been unusually poor, and you recently observed her being rude and unprofessional toward patients. Yesterday, she told you that she had just been given a verbal warning. This morning, she is late again and has called to ask you to cover for her until she can report to work.

1. How would you handle this situation?
2. What do you think should be your employer's next step in addressing your coworker's behavior?

Emotional Intelligence and Quotient

An important component of professionalism is **emotional intelligence (EI)**, sometimes referred to as **emotional quotient**, although emotional quotient is a measure of emotional intelligence. EI is one's ability to perceive, understand, reason with, and manage his or her emotions and the emotions and behaviors of others. It allows us to be self-aware, self-confident, socially competent, and able to get along with others. Employees with high EI work well on teams and are often more flexible in dealing with change. A higher EI will reflect in positive relationships with coworkers and patients and a staff that is productive and effective.

Ideally, all healthcare professionals should possess a high level of professionalism and EI. Healthcare professionals with higher EI have a better understanding of their emotions and how to manage them and the emotions of others, which is an essential skill when managing patients. As a result, EI is an important consideration in human resources planning, job profiling, recruitment, interviewing, selection, and management development. In fact, employment applications and admission examinations to medical and nursing schools have included emotional quotient testing to better identify candidates with high EI. Healthcare organizations have also developed EI training for staff members, which will result in improved workplace environment, better patient retention, and better outcomes.

EMPLOYMENT CONTRACTS

Once hired, it is preferable that an individual receives a written **contract** indicating the job description, salary offered, and start date of the position. However, some agencies or positions are still based on verbal or implied contracts, which are a bit riskier for both sides. Another variation is the practice of hiring an employee "at will." An **employment-at-will** is designed so that either party may discontinue the employment agreement at any time. These may be found and even presented as a contract, for example, in a per diem (paid per day) or temporary employment. For employment-at-will employees, there is no need to follow protocols for termination; instead, the agreement itself dictates that this type of employee may end without cause. Reasons for firing or terminating a regular employee, however, should be explicitly described in the policies and procedures of the employee handbook.

Almost every state recognizes employment-at-will employment, although many states place limitations on it. Courts may also consider an employee handbook to be a binding contract, even if the employment relation is employment-at-will. Thus, a well-structured, detailed employee handbook may protect both the employee and the employer because it sets forth certain rules and structures whenever an issue arises.

EMPLOYMENT HANDBOOKS

One of the most important tools any organization can have is an employee handbook. An employee handbook is an indispensable tool in communication between an employer and employee. A well-written employee handbook will include information about work schedules, benefits, and pay, as well as promote the culture of the company. It can help an employee understand what is expected and improve morale by ensuring that employees are treated consistently and fairly.

An employee handbook should detail specific employee policies and procedures that can resolve disputes before they arise and protect both the employer and the employee from any sort of misperception and the potential of litigation.

Policies and procedures outlined in an employee handbook should include specific steps in the process for both hiring and job termination for the organization. Hiring policies should address interviewing and orienting new employees, starting with employment application requirements and any required documentation needed for employment (e.g., licenses). Company policy regarding advancement and hiring from within the organization should also be addressed in the handbook.

Although an employee handbook may vary with organization and industry, most will include the following:

- Introduction
- Company's history, business philosophy, or mission statement
- Hours of work, with normal working hours for full-time employees, part-time employees, and overtime compensation
- Compensation, including raises and bonus program
- Benefits, including vacation pay, sick leave, unpaid leave, and other benefits (i.e., health benefits, insurance benefits, retirement benefits, and employee referral benefits)
- Harassment
- Attendance, including unexplained absences or repeated tardiness
- Complaints
- Use of electronic gadgets
- Disciplinary and termination policy
- Employee conduct

Due Process

It is essential for all employees to feel assured that they will be treated fairly and that they should have a right to **due process**, which means that an employee has the right to require that all specified procedures outlined in the employee handbook be followed if that employee's employment is in jeopardy. For example, if an employee is given a verbal warning for a violation and the next step, per the policy, would be a written warning, then the employer cannot just fire the employee arbitrarily without following the steps defined in the policy.

Most employers have a series of steps that must be taken before an employee can be terminated. For instance, policy may dictate that a first offense incurs a verbal warning; the second offense involves a written or more formal warning; and a third offense will result in termination. The employer must accurately document each step in the employee's file to show that due process was followed and that the policy of the institution was observed. However, some employers identify offenses that would be "grounds for immediate dismissal," and these include extreme offenses such as Health Insurance Portability and Accountability Act (HIPAA) violations or embezzlement.

Failure to provide written policies can be a dangerous position for both employee and employer. With no written policy of expectations, how does an employee know how to meet his or her expectations? Similarly, how does the employer have any power to reprimand or impose sanctions on an employee when no policy is in place to explain the expectations? Therefore, a clear and detailed policy and procedures manual or employee handbook is necessary to protect both employee and employer.

APPLY THIS

A medical assistant has been making errors in documenting in patients' charts and is given a verbal warning. She is placed on a corrective action plan, which includes mandatory training on the proper method of documenting. The medical assistant does not comply with the corrective action plan, and, as a result, the employer fires her.

1. Did the employer take the correct steps in terminating the medical assistant?
2. Does the medical assistant have the right to fight the termination of employment based on due process?
3. What could the employer or the employee have done differently in this case?

EMPLOYEE PROTECTION AND LABOR LAWS

There are many federal agencies that administer and oversee laws that protect employees in the workplace, with the two primary agencies being the U.S. Department of Labor and the U.S. Equal Employment Opportunity Commission. Additionally, every state implements their own labor laws while also complying with federal laws.

The U.S. Department of Labor (DOL), in coordination with state labor departments, enforces more than 180 employee protection laws. The objectives of the DOL are to help foster, promote, and develop the welfare of the wage earners, job seekers, and retirees of the United States; improve working conditions; advance opportunities for profitable employment; and assure work-related benefits and right. There are a number of different agencies under the DOL that administer the different employee rights and labor laws that range from defining hours of minors to requiring employers to carry unemployment insurance (Box 8.1).

Fair Labor Standards Act

The Fair Labor Standards Act prescribes standards for wages and overtime pay, which affect most private and public employment. Requirements include employers to pay covered employees who are not otherwise exempt at least the federal minimum wage and covered nonexempt employees must receive overtime pay of one-and-one-half-times the regular rate of pay for hours worked over 40 per work week. In most workplace settings, including health care, it restricts the hours that children under age 16 can work and forbids the employment of children under age 18 in certain jobs deemed too dangerous.

Family Medical Leave Act

The Family Medical Leave Act (FMLA), enacted in 1993, required employers with 50 or more employees to allow eligible employees to take up to 12 weeks of unpaid, job protected leave to stay at home after the birth or adoption of a child or help care for a family member's illness of the employee or a spouse, child, or parent. Similar to a short-term disability, the FMLA is an insurance that is paid for by the employees.

New York is one of few states that offers an additional policy for employee protection and expands on the state's disability insurance program. Effective on January 1, 2018, employees of most private companies in New York State will be eligible for the Paid Family Leave program. Employees are able to maintain job security while able to take paid leave after having a new child, care for a family member with a serious health condition, or when someone is deployed abroad on active military service. They are able to take 8 weeks of paid time off to take care of a newborn, a sick relative, or if a military family member is deployed. Eligible employees in the state are able to take up to 8 weeks of paid family leave and receive 50% of their average weekly wage, capped at 50% of the New York State Average Weekly Wage.

BOX 8.1 Scope of U.S. Department of Labor Employment Rights and Labor Laws

- Wages and hours
- Workplace safety and health
- Workers' compensation
- Employee benefit security
- Unions and membership
- Employee protection
- Family and medical leave

APPLY THIS

A veterinary assistant was originally hired for a full-time position, with the employee handbook defining "full time" as working 35 h per week with 1 h each day for unpaid lunch breaks. After 4 months, a new supervisor is hired at the facility and begins scheduling the full-time employees for 30 h per week. As a result, the veterinary assistant will suffer a deduction in pay for 5 h loss of time and will lose her health insurance benefits because coverage requires her to be a full-time employee. When she complains, the supervisor says that the facility is cutting back department costs and hours need to be reduced for all staff.

1. What recourse do the employees have?
2. Is the supervisor justified in her actions? Are the supervisor's actions legal?

Workers' Compensation

Workers' compensation is a mandated insurance program that covers medical costs and wage replacement for employees injured on the job. All states provide insurance to pay the expenses of employees who are harmed while performing job-related duties. Employees can recover lost wages, medical expenses, disability payments, and costs associated with rehabilitation and retraining.

When injured, the most important thing for the employee to do is report the injury even if immediate medical attention is not required. Failing to report an incident when it happens can lead an employer and the workers' compensation carrier to question whether the injury occurred on the job or not. An incident report would include the details of the injury and how it occurred, statements from any witnesses, and a description of medical treatment from the treating healthcare provider.

In most states, an injured employee receiving workers' compensation waives the right to sue the employer for negligence. However, some states do allow the employee to seek further damages if the employer is found to have intentionally caused harm. It is important to note that in most of the United States it is illegal for an employer to fire or fail to hire an employee based on his or her having filed a workers' compensation claim.

OCCUPATIONAL SAFETY AND HEALTH ACT

Employers are responsible for ensuring that all areas of the workplace are safe for both employees and patients. To ensure that, Congress passed the Occupational Safety and Health (OSH) Act of 1970, which required that employers provide employees with an environment free from recognized hazards, such as exposure to toxic chemicals, excessive noise levels, mechanical dangers, heat or cold stress, or unsanitary conditions. The OSH Act also created the Occupational Safety and Health Administration (OSHA), whose function is to "assure safe and healthful working conditions for working men and women by setting and enforcing standards and by providing training, outreach, education and assistance."

Regulations under OSHA encompass everything from ergonomic workstations to lumbar support braces for heavy lifting, protective gloves, eye-wash stations, goggles and gowns, and establishing standards for all employees who are at risk for injury or infection. OSHA requires personal protection equipment that is designed to protect healthcare workers from exposure to contagious illnesses, as well as injuries from equipment or instruments that can be sharp or dangerous (Fig. 8.2). OSHA also mandates that healthcare workers who are at risk of exposure should be immunized for various diseases, such as hepatitis B and HIV.

Other guidelines include mandatory annual inservice training for those staff regularly exposed to blood-borne pathogens and infectious diseases, and most healthcare facilities must include mandatory fire safety and first aid/cardiopulmonary resuscitation training. All employees should follow the guidelines for their specific area from the OSHA mandates to ensure the health and well-being of themselves and their patients.

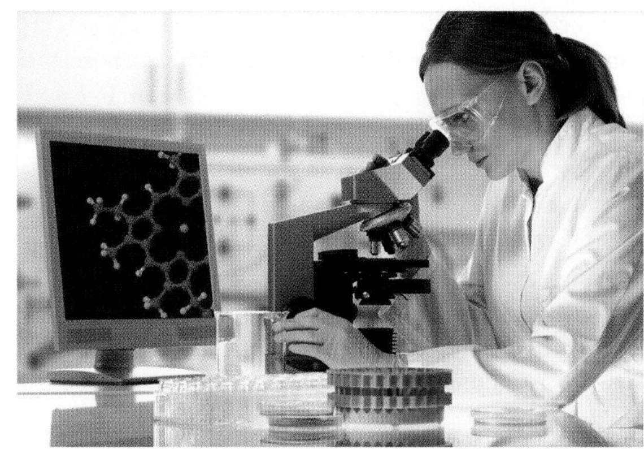

Fig. 8.2 All physical hazard spaces, medical waste, and medical biohazards (such as used sharps) must be handled following specific guidelines initiated by OSHA. (http://www.thinkstockphotos.com/image/stock-photo-laboratory/133696775/popup?sq=alexraths%20lab/f=CPIHVX/s=DynamicRank.) (iStock.com/AlexRaths.)

DISCUSSION

According to the Occupational Health and Safety Act, all employees are entitled to three fundamental rights:

- The right to know about health and safety matters.
- The right to participate in decisions that could affect their health and safety.
- The right to refuse work that could affect their health and safety and that of others.

1. What role do you think the government should have in protection employees in the workplace?
2. What if it is too costly for the employers to train and install systems and processes to fully protect an employee? What level of risk should be acceptable?
3. In the healthcare setting, describe activities that may be considered high risk for injury and safety.

Workplace Violence

According to OSHA, more than 2 million American workers report having been victims of workplace violence each year. Homicide is one of the leading causes of occupational fatalities in the United States. Workplace violence is any act or threat of physical violence, harassment, intimidation, or other threatening disruptive behavior that causes fear for personal safety in the workplace. It can be a verbal threat or a physical altercation and can involve employees, clients, customers, or visitors. Violence can arise from any number of situations, both real and perceived, such as anger over a disciplinary action, the belief that an employee was passed over for a promotion, or disapproval of a new regulation. It may originate with an unsatisfied customer, an abusive manager, or a domestic problem that carries over to the workplace. Regardless of the reason behind the violent threat or act, it is important that it not be tolerated. Some of the employees who are at the highest risk for potential workplace violence include those who exchange money with the public, law enforcement, delivery drivers, and healthcare workers.

Serious workplace violence is four times more likely to occur in a healthcare setting than any other place of employment, with patients being the largest source of this violence. Many healthcare workers are at risk from violence due to involuntary actions from patients, either while moving or subduing patients or from patients with mental disorders. Other violent situations may stem from disgruntled coworkers, visitors, or other people who come into the facility. Despite the high number of reported incidents, it is believed that many acts of workplace violence go unreported because of fear of retaliation.

Although OSHA does not have specific regulations that address workplace violence, employers have a general duty to provide a safe work environment where an employee is free from the threat of harm. Unfortunately, it is difficult to predict when and where violence can happen on the job. The best precaution an employer can make is to have a zero-tolerance policy that includes employees, patients, clients, visitors, contractors, and anyone else who may interact with employees. In addition, employers should include policies on workplace violence in the employee handbook and any other operating manual. It is critical to ensure that all workers know the policy and understand that all claims of workplace violence will be investigated and promptly addressed. Additional training in how to handle an active shooter situation is highly recommended.

APPLY THIS

Sandra is a nurse in a medical office, and she has just assisted the physician with a suturing procedure. As she is cleaning up afterward, she accidently punctures her finger by the suture needle.

1. What procedures should be followed?
2. Is the employer responsible even though Sandra made the mistake?
3. Would the employer be responsible if Sandra was not wearing gloves while cleaning the room?

CIVIL RIGHTS ACT

The **Civil Rights Act of 1964**, sometimes referred to as Title VII, is a law making it illegal to discriminate against someone on the basis of race, color, religion, national origin, or sex. In addition to these protected classes, there are now also protections for physical or mental disability and, most recently added, sexual orientation.

The law also makes it illegal to retaliate against a person because the person complained about discrimination, filed a charge of discrimination, or participated in an employment discrimination investigation or lawsuit. The law also requires that employers reasonably accommodate the sincerely held religious practices of applicants and employees, unless doing so would impose an undue hardship on the operation of the employer's business.

Equal Employment Opportunity Commission

The Civil Rights Act of 1964 also created the Equal Employment Opportunity Commission (EEOC), which is another independent federal agency responsible for enforcing the Act and other employment laws to protect employees from discrimination and discriminatory practices. In 1972, Congress passed the **Equal Employment Opportunity Act of 1972**. This made the EEOC responsible for enforcing federal laws that make it illegal to discriminate against a job applicant or an employee because of the person's race, color, religion, sex (including pregnancy, transgender status, and sexual orientation), national origin, age (40 or older), disability or genetic information.

Most employers with at least 15 employees are covered by EEOC laws (20 employees in age discrimination cases). Most labor unions and employment agencies are also covered. The laws apply to all types of work situations, including hiring, firing, promotions, harassment, training, wages, and benefits.

Pregnancy Discrimination Act

The Civil Rights Act has also been amended several times to protect other groups. For example, the Pregnancy Discrimination Act of 1978 amended the Civil Rights Act and prohibited discrimination based on pregnancy and other related medical conditions. Pregnancy is considered a short-term disability, and employers must treat pregnant employees as they would any other employee with a short-term disability. This includes making accommodations to their duties and work assignments, as well as allowing them disability leave. The law also makes it illegal to retaliate against a person because the person complained about discrimination, filed a charge of discrimination, or participated in an employment discrimination investigation or lawsuit.

Discrimination

Many laws and regulations enforced by the EEOC are created to prevent the discrimination of protected groups of people, especially during the process of hiring (Fig. 8.3). These include specific restrictions for interview and employment application questions. The below box lists questions that cannot be asked of a candidate during a job interview.

EXAMPLES OF ILLEGAL INTERVIEW QUESTIONS

- **Age:** You may ask if a person is between 17 and 70 years old but not specifically ask the person's age.
- **Religion:** You may not ask the candidate's religious background.
- **Race or color:** You may not ask a candidate's race, color, nationality, or heritage.
- **Children:** It is illegal to ask whether the candidate has children or daycare issues.
- **Height and weight:** It is illegal to ask questions about a candidate's height or weight, although equipment restrictions can be shared and explained.
- **Disabilities:** It is illegal to ask whether the candidate has a disability or disease. But it is legal to ask if the candidate has any physical impairment that would prevent him or her from performing the position for which he or she has applied.
- **Arrest records:** A person may have been arrested but not convicted of a crime, so it is illegal to ask whether he or she has ever been arrested. It is permissible to ask whether someone has been convicted of a felony.
- **Maiden name:** This should be requested only if there is a need to clarify a difference in name on review of licenses or educational verifications; otherwise, it is an illegal question.

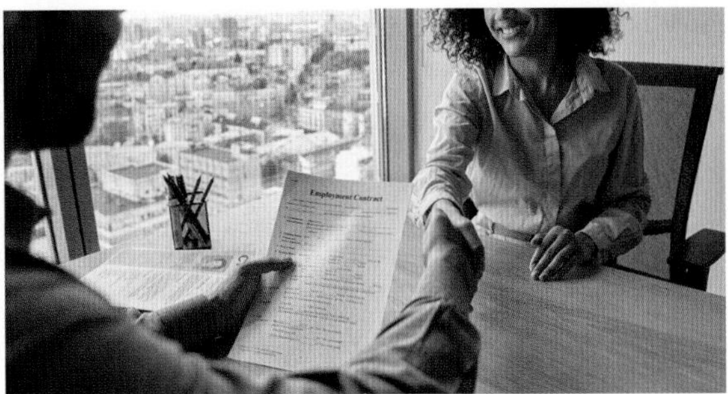

Fig. 8.3 Many laws and regulations enforced by the EEOC are created to prevent the discrimination of protected groups of people, especially during the process of hiring. (iStock.com/Insta_Photos.)

Areas that the candidate can be lawfully asked about but should be asked only as they relate to the position include languages spoken, birthplace, marital status, citizenship, organizations or affiliations, and military experience. In general, it is a good practice to avoid asking questions that do not directly pertain to the ability of the candidate to perform the duties of the position for which he or she is applying.

Sexual Harassment

Sexual harassment is a form of sex discrimination that violates the Civil Rights Act of 1964. Sexual harassment is the intimidation of another or unwanted advances or sexual comments that cause another person to feel uncomfortable. Unwelcome sexual advances, requests for sexual favors, and other verbal or physical conduct of a sexual nature constitute sexual harassment when this conduct affects an individual's employment; unreasonably interferes with an individual's work performance; or creates an intimidating, hostile, or offensive work environment.

The offender can be a male or a female, and the offense can be committed by either an opposite or a same-sex individual. Per the EEOC guidelines, the victim should make it clear to the harasser that the actions are unwanted and unacceptable. If the action does not stop immediately, the victim should then inform management and follow internal complaint policies. For the offender, it may result in corrective action and even dismissal, depending on the offense.

Most employers have policies and procedures in place to follow when such incidents occur. These procedures include steps for reporting, following up, and discontinuing any harassment conduct, as well as provisions for disciplining or terminating an offender. It is important to note that sexual harassment may involve patients, both as the victim and as the harasser. Healthcare employers must also address these situations when establishing protocols for addressing harassment.

Guidelines related to sexual harassment can be reviewed at https://www.eeoc.gov/eeoc/publications/fs-sex.cfm.

Other Employment Right and Laws

There are a number of other employment laws protected by the EEOC.

- The Equal Pay Act of 1963 (EPA) is a law that makes it illegal to pay different wages to men and women if they perform equal work in the same workplace.
- The Age Discrimination in Employment Act of 1967 (ADEA) protects people who are 40 or older from discrimination because of age.
- The Genetic Information Nondiscrimination Act of 2008 (GINA) went into effect on November 21, 2009 and makes it illegal to discriminate against employees or applicants because of genetic information. Genetic information includes information about an individual's genetic tests and the genetic tests of an individual's family members, as well as information about any disease, disorder, or condition of an individual's family members (i.e., an individual's family medical history).

All EEOC laws make it illegal to retaliate against a person because the person complained about discrimination, filed a charge of discrimination, or participated in an employment discrimination investigation or lawsuit.

In addition, many states also have their own antidiscrimination laws and policies that may be broader than the federal statutes. This means that state laws may protect more people than perhaps the federal laws do. For example, some state laws also protect people on the basis of political ideology and service in a state militia. State laws may provide more protections than federal laws; however, they cannot give fewer protections than federal laws.

Private employers may also have policies in place to protect their employees from discrimination or harassment in the workplace based on certain statuses, such as marital status, gender, or sexual orientation.

DISCUSSION

Although discrimination can exist in all types of groups, not every group is considered a protected class under the law. Unfortunately, if a person is not a member of a protected class, that person may not be protected under federal or state antidiscrimination laws. For example, groups that are not considered protected classes include education level, economic class, social membership, undocumented or citizenship, and people with criminal records.

1. Should any of these groups be considered a legally protected class?
2. Describe some examples of how each of these groups could be discriminated against.
3. What other groups should be added to the list of protected classes?

AMERICANS WITH DISABILITIES ACT

Over the latter half of the 20th century, the disability rights movement grew in the United States, prompting the enactment of the Americans with Disabilities Act (ADA) of 1990, sometimes referred to as Title I, and its predecessor, the Rehabilitation Act of 1973. Under these laws, if an individual applies for enrollment to an educational institution or for employment, ADA requires that the individual receives "reasonable" accommodations if necessary and should not be discriminated against in the pursuit of employment, education, or access to public places because of the disability. "Reasonable accommodations" refers to necessary and appropriate changes to any system or structure that would make the environment equal and fair. These standards also apply to healthcare facilities and equipment, especially regarding patient care and access. Doorways, parking lots, building access, drinking fountains, and all other physical aspects of the facility must meet code requirements for accessibility.

Signage must incorporate Braille. Examination tables must be designed to be accessible to patients in wheelchairs. Mobility aids must be available to help transfer patients safely. Even mammography equipment and scales need to be designed with wheelchairs in mind. Staff and providers must be trained to communicate effectively with patients who may have cognitive, vision, hearing, and speech disabilities.

The full listing of and complete guidelines for reasonable accommodations can be found on the EEOC website: https://www.eeoc.gov/policy/docs/accommodation.html.

DISCUSSION

Several coworkers are in the lunchroom during their lunch break. Two of your coworkers, Sam and George, are having a rather loud conversation about a party they attended over the past weekend. George retells a joke that he heard at the party, which is sexually explicit and includes several words that offend Sally. Sally is upset and offended and confronts them about the nature of the conversation that they are having and how it is offensive to her. George and Sam tell her that she is overreacting and dismiss her complaint.

1. Is this considered sexual harassment because the conversation did not involve Sally?
2. What actions can be taken to address this incident?

COLLECTION STANDARDS

As with any business, healthcare providers and organizations are held to federal laws that will shape their credit and collection policies. Ideally, any portion of a bill that reflects a patient's out-of-pocket responsibility will be collected at the time of service. However, physicians in some specialties, such as radiology and anesthesiology, do not see patients in an office setting and are unable to collect at the time of service. Other medical bills, such as hospital bills for inpatient stays and other large-ticket services, are simply too large to expect patients to pay for in one lump sum. Thus, payment plans and credit card billing are often offered as a way to assist patients with their bills.

Many laws protect patients and how they are treated with regard to payments and credit:

- The **Fair Debt Collection Practices Act** prohibits debt collectors, including physician office staff, from using deceptive or abusive practices in the collection of consumer debts. This would include contacting patients at odd hours and harassing them with repeated phone calls and threats.
- The **Fair Credit Reporting Act** protects patients from inaccurate information on their credit reports.
- The **Consumer Credit Protection Act (1968)** requires providers to be up front about fees and finance charges when offering credit.
- The **Fair Credit Billing Act** requires prompt written response to billing complaints and investigation of possible billing errors.

Failure to follow these laws when collecting money owed to a medical practice can lead to significant fines and penalties.

CONCLUSION

Medical offices and healthcare organizations operate the same as any other business with different federal, state, and workplace laws and regulations. Employment protection laws are in place to protect the workers' rights by making discrimination illegal and requiring a certain level of compensation. Other legislation is in place to protect an employee in case of injury and to ensure the employer offers standard benefits. Maintaining clear and concise policies and procedures in any organization is essential. All individuals employed will have security in knowing and understanding their employer's policies and procedures.

A hostile or uncomfortable workplace is difficult, at best, to handle, but proper procedures and policies should help to defend the employee and protect the employer in all situations that might arise. In the healthcare profession, this should be especially true, and indeed the highest standards of professionalism and ethical behavior are expected and should be upheld.

CHAPTER REVIEW QUESTIONS

1. Which organization oversees the enforcement of equal rights and fights discrimination?
   A. CMS
   B. OSHA
   C. EEOC
   D. HIPAA
2. Which organization oversees and protects employment labor laws, such as workers' compensation?
   A. OIG
   B. OSHA
   C. EI
   D. DOL

3. Which agency oversees the safety of all workplaces?
   A. CMS
   B. OSHA
   C. EEOC
   D. HIPAA
4. The right of an employee to have certain policies and procedures followed if he or she thinks his or her rights are in jeopardy is called
   A. utilitarianism.
   B. due process.
   C. workers' compensation.
   D. HIPAA.
5. Insurance that covers medical costs and wage replacement if an employee is injured on the job is
   A. Workers' compensation.
   B. Equal Employment Opportunity Act.
   C. Family Medical Leave.
   D. OSHA.
6. This law prohibits sexual harassment and defines it as an act of sexual discrimination.
   A. Civil Rights Act
   B. Occupational Safety and Health Act
   C. Patient Protection and Affordable Care Act
   D. Fair Labor Standards Act
7. The ability to perceive, understand, reason with, and manage one's motions and the behaviors of others is
   A. professionalism.
   B. emotional quotient.
   C. emotional intelligence.
   D. discrimination.
8. Which of the following would not be covered in an employee handbook?
   A. Bullying and harassment policy
   B. Job duties and responsibilities
   C. Vacation and personal time-off
   D. Company's mission statement
9. Which of the following is *not* a protected class, according to the Civil Right Act?
   A. Age
   B. Economic
   C. Race
   D. Sexual orientation
10. The Consumer Credit Protection Act protects consumers for which of the following:
    A. requiring providers to disclose any fees and finance chargers when offering credit.
    B. requiring prompt written response to billing complaints.
    C. prohibiting any inaccurate information on a patient's credit report.
    D. prohibiting debt collectors from using any deceptive or abusive practices when attempting to collect a debt.

SELF-REFLECTION QUESTIONS

1. What discriminations, if any, have you felt victim of in the past? What would you do if you were a witness to another employee being subjected to discrimination?
2. How does OSHA guidelines directly affect you in the workplace?
3. If you were designing an employee handbook, what would be some important items you would want to be sure were included?

INTERNET ACTIVITIES

1. Using https://www.eeoc.gov/eeoc/publications/fs-sex.cfm, find the EEOC guidelines regarding sexual harassment and investigate the different forms.
2. Investigate one or more of the following laws and write an assessment of how they relate to your place of employment:
   - Drug-Free Workplace Act of 1988
   - Fair Labor Standards Act (FLSA) of 1938
   - Family Medical Leave Act (FMLA) of 1994
   - Americans with Disabilities Act
   - Equal Employment Opportunity Act of 1972
   - The National Labor Relations Act (NLRA) of 1935
   - Occupational Safety and Health Act (1970)

ADDITIONAL RESOURCES

https://www.dol.gov/general/topic/disability/ada
https://www.uslegal.com
https://www.eeoc.gov
https://www.ada.gov
https://www.eeoc.gov/eeoc/publications/fs-sex.cfm
https://www.osha.gov
https://www.dol.gov
https://www.ada.gov/medcare_mobility_ta/medcare_ta.htm
https://www.eeoc.gov/facts/health_care_workers.html
https://www.hhs.gov/sites/default/files/2016-06-07-section-1557-final-rule-summary-508.pdf
http://civilrights.findlaw.com/discrimination/health-care-discrimination.html

9

Medical Records and HIPAA

CHAPTER OBJECTIVES

1. Outline the purpose of medical records.
2. List the organization and contents within a medical record.
3. Describe the importance of correct documentation in a patient medical record.
4. Name key guidelines for storage, retention, and maintenance of medical records.
5. Discuss the confidentiality and consent forms for release of medical records.
6. Discuss HIPAA privacy and security for medical records.
7. Discuss the different types of safeguards for medical records.

KEY TERMS

Active patient files Files of patients who are being actively seen within the specific healthcare facility.

CHEDDAR A type of organization of medical record documentation that breaks down information into chief complaint, history, examination, details, drugs, assessment, and return visit plan.

Chief complaint (CC) A specific reason the patient is being seen by the healthcare provider.

Clearinghouses Entities that process electronic transactions into HIPAA standardized transactions for billing submission.

Closed-ended questions Types of questions that can be answered by a simple "yes" or "no."

Continuity of care record (CCR) A patient's medical health record that is accurate to ensure continuity of care when a patient is transferred to another healthcare provider or to a medical specialist.

Covered entity (CE) Health plans, healthcare clearinghouses, and healthcare providers under HIPAA who electronically transmit any health information.

Differential diagnosis A list of possible diagnoses that may likely be the cause of the presenting symptoms.

Double lock system A safeguard that requires passing through two systems of security to access any confidential patient information.

Electronic medical record (EMR) Electronic medical records that contain medical and health records of individual patients, maintaining the HIPAA standards for privacy and security.

Electronic health record (EHR) Electronic medical records that can be shared, created, managed, and consulted by authorized healthcare providers, professionals, and staff across more than one healthcare organization

Firewalls Network security devices that monitor incoming and outgoing network traffic and decide whether to allow or block specific traffic based on a defined set of security rules.

Health Insurance Portability and Accountability Act of 1996 (HIPAA) Federal legislation that provides data privacy and security provisions for safeguarding medical information.

Inactive patient files Files of patients who have not been seen within the specific healthcare facility over the preceding 3 years.

Open-ended questions Types of questions that require more thought and more than a simple one-word answer.

Protected health information (PHI) Any information about a patient's health status, provision of health care, or payment for health care that is created or collected by a covered entity (or a business associate of a covered entity) and can be linked to a specific individual.

SOAP An acronym used to document in patient's medical chart meaning: Subjective, Objective, Assessment, and Plan.

INTRODUCTION

Medical records and documentation play an intricate and critical function in providing quality patient care. They allow for the continuity of care of patients by detailing the evaluation, management, and treatment of patients by healthcare professionals. Medical records also allow healthcare professionals to accurately reconstruct each patient's medical encounters from the past to the present. Not only does medical records play an important role in patient care, but they are also often used as a central piece of evidence in a medical malpractice lawsuit, professional ethics breaches, and billing fraud cases.

All healthcare professionals must be trained in proper documentation and maintenance of medical records and follow federal and state laws and guidelines. This chapter will outline the necessary components of documentation and the critical guidelines, standards, and laws to follow.

PURPOSE OF MEDICAL RECORDS

The primary purpose of a medical record is to provide a complete and accurate description of the patient's medical history, including medical conditions, diagnoses, the care and treatment received, and results of such treatments. Medical records include important components in a patient's health care and play a role in:

- providing the patient's past and present medical history as a **Continuity of Care Record (CCR)**,
- allowing members of the healthcare team to communicate with one another,
- protecting both the patient and healthcare professional in cases of negligence and malpractice,
- serving as research and quality control, and
- providing documentation for billing and coding purposes for insurance claims.

As a result, it is vital that all healthcare professionals and staff realize the seriousness of their effect on patients' current and future treatment and progress when documenting medical records.

When using paper medical records or charts, all documentation must be initialed or signed and dated by the healthcare professional. For initialing or signing the medical record, follow the procedure or standard for the appropriate protocol of that healthcare facility. All entries in the patient medical records should be documented as a legal entry that would uphold in a court of law.

With the passage of the **Health Insurance Portability and Accountability Act of 1996 (HIPAA)**, almost all medical offices and healthcare facilities have transitioned from paper medical records to electronic. This would allow for easier transferability when patients requested their medical records to share or transfer to a **covered entity (CE)**, which is any healthcare plans, healthcare **clearinghouses**, and healthcare providers who electronically transmit any health information. CEs can be institutions, organizations, or persons. For example, hospitals, academic medical centers, physicians, and other healthcare providers who electronically transmit claims transaction information directly or through an intermediary to a health plan are covered entities.

One of the most important federal laws that establishes standards to protect medical records is HIPPA, which will be discussed in further detail later in this chapter. As a result of the passage of HIPAA, healthcare professionals now have computer-generated charts called **electronic medical records (EMRs)**. EMRs are digital versions of paper charts that contain the patient's medical records, including all laboratory results, test results, diagnoses, and treatment plans in the healthcare provider's office or at one organization. EMRs have advantages over paper records in that they allow healthcare providers to monitor patients over time

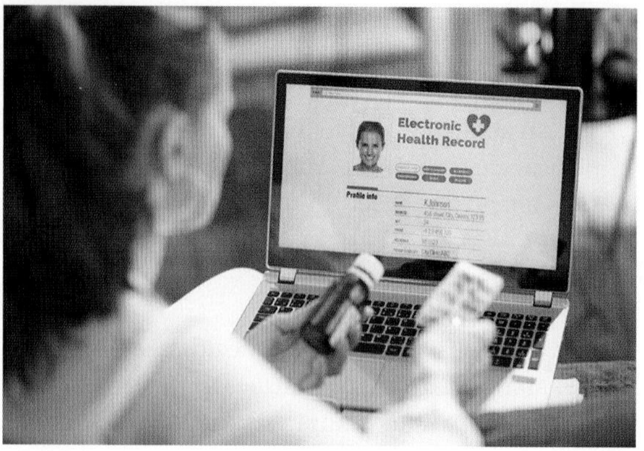

Fig. 9.1 Electronic health records (EHRs) are electronic medical records (EMR) that can be shared beyond the healthcare organization that originally collected and compiled the patient information. (iStock.com/CentralITAlliance.)

and identify which patients are due for any preventative screenings or check-ups. However, EMRs are not shared with other healthcare professionals outside of that practice.

Although often used interchangeably, there are differences between EMR and electronic health records (EHR). **EHRs** are medical records that can be shared, created, managed, and consulted by authorized healthcare providers, professionals, and staff across more than one healthcare organization (Fig. 9.1). EHRs are designed to extend beyond the health organization that originally collects and compiles the patient information. They are built to share information with other healthcare providers, such as laboratories and specialists, so they contain information from all the providers involved in the patient's care. With a functional EHR, for example, patient information gathered by the primary care provider about the patient's life-threatening allergy can be transmitted to the emergency department physician, so that care can be adjusted appropriately, even if the patient is unconscious. Or the physician's notes from the patient's hospital stay can help inform the discharge instructions and follow-up care to the patient's primary care provider.

ELEMENTS OF MEDICAL RECORDS

The main elements of a medical record are usually standard for most healthcare organizations, although there may be some variation based on the facility and the type of specialty practice. For example, a cardiology practice may have additional questions about family history of cardiac diseases and history of any cardiac procedures. Regardless, each type of healthcare facility will include the patient's basic information, which is often compiled using a patient intake form (Fig. 9.2) or patient registration form. Patient information in a medical record should include the following:

- *Demographics:* Patient information, including name, contact information, date of birth, occupation, and emergency contact information. In some cases, the Social Security number may be requested.
- *Insurance information:* This includes the name of the insurance provider and number, the subscriber's information, and any financial liabilities, such as a copay.
- *Consent forms:* HIPPA agreement and release of information form.
- *Medical history:* A detail of the patient's past health history and family history.
- *Medications:* Currently taken or currently prescribed medications and any vitamins or other health supplements.
- *Examination and notes:* Include observations, examination findings, diagnosis, and treatment plans.
- *Laboratory and test results:* Laboratory and blood results and any imaging studies, such as radiographic images and magnetic resonance imaging (MRI), computed tomography (CT), or positron emission tomography (PET) scans.
- *Communication:* Notes from any communication with the patient by phone, email, or other types of communication.

Often the financial records are kept separate from the patient's medical records to safeguard against data breaches.

Many healthcare professionals and facilities communicate information to patients via email or through a secure patient portal system. The patient portal system can be accessed anywhere and at any time by the patient and is password protected. Thus, the patient portal system is an efficient and secure method of communicating with patients.

Text continued on p. 109

Patient Navigator Outreach and Chronic Disease Prevention Program

Patient Intake Form

Study ID: ______________ Navigator: ______________

Enrollment Date: ______________ Subsite: ______________

Local Identifiers (site use only)

Demographics

Gender *(Check one)* *
- ❑ Male
- ❑ Female
- ❑ Transgender

Birth year * _ _ _ _

Education *(Check one)*
- ❑ No formal education
- ❑ Primary education only
- ❑ Some HS/secondary education
- ❑ HS Diploma/GED/other secondary education
- ❑ Some college/vocational school/ other post-secondary education
- ❑ Completed college, post-secondary or vocational school
- ❑ Post-college/graduate school
- ❑ Refused

Ethnicity *(Check one)* *
- ❑ Hispanic or Latino
- ❑ Non-Hispanic

Race *(Check all that apply)*
- ❑ White
- ❑ Black/African American
- ❑ Asian
- ❑ Native Hawaiian/Pacific Islander
- ❑ American Indian/Alaska Native
- ❑ Refused

Optional race coding:

Primary/preferred language *
(Check one)
- ❑ English
- ❑ Spanish
- ❑ Chinese
- ❑ Fijian
- Filipino → ❑ Tagalog ❑ Ilocano ❑ Visayan ❑ Other
- ❑ French
- ❑ Haitian Creole
- ❑ Hmong
- ❑ Japanese
- ❑ Korean
- Micronesian → ❑ Chuukese ❑ Kosraean ❑ Marshalese ❑ Pohnpeian ❑ Yapese
- ❑ Mixteco
- ❑ Navajo
- ❑ Samoan
- ❑ Somali
- ❑ Tongan
- ❑ Vietnamese
- ❑ Other
  - ↳ *Specify*: ______________

** Required for registration*

Household

3-digit zip prefix _ _ _
❑ Refused

Household size _ _
❑ Refused

(# in household, Including patient)

Household income *(Check one)*
- ❑ Less than $10K
- ❑ $10K to $19,999
- ❑ $20K to $29,999
- ❑ $30K to $39,999
- ❑ $40K to $49,999
- ❑ $50K or more
- ❑ Refused

Utilization

 # Hospital stays, past year
- ❑ None
- ❑ One stay
- ❑ More than 1 stay
- ❑ Not Available

 # ER visits, past year
- ❑ None
- ❑ One ER visit
- ❑ More than 1 visit
- ❑ Not Available

Coverage

Pharmacy assistance
- ❑ No
- ❑ Yes
- ❑ Not Available

Heath care coverage
(Check all that apply)
- ❑ No coverage
- ❑ Medicare
- ❑ Medicaid
- ❑ IHS (Indian Health Service)
- ❑ Private insurance
- ❑ Other Government plan
- ❑ Single service plan
- ❑ Reduced-fee/sliding scale
- ❑ Free care
- ❑ Other
  - ↳ *Specify*: ______________

Navigated Condition(s)

Check all that apply

Asthma _ _/_ _/_ _ _ _
- ❑ Asthma, at risk/pre-asthma
- ❑ Asthma, diagnosed

CHF _ _/_ _/_ _ _ _
(Congestive Heart Failure)
- ❑ CHF, diagnosed

CVD _ _/_ _/_ _ _ _
(Cardiovascular Disease)
- ❑ CVD, at risk/family history
- ❑ CVD, diagnosed

Depression _ _/_ _/_ _ _ _
- ❑ Depression, positive screen
- ❑ Depression, diagnosed

Diabetes _ _/_ _/_ _ _ _
- ❑ Diabetes, at risk/family history
- ❑ Diabetes, pre-diabetes
- ❑ Diabetes, diagnosed
- ❑ Gestational diabetes

Hyperlipidemia _ _/_ _/_ _ _ _
- ❑ Hyperlipidemia, diagnosed

Hypertension _ _/_ _/_ _ _ _
- ❑ Hypertension, positive screen
- ❑ Hypertension, diagnosed

Obesity _ _/_ _/_ _ _ _
- ❑ Obesity (adult)
- ❑ Obesity (pediatric)

Other _ _/_ _/_ _ _ _
- ❑ Other
  - ↳ *Specify*: ______________

Cancer _ _/_ _/_ _ _ _

Type of cancer: ______________
- ❑ Cancer, screening
- ❑ Cancer, abnormal finding
- ❑ Cancer, diagnosed
  - ↳ Stage*:* 0 1 2 3 4 N/A

Rev. 19-Sep-2011 **Entered:** _ _/_ _/_ _ **By:** ______

Fig. 9.2 Patient intake form. (From https://www.reginfo.gov/public/do/DownloadDocument?objectID=29355301. Accessed 05.07.2018.)

Continued

Patient Navigator Outreach and Chronic Disease Prevention Program

Patient Intake Form *(cancer only)*

Study ID: ______________ Navigator: ______________

Enrollment Date: ______________ Subsite: ______________

Local Identifiers (site use only)

Demographics

Gender *(Check one)* *
- ❑ Male
- ❑ Female
- ❑ Transgender

Birth year * _ _ _ _

Education *(Check one)*
- ❑ No formal education
- ❑ Primary education only
- ❑ Some HS/secondary education
- ❑ HS Diploma/GED/other secondary education
- ❑ Some college/vocational school/ other post-secondary education
- ❑ Completed college, post-secondary or vocational school
- ❑ Post-college/graduate school
- ❑ Refused

Ethnicity *(Check one)* *
- ❑ Hispanic or Latino
- ❑ Non-Hispanic

Race *(Check all that apply)*
- ❑ White
- ❑ Black/African American
- ❑ Asian
- ❑ Native Hawaiian/Pacific Islander
- ❑ American Indian/Alaska Native
- ❑ Refused

Optional race coding:

Primary/preferred language *

(Check one)
- ❑ English
- ❑ Spanish
- ❑ Chinese
- ❑ Fijian
- Filipino → ❑ Tagalog ❑ Ilocano ❑ Visayan ❑ Other
- ❑ French
- ❑ Haitian Creole
- ❑ Hmong
- ❑ Japanese
- ❑ Korean
- Micronesian → ❑ Chuukese ❑ Kosraean ❑ Marshalese ❑ Pohnpeian ❑ Yapese
- ❑ Mixteco
- ❑ Navajo
- ❑ Samoan
- ❑ Somali
- ❑ Tongan
- ❑ Vietnamese
- ❑ Other
  - ↳ *Specify*: ______________

** Required for registration*

Household

3-digit zip prefix _ _ _

❑ Refused

Household size _ _

❑ Refused

(# in household, Including patient)

Household income *(Check one)*
- ❑ Less than $10K
- ❑ $10K to $19,999
- ❑ $20K to $29,999
- ❑ $30K to $39,999
- ❑ $40K to $49,999
- ❑ $50K or more
- ❑ Refused

Utilization

 # Hospital stays, past year
- ❑ None
- ❑ One stay
- ❑ More than 1 stay
- ❑ Not Available

 # ER visits, past year
- ❑ None
- ❑ One ER visit
- ❑ More than 1 visit
- ❑ Not Available

Coverage

Pharmacy assistance
- ❑ No
- ❑ Yes
- ❑ Not Available

Heath care coverage

(Check all that apply)
- ❑ No coverage
- ❑ Medicare
- ❑ Medicaid
- ❑ IHS (Indian Health Service)
- ❑ Private insurance
- ❑ Other Government plan
- ❑ Single service plan
- ❑ Reduced-fee/sliding scale
- ❑ Free care
- ❑ Other
  - ↳ *Specify*: ______________

Navigated Condition(s)

- ❑ Cancer, screening
- ❑ Cancer, abnormal finding
- ❑ Cancer, diagnosed

Date: _ _ / _ _ / _ _ _ _

Type of cancer: ______________

Diagnosed cancer only

Stage: 0 1 2 3 4 N/A

Substage (optional): A B C

TNM Staging (optional): ______________

Histology(optional):

Rev. 14-Oct-2011

Entered: _ _ / _ _ / _ _ **By:** ______

Fig. 9.2, cont'd

Patient Navigator Outreach and Chronic Disease Prevention Program

Navigation Target Form

Local Identifiers (site use only)

Study Data

Study ID: ______________

Navigator ID: ______________

Date Identified: ______________

Date Scheduled: ______________

❑Unscheduled Service

Location *Check one*

❑ Internal
❑ External

Location Notes:

Status Options

Open target:	**Closed target:**
Scheduled	Services received
Rescheduled	Ineligible
Canceled	Unable to access
No show	No longer relevant
Paperwork complete	Refused

Type of Service *Check one*

Medical visit for cancer
❑ Screening
❑ Diagnostic test
❑ Cancer treatment

Medical visit for other conditions
❑ Lab or diagnostic test
❑ Primary care
❑ Medical specialist (MD or DO)
Optional: ______________________

Health education
❑ Certified diabetes educator
❑ Nutritionist
❑ Other health education/disease management

Social services and assistance
❑ Health care coverage
❑ Pharmacy assistance
❑ Medical equipment
❑ Other service (Government agency)
❑ Other service (nonprofit/charitable org)

Other services
❑ Behavioral/mental health services
❑ Clinical trials
❑ Other
↳ *Specify:* ______________________

Notes

Use the table below to record scheduling changes and/or target resolution.

Date	Status	Notes (optional)

Rev. 20-Sep-2011

Entered: __ __ / __ __ / __ __ **By:** _______

Fig. 9.2, cont'd

Continued

Navigation Target Form (page 2)

Use the table below to record scheduling changes and/or target resolution.

Date	**Status**	**Notes (optional)**

Notes:

Rev. 20-Sep-2011

Entered: __ __ / __ __ / __ __ By: ______

Fig. 9.2, cont'd

DOCUMENTATION OF MEDICAL RECORDS

Documentation of all patient encounters is one of the most important parts of the healthcare delivery process. It protects all parties—the patient, the healthcare professional and facility, and insurer—by recording the details of each patient encounter or visit, and the procedures and treatment performed. What is documented in the patient's medical record may also include any observations, diagnoses, laboratory and test results, and treatment plans, which aid in the patient's overall health by providing a continuity of care.

All healthcare providers and staff must be diligent and accurate in their documentation or dictation of the events of all encounters and must understand that the thoroughness of that record is essential. This includes any conversation with the patient in the facility that is in-person or by telephone, fax, or email. The patient's medical record is considered a legal record and can be requested, or subpoenaed, in court, for example, in cases of malpractice and negligence. When it comes to medical records, the golden rule is "If it is not documented, it did not happen."

The completeness, timeliness, and accuracy of the medical records are critical to the protection of the patient and the healthcare professional. Any individual who is documenting data into the medical record needs to appreciate the importance of maintaining the credibility of the record.

Documentation of Patient Encounters

During the patient's visit to the medical office or healthcare facility, a healthcare professional will document information given by the patient, as well as findings during the physical examination. There are different methods that healthcare providers may use to document: written documentation in the patient's chart, inputting information electronically, or dictating the information for a transcriber. Occasionally, a healthcare provider will have a staff member, such as a medical assistant, in the treatment room inputting information while the provider examines and speaks to the patient. Regardless of the method of documentation, the format or guidelines used to document information need to be in a consistent and organized manner. There are several standard formats for documentation used in the healthcare setting, with the most common being SOAP and CHEDDAR.

"SOAP" Format

One common method of documenting a patient's medical information is the SOAP notes format (Box 9.1). SOAP is an acronym that stands for **S**ubjective, **O**bjective, **A**ssessment, and **P**lan:

S—Subjective: Patient's health history given by the patient, usually a brief statement on the purpose of the visit and should include the chief complaint (CC), history of present illness (HPI), and any past, family, and social history taken (PFSH).

During the review of the patient's information, it is important for the healthcare professional to ask open-ended questions to encourage the patient to give more information instead of closed-ended questions with a "yes" or "no" answer. Closed-ended questions do not provide detailed information from the patient, but they allow for quicker responses when details are not necessary. For example, an open-ended question would be: "Describe the pain." An example of a close-ended question is: "Did that injury hurt?"

- O—Objective: Includes information that healthcare professionals can observe or measure, such as the review of systems and any test results. Examples include the patient's vital signs, height and weight, findings from the physical examinations, and results of any laboratory or diagnostic test.
- A—Assessment: Summation of the healthcare provider's impressions is recorded that includes the differential diagnosis, or the list of possible diagnoses based on the presenting signs and symptoms.

BOX 9.1 SOAP Notes Format and Examples

- **S**: Subjective—Headache, stomach pain, feeling exhausted, can't sleep
- **O**: Objective—Weight, temperature, physical exam findings, laboratory results, X-rays, and other imaging studies
- **A**: Assessment—Patient continues to have uncontrolled blood glucose levels despite being referred to a dietician and starting new medication.
- **P**: Plan—Patient plans to see a therapist next week; referred to a cardiologist; prescribed metformin

- P—Plan: Outlines the next step, which may include additional diagnostic tests, treatments or procedures, referrals, and follow-up plans for the patient. This section should also include any patient education provided or any other relevant interactions with the patient or family member.

"CHEDDAR" Format

Another common type of medical record documenting format used is CHEDDAR. The CHEDDAR format expands on the SOAP format by providing a more detailed report. This format is used to document the following:

- **C:** Chief complaint (CC)—Examination findings and any test results reviewed, including chief complaint, presenting problems, and any statements from the patient.
- **H:** History—History of present illness (HPI) and past illness, including hospitalization, surgeries, and physical history.
- **E:** Examination—All findings during the physical examination, including the review of systems, vital signs, and any tests results.
- **D:** Details—Patient complaints or detailed information about specific concerns regarding the current visit.
- **D:** Drugs and dosages—All medications that the patient is currently taking, including herbal supplements and vitamins, and any allergies to medications.
- **A:** Assessment—Detailed documentation regarding the assessment of the patient, including diagnostic process, differential diagnosis, and any future treatment plans.
- **R:** Return to office—A schedule of future appointments or referral to a specialist.

Regardless of the format used, the healthcare professional's documentation must be accurate and completed in an organized, thorough manner to prevent the omission of any pertinent information.

Corrections and Amendments to the Medical Record

Occasionally, errors are made during the documentation in a medical record by the healthcare professional or pertinent information was mistakenly omitted. In these cases, there are acceptable and legal ways to correct a written document, a dictated document, or typed information submitted into the patient's electronic chart. Under no circumstance should the original entry be erased, removed, or deleted from the patient's medical record. It is ultimately the responsibility of healthcare providers to review carefully all their patients' documentation on the medical record for completeness and accuracy of medical records, including the information submitted by members of their staff.

State laws vary on how medical records can be amended. If corrections need to be documented, the only permissible corrections are outlined in the sections that follow.

Correcting Written Medical Records

- Draw a single line through the error.
- Write the corrected entry above the mistake.
- A written addendum may be added for additional information.
- Initial or sign and date the correction or addendum.
- All written corrections or addenda must be reviewed, initialed or signed, and dated by the supervising healthcare provider.

Correcting Electronic Medical Records

- Correcting errors in EMRs should follow the same principles as correcting paper medical records.
- When correcting or making a change to an entry, the original entry should be viewable, the current date and time should be entered, the person making the change should be identified, and the reason for making the change should be noted.
- The amended EMR record should be flagged to indicate that it has been corrected from the original entry. A process or mechanism should be put in place to retain and easily access copies of the original.
- A narrative entry or comment should be added to the medical record statement indicating that an error has been made and is being corrected.
- The EMR system should allow for error corrections, and every medical office or healthcare organization should establish a process for making correction.

Correcting Dictated or Typed Medical Record

- For paper medical records, an addendum may be added to correct or add information by the medical transcriptionist who typed it. The changes must be approved by the healthcare provider, who must initial or sign and date the correction.
- For electronic medical records, an addendum may be added electronically, or the information corrected into the electronic documentation and then approved, initialed, or signed, and dated by the healthcare provider.

OWNERSHIP OF MEDICAL RECORDS

Determining who owns a patient's medical record seems like an easy answer with patients owning their medical records. In fact, ownership is more complicated. Patient data ownership can generally be broken into the ownership of the data vs. the medical records and the ability of patients to access their data.

As discussed earlier, medical records are legal documents generated by the healthcare provider or facility. Because it is a legal document and even though the information in the medical records pertains to the patient, the patient's original medical records must remain with the healthcare facility and the healthcare provider is the owner of the medical records.

However, based on HIPAA, the information that is in the medical record belongs to the patient. Thus, with few exceptions, patients have the right to inspect, review, and receive a copy of their medical records and billing records that are held by health plans and healthcare providers. In addition, only the patient and any of their authorized representatives, such as a family member with the patient's consent, have the right to access the patient's medical record.

DISCUSSION

According to HIPAA, patients have access to their medical records, with few exceptions. One of these exceptions is a healthcare provider's psychotherapy notes, which are notes taken by mental health professionals during a conversation or an appointment with a patient. They are kept separate from the patient's medical and billing records.

1. Why do you think this exception exists for psychotherapy notes?
2. What liability could occur if patients would be able to access these notes? What liability could occur if they were not able to?
3. Are there other medical records that should not be accessed by patients?

Release of Information

Patients may also request release of medical records or to receive copies of their medical records from the healthcare provider with a signed release form. This signed release form ensures that the confidentiality of the medical record is protected and can be shared only with an approved and authorized healthcare provider or entity. For example, if a patient transfers to another healthcare provider, the new healthcare provider may obtain the medical records only after the patient signs a release form.

Once authorized by the patient, the medical records are then copied and sent to the new healthcare provider. Most healthcare providers or facilities do not charge for this service but offer it as a courtesy to the patient; others will charge a nominal fee, such as 25 cents per page for the copies.

When medical records are sent electronically, the healthcare provider or facility must check with the state and federal laws pertaining to patient confidentiality and the transmission of medical records. For example, some healthcare providers or facilities will not send medical records through the public Internet but will use a virtual private network (VPN) or will encrypt the files for better safeguarding. In most cases, HIPAA requires the copies to be sent within 30 days of the request. Releasing the patient's medical information without authorization is a violation of HIPAA laws that can result in fines and penalties ranging from up to \$100 to \$50,000 per incident.

There are a few exceptions that would allow for the release of medical records without the patient's authorization or a signed release form from the patient. These exceptions include:

- Criminal acts: Evidence used in abuse cases, stabbings, gunshot wounds, or sexual assaults.
- Legally ordered: Court orders or subpoena of records, regardless of criminal cases.
- Communicable diseases: The Centers for Disease Control and Prevention or local health departments can require release of information in case of the possibility of diseases that potentially could cause a pandemic or sexually transmitted diseases, such as human immunodeficiency virus (HIV), syphilis, bubonic plague, severe acute respiratory syndrome (SARS), whooping cough, or tuberculosis.
- Mandated examinations: Ordered by employers' insurance companies for workers' compensation cases.

RETENTION OF MEDICAL RECORDS

Although the data in the medical record are owned by the patient, the storage and maintenance of these data is the responsibility of the healthcare provider and facility that collected the data. As the laws and guidelines for the storage and maintenance of medical records vary among each state, healthcare professionals and facilities must be aware of the various statutes of limitations that apply to their respective state. The statutes of limitations outline the minimum number of years patients' medical records must be retained. State medical record laws can be found in Appendix C. However, there are specific government health plans that require a healthcare professional to maintain medical records for a specific period of time (Box 9.2).

In general, most states require that healthcare facilities retain medical records for a minimum of 10 years, with some states requiring imaging studies to be kept even longer. In several states, electronic and paper medical record charts must be kept as **active patient files** for a certain amount of time after the last visit by the patient. **Active patient files** are medical records consulted or used on a routine basis. **Inactive patient files** are medical records rarely used but must be retained for reference or to meet the full retention requirement. Inactive patient files usually involve a patient who has not sought treatment for a period of time or one who completed his or her course of treatment, usually longer than 3 years.

Fortunately, with most healthcare facilities already transitioned to an EHR system, the storage and retention of EMRs is much easier compared with maintaining paper medical records. If a healthcare facility is transitioning from paper medical records to electronic, the medical records need to be scanned as electronic files, and the original paper documents must be shredded.

BOX 9.2 Examples of State Government Laws That Specify a Retention Period for Medical Records

- Welfare and Institutions Code Section 14124.1 relates to Medi-Cal patients.
- Health and Safety Code Section 1797.98(e) relates to services reimbursed by the Emergency Medical Services Fund.
- Health and Safety Code Section 11191 relates to situations in which a physician prescribes, dispenses, or administers a Schedule II controlled substance.
- The Knox–Keene Act requires that HMO medical records be maintained a minimum of 2 years to ensure that compliance with the act can be validated by the Department of Corporations.
- In Workers' Compensation Cases, qualified medical evaluators must maintain medical-legal reports for 5 years.
- Health and Safety Code Section 123145 indicates that providers who are licensed under Section 1205 as a medical clinic shall preserve the records for 7 years.

HEALTH INSURANCE PORTABILITY AND ACCOUNTABILITY ACT OF 1996

In 1996, the Health Insurance Portability and Accountability Act of 1996 (HIPAA) was passed with the objective to make it easier for patients to keep their health insurance by providing portability and continuity, protecting the confidentiality and security of healthcare information, and helping the healthcare industry control administrative costs. In addition, HIPAA was designed to:

- protect the privacy of sensitive patient information,
- combat fraud in the healthcare industry,
- simplify administration of health insurance, and
- promote the use of medical savings plans for employees.

HIPAA consists of five titles:

- Title I: Health Care Access, Portability, and Renewability
- Title II: Preventing Health Care Fraud and Abuse; Administrative Simplification; Medical Liability Reform
- Title III: Tax-related health provisions governing medical savings accounts
- Title IV: Application and enforcement of group health insurance requirements
- Title V: Revenue offset governing tax deductions for employers

For healthcare professionals and organizations, Title II of HIPAA is the most relevant because it focuses on privacy and security of health information.

Title II: HIPAA Administrative Simplification

The purpose of Title II: Administrative Simplification is to improve the efficiency and effectiveness of the healthcare delivery system; to improve the Medicaid and Medicare programs; to address fraud and abuse; and to simplify the administrative processes involved with healthcare delivery. In addition, it is crucial to have specific laws and guidelines to help safeguard the patient's medical information with the adoption of electronic medical records. Title II of HIPAA also establishes national standards for processing electronic healthcare transactions and requires healthcare facilities to implement secure electronic access to health data and to remain in compliance with privacy regulations. Under Title II, the most important provisions are the Privacy Rule and Security Rule.

Privacy Rule

The *Standards for Privacy of Individually Identifiable Health Information,* commonly known as the HIPAA Privacy Rule, establishes the first national standards in the United States to protect patients' **protected health information (PHI)**. PHI is defined as "individually identifiable health information" and generally refers to medical history, test and laboratory results, insurance information, demographics, and other data that a healthcare professional collects to identify an individual and determine appropriate care. Examples of PHI include the following:

- Patient's name
- Dates, such as birth, admission, discharge, and death
- Social Security number
- Address, including street address, city, county, and zip code
- Telephone number
- Fax number
- Email address
- Web universal resource locator (URL)
- Internet protocol (IP) address number
- Medical record numbers
- Health plan beneficiary number
- Certification/license numbers
- Biometric identifiers, such as finger and voice prints
- Photographic images

An important provision of the HIPAA Privacy Rule is to limit the use and disclosure of sensitive PHI. It also sought to protect the privacy of patients by requiring healthcare providers to provide patients with an account of each entity to which the provider discloses PHI for billing and administrative purposes, while still allowing relevant health information to flow through the proper channels. Based on the HIPAA Privacy Rule, patients are provided the following:

- The right to obtain a notice of privacy practices that explains how a provider or health plan uses and discloses their health information, outlined in a Notice of Privacy Practices (NPP). The NPP must describe how the HIPAA Privacy Rule allows the CE to use and share PHI. If the CE uses PHI for any other reason, it must obtain the patient's authorization.
- The right to ask for and obtain a copy of their medical records, including electronic records. A patient may authorize a third party, such as a family member or attorney, to receive his or her medical records. In specific situations, a patient may be denied access to these records based on circumstances.
- The right to ask for an amendment to his or her medical records if the patient believes his or her information is incorrect.
- The right to appeal for special privacy protection for PHI.
- The right to an accounting of disclosures. HIPAA allows a patient to learn to whom the CE has disclosed his or her PHI, the reason for the disclosure, a brief description of the PHI that was provided, and the date the disclosure was made.
- The right to access a minor child's medical records, as long as the parent who is acting as the child's "personal representative" and release of the minor child's PHI are consistent with state and other law.

These HIPAA standards specifically target PHI that are electronically submitted from healthcare providers to **clearinghouses** and then to the individual carriers. Both carriers and healthcare providers are mandated to update language and software to be compliant with the universal format. In fact, HIPAA requires that all **covered entities** or business associates in the healthcare field convert all electronic transmission to this universal format, and the transmission of any electronic files or patient information be sent under the secure code in order to de-identify the patient's information.

Security Rule

The second provision of the Title II: Administrative Simplification is the Security Standards for the Protection of Electronic Protected Health Information, commonly known as the HIPAA Security Rule, which required all CEs submitting electronic information to be in compliance with the electronic code set and the security guidelines for physical and electronic devices by April 14, 2003. The HIPAA Security Rule affects covered entities, including health plans, healthcare clearinghouses, and any healthcare provider who transmits health information in electronic form in connection with a transaction. As a result, covered entities are required to take reasonable and suitable steps in protecting PHI by:

- ensuring the confidentiality, integrity, and availability of all e-PHI they create, receive, maintain, or transmit;
- identifying and shielding against realistic anticipated threats to the safety or integrity of the information;
- protecting against reasonably predictable, unallowable uses or disclosures; and
- guaranteeing compliance by their workforce.

To ensure security of PHI and to prevent breaches of confidentiality, HIPAA has recommended implementing the following: administrative safeguards, physical safeguards, and technical safeguards (Fig. 9.3).

Administrative safeguards. Administrative safeguards refer to the policies and procedures documented in writing that show how covered entities will comply with HIPAA. The administrative safeguards should include the covered entities' method for clearing or authorizing someone for access to PHI during the hiring process, modification of access during employment, and discontinuation of access on termination. If the CE employs a third party for any service, it must determine what, if any, PHI is necessary for the services rendered, and that the third party also has a plan in place to comply with HIPAA.

Most medical staff members who have access to the electronic files have a password to enter the files in the computer system. In most cases, computer software programs have the capability to document any person who accesses the patient files. According to HIPAA regulations, there needs to be a significant reason, or "need to know," for a staff member to access specific patient medical records. This would include, but not be exclusive to, any medical information, test results, patient treatment plans, financial information, and appointment scheduling.

Fig. 9.3 HIPAA requires implementing administrative, physical, and technical safeguards to protect patient medical records. (Copyright © cyano66/iStock/Thinkstock.com.)

Administrative safeguards should also include a plan for continuing training and education of employees. As with any compliance-related area, training is necessary and creates a culture of compliance when it has demonstrated priority within a company. Training can be driven by internal audits that monitor HIPAA compliance in the business, which may uncover areas of weaknesses and compliance risk and where further training is needed. In addition, many healthcare facilities may appoint a staff member as a security officer, who is responsible for training, performing internal audits, and monitoring the facility's security.

Physical safeguards. Physical safeguards are the second area covered by the HIPAA Security Rule and refer to the physical monitoring and access to PHI. This guideline demands that hardware and software used by CEs be installed and removed properly to protect PHI. This rule also refers to physical information storage, such as files and records, and the control mechanisms in place to protect that data. Many healthcare facilities use a "**double lock system**," which requires passing through two systems of security to access any PHI. For example, the "double lock system" may be a locked room and a locked filing cabinet. This not only includes the storage of information, but also the destruction of information once it is no longer needed. Important factors to consider when physically safeguarding PHI in the healthcare facility include the following:

- Keeping workstations with PHI out of high-traffic areas
- Having appropriate documentation of visitor sign-ins
- Restricting access to client data from third parties using facility equipment
- Properly removing all client data from hardware or software before disposing of it
- Record storage and maintenance
- Employee access granted to areas where PHI is located
- Controlling and securing areas with PHI from third parties, such as janitorial services

- Verifying appropriate training of third-party vendors
- Preventing the visibility of computer screens to unauthorized users

Paper charts that contain patients' medical records or financial information, including insurance information, must be kept in a fireproof filing cabinet that must be closed and locked at the end of the day or when the front office staff is not present.

Technical safeguards. Technical safeguards are the final area and one of the most important provisions of the HIPAA Security Rule and refer to the responsibility of the healthcare provider to monitor and safeguard PHI through all technology-related items and uses. With the advent and increased adoption of EHRs, every healthcare provider and CE should have a documented system for technical safeguards and a plan for internal monitoring to make sure that it is operational, effective, and sufficient in protecting patient data.

Technology includes all facets of the business using technical means of data storage of communication, including emails, faxes, phones, and computer systems. Not only should data be secured at the point of use in the healthcare facility, but must also be secured and verified that they are received by the intended recipient. A common way to do this is to use a data encryption system that would secure the patient information and only the intended recipient with the appropriate corresponding system for decoding the information can access the data. For example, if a patient's medical chart is sent to a medical office via email, the email can be opened or decrypted only by providing a code, which was sent in a separate email to the healthcare provider.

In addition, the healthcare organization should maintain a current antivirus protection software to safeguard confidential information. Most healthcare organizations also install firewalls if their computer systems are connected to the Internet. Firewalls are computer network security devices that monitor incoming and outgoing network traffic and decide whether to allow or block specific traffic based on a defined set of security rules. Computer software for the healthcare organization must also have a system and process in place to back up patient records. To protect the electronic files, patient files must be backed up each day, and, in some cases, files are backed up in two different locations: the healthcare organization and an offsite medical records storage facility. All these sites must follow the same HIPAA standards and guidelines.

HIPAA Violation Penalties

Violators of the HIPAA may face both criminal and civil penalties if a patient's privacy rights are compromised. There are four categories of HIPAA violations:

- **Category 1:** A violation that the CE was unaware of and could not have realistically avoided had a reasonable amount of care been taken to abide by HIPAA rules
- **Category 2:** A violation that the CE should have been aware of but could not have avoided even with a reasonable amount of care
- **Category 3:** A violation suffered as a direct result of "willful neglect" of HIPAA Rules, in cases in which an attempt has been made to correct the violation
- **Category 4:** A violation of HIPAA rules constituting willful neglect, where no attempt has been made to correct the violation

Under the U.S. Department of Health and Human Services (HHS), the Office for Civil Rights (OCR) and state attorneys general have the authority to administer financial penalties in cases of HIPAA violations. Before imposing a financial penalty for the violation, however, the OCR takes into consideration the nature of the PHI exposed, the length of time a violation was allowed to continue, and the number of people affected. These factors could increase or decrease the financial penalty issued based on the violation. Each category of violation carries a separate HIPAA penalty:

- **Category 1:** Minimum fine of $100 per violation up to $50,000
- **Category 2:** Minimum fine of $1000 per violation up to $50,000
- **Category 3:** Minimum fine of $10,000 per violation up to $50,000
- **Category 4:** Minimum fine of $50,000 per violation

Financial penalties are issued per violation category, per year that the violation was allowed to persist. The maximum penalty per violation category is $1,500,000 per year. In addition, criminal penalties for HIPAA violations are classified into three tiers:

- Tier 1: Reasonable cause or no knowledge of violation—up to 1 year in jail
- Tier 2: Obtaining PHI under false pretenses—up to 5 years in jail
- Tier 3: Obtaining PHI for personal gain or with malicious intent—up to 10 years in jail

APPLY THIS

A famous singer is brought to the emergency department where you are currently working as a patient care technician. The singer was brought in by an ambulance after being in a car accident and being under the suspicion of driving while being intoxicated. Photographers and news crews start arriving and medical staff throughout the hospital start coming to the emergency department hoping to catch a glimpse of the singer. You notice one of the hospital staff take a picture with his phone of the unconscious singer.

1. Which laws or standards did the hospital staff member violate?
2. What penalty could he face for his action?
3. Since you witnessed this, what should you do?

CONCLUSION

Technology has rapidly changed the way we document, store, and transmit patient information. With most healthcare providers having transitioned to electronic medical records, it is imperative to always follow the ethical and legal methods and standards in practicing and delivering health care for all patients. Obtaining and accurately documenting all the information from the patient is of the utmost importance to ensure continuity of care, quality patient care, and compliance. Furthermore, HIPAA guidelines must be followed to ensure patients' confidentiality and the security of the medical records.

CHAPTER REVIEW QUESTIONS

1. Which organization established standards in privacy, security, and electronic healthcare transactions?
   A. Centers for Medicare and Medicaid Services
   B. Department of Health and Human Services
   C. Food and Drug Administration
   D. National Council for Prescription and Drug Programs
2. All the following are examples of protected health information (PHI) *except*
   A. biometric identifiers.
   B. patient's medical record number.
   C. patient's gender.
   D. patient's Social Security number.
3. Which of the following is a patient's right under HIPAA?
   A. The right to access and request a copy of his or her medical records
   B. The right to make changes in his or her medical records if the patient believes an item is incorrect
   C. The right to be provided an accounting of all disclosures
   D. All the above
4. If an individual believes his or her rights under HIPAA were violated, he or she would contact the
   A. Attorney General of the United States.
   B. Centers for Medicare and Medicaid Services.
   C. Office for Civil Rights.
   D. Office of the Inspector General.
5. All the following are types of safeguards as outlined by the HIPAA Security Rule *except*
   A. physical safeguards.
   B. security safeguards.
   C. technical safeguards.
   D. administrative safeguards.
6. Your new laptop comes with a software that monitors incoming and outgoing traffic and either allows it or blocks it is an example of a/n
   A. clearinghouse.
   B. Inactive patient files.
   C. administrative safeguard.
   D. firewall.
7. Using the SOAP format, a patient complaining about having a pain in his stomach would have it documented under
   A. S.
   B. O.
   C. A.
   D. P.
8. To correct a mistake made in an electronic medical record, you would do which of the following:
   A. Draw a single line through the error.
   B. Delete it and make a note as an addendum.
   C. The record should be flagged, and a narrative entry or comment should be added.
   D. The transcriptionist should be notified to make and approve the correction.

9. In which of the following situations would a patient have to authorize the release of her medical records?
   A. She is relocating and needs to find a new healthcare provider.
   B. She is being investigated for elder abuse.
   C. She has been exposed to tuberculosis and contact tracing must occur.
   D. She has filed for workers' compensation.

10. Which of the following is an example of a technical safeguard, according to HIPAA?
   A. Removing a medical administrative staff's log-in access after being terminated.
   B. Data encryption of a patient's medical record being sent to another medical office.
   C. Using computer privacy screens or filters to prevent nonauthorized users from seeing confidential medical information.
   D. Locating computer workstations in a secure and private area away from public access.

SELF-REFLECTION QUESTIONS

1. Why was the passage of the HIPAA guidelines necessary?
2. When you work within an organization that violates HIPAA compliance guidelines, how would you address your concerns?
3. When is it permissible to access the patient files of a former patient to whom you were previously assigned?
4. What would be some of the negative consequences if your personal information was sent to an unintended entity?

INTERNET ACTIVITIES

1. Determine the laws in your state that are specific to the HIPAA guidelines: https://www.hhs.gov/hipaa/newsroom/index.html.
2. Search the HIPAA News Releases & Bulletins for violations and select a case for discussion: https://www.hhs.gov/hipaa/newsroom/index.html.
3. How does your current or future healthcare profession comply with the HIPAA guidelines? https://www.hhs.gov/hipaa/for-professionals/special-topics/index.html

BIBLIOGRAPHY

Centers for Medicare and Medicaid Services, U.S. Department of Health and Human Services. *HIPAA basics for providers: Privacy, security, and breach notification rules.* Available from: https://www.cms.gov/Outreach-and-Education/Medicare-Learning-Network-MLN/MLNProducts/Downloads/HIPAAPrivacyandSecurity.pdf.

Centers for Medicare and Medicaid Services, U.S. Department of Health and Human Services. *Transactions overview.* Available from: https://www.cms.gov/Regulations-and-Guidance/Administrative-Simplification/Transactions/TransactionsOverview.html.

Centers for Medicare and Medicaid Services, U.S. Department of Health and Human Services. *Code sets overview.* Available from: https://www.cms.gov/Regulations-and-Guidance/Administrative-Simplification/Code-Sets/index.html.

Centers for Medicare and Medicaid Services, U.S. Department of Health and Human Services. *HPID.* Available from: https://www.cms.gov/Regulations-and-Guidance/Administrative-Simplification/Unique-Identifier/HPID.html.

Centers for Medicare and Medicaid Services, U.S. Department of Health and Human Services. *Electronic data interchange system access and privacy.* Available from: https://www.cms.gov/Medicare/Billing/ElectronicBillingEDITrans/SystemAccess.html.

Centers for Medicare and Medicaid Services, U.S. Department of Health and Human Services. *Regulations & guidance.* Available from: https://www.cms.gov/Regulations-and-Guidance/Regulations-and-Guidance.html.

HIPAA Journal. *What are the penalties for HIPAA violations?.* Available from: http://www.hipaajournal.com/what-are-the-penalties-for-hipaa-violations-7096/.

Privacy Rights Clearinghouse. *The HIPAA privacy rule: Patients' rights.* Available from: https://www.privacyrights.org/consumer-guides/hipaa-privacy-rule-patients-rights.

U.S. Department of Health and Human Services. *Summary of the HIPAA security rule.* Available from: https://www.hhs.gov/hipaa/for-professionals/security/laws-regulations/index.html.

10

Mandatory Reporting and Public Health

CHAPTER OBJECTIVES

1. Describe what is meant by mandatory reporting duties required of healthcare professionals.
2. Explain the reasons for documentation of vital statistics.
3. Explain the importance of birth and death certificates and describe when a physician, medical examiner, or coroner needs to sign one.
4. Identify the communicable and sexually transmitted diseases that must be reported.
5. Describe child, spousal, elder, and sexual abuse, and possible signs of abuse.
6. Explain addiction and regulations of controlled substances and the U.S. Drug Enforcement Administration (DEA) schedule of drugs.

KEY TERMS

Abuse A misuse or a maltreatment. In relationships, it is the systematic pattern of misuse or inappropriate treatment to gain control and power over another individual.

Addiction Habit or a compulsive behavior in which a person engages in a habit or action despite its negative consequences and effect.

Birth certificate An official record declaring a live birth of a baby.

Case investigation The process of identifying and investigating individuals with confirmed and probable diagnoses of a reportable communicable disease.

Certificate of live birth An unofficial record of a live birth that is signed by the healthcare provider in attendance at the birth and includes information on the baby, parents, and the events at the time of the birth.

Communicable disease Specific disease or illness that can cause an epidemic or pandemic to the general public.

Contact tracing The process to identify, monitor, and support individuals who may have been exposed to a person with a communicable disease, often follows case investigation.

Controlled Substances Act Federal drug policy regulating the manufacture, importation, possession, use, and distribution of certain substances.

Coroner An elected or appointed position, often not a physician, to perform autopsies and testing to determine cause of death and time of death in suspicious deaths or under circumstances when no person was in attendance of the death.

Domestic violence Any abusive act between family members, ex-spouses, intimate cohabitants, former intimate cohabitants, dating couples and former dating couples in which one party seeks to gain/maintain power and control over the other partner.

Employee Assistance Program (EAP) Program designed to help employees receive counseling for substance abuse or other issues of abuse, without fear of losing their jobs; may offer legal and financial counseling as well.

Intimate partner violence (IPV) A form of domestic violence or abuse resulting in physical, sexual, or psychological harm caused by a current or former partner or spouse; can occur among either heterosexual or same-sex couples.

Inquest Investigation into a suspicious death, including autopsy and other investigation, to determine time and cause of death.

Mandatory reporting The legal responsibility of healthcare professionals to report vital information and incidence to the appropriate agencies for the protection and welfare of the general public and specific vulnerable populations.

Nonintimate partner violence A form of domestic violence between individuals who are not intimate partners, but have a familial relationship, such as mother/adult son, or brother/sister.

Older Americans Act of 1987 (OAA) Legislation passed to protect adults older than the age of 60 from abuse, neglect, abandonment, and exploitation.

Medical examiner An elected or appointed position to perform autopsies and testing to determine cause of death and time of death, often a physician with training in forensic pathology.

Postmortem Examination that is performed on an individual after death.

Vital statistics Community-wide recording of individual key human events such as births, deaths, marriages, or divorces.

INTRODUCTION

State and federal guidelines and statutes require all facilities and businesses connected to the general public to maintain standards to ensure public safety. For example, a restaurant needs to be inspected regularly for cleanliness and compliance to food storage guidelines to ensure that the general public is safe from possible diseases and illnesses. In the area of medicine and healthcare professions, there are even more guidelines, laws, and statutes to follow. If these guidelines and standards are not met, a healthcare facility or clinic can be cited and/or closed for noncompliance.

Those in the healthcare field must be aware that they are held to the highest professional standards and that the lives and well-being of their patients and the general public must always be their utmost concern. For that reason, it is the duty of the healthcare professional to report and document incidents of concern for a patient's safety and for the safety of the public at large.

Healthcare professionals also have a duty to maintain strict and accurate documentation of events that affect and contribute to the vital statistics of the public, such as birth and death rates. This chapter will discuss some of the general guidelines and expectations of healthcare professionals' responsibility and duty to both their patients and the general public.

MANDATORY REPORTING DUTIES

In the healthcare field, mandatory reporting duties refer mainly to the responsibility of healthcare professionals to report vital information and incidence to the appropriate agencies for the protection and welfare of the general public, as well as specific vulnerable populations. Although these mandatory reporting guidelines may vary by state, prompt reporting of the following is mandatory:

- Births
- Deaths
- Communicable diseases
- Assaults or criminal acts
- Abuse—child, elder, and intimate partner
- Substance abuse

Vital Statistics and Public Health Records

Statistical tracking over the centuries has long included the recording of births, deaths, causes of deaths, and illnesses. In fact, monitoring the trends of diseases and illnesses that cause mortality (death) or morbidity (illnesses) has existed since the 17th century. It was this early tracking and monitoring of health records that was used to create the International Classification of Diseases (ICD), or the code set that is used by healthcare professionals to collect, process, and classify health information for statistical analysis and reimbursements.

The health data compiled by ICD are maintained by the Centers for Medicare and Medicaid Services (CMS) and the U.S. Department of Health and Human Services. Thus, accurate coding of the diagnoses is mandated for all healthcare facilities and providers by local and individual states' health departments, as well as the federally operated Centers for Disease Control and Prevention (CDC). Although many healthcare professionals may assist in the completion and documentation of these events, it is ultimately the legal responsibility of the physician or another authorized healthcare provider to sign the documentation to verify that the information is accurate and complete.

Births

A birth record is a permanent and legal record. Throughout an individual's life, a person will use this birth record or certificate to acquire a Social Security number, register for school, apply for a driver's license or passport, get a marriage license, and register to vote. For that reason, it is easy to see that the accurate reporting of a person's birth is very important to each individual because it can affect so many areas of a person's life. In addition, birth records are compiled annually to track and monitor the number and rate of births based on specific characteristics, such as place of birth, place of residence of the mother, age of mother, plurality, and birth weight. Local, state, and federal governments, as well as private industries, use this data to plan and evaluate programs in public health and other important areas, such as urban planning and resource allocation.

According to the World Health Organization, "live birth" refers to the complete expulsion or extraction from its mother of a product of conception, irrespective of the duration of the pregnancy, which, after such separation, breathes or shows any other evidence of life, such as beating of the heart, pulsation of the umbilical cord or definite movement of voluntary muscles, regardless of if the umbilical cord has been cut or the placenta is attached. Each product of such a birth is considered a live birth or born.

The reporting and documentation of births are the responsibility of the healthcare provider assisting with the birth. Generally, the information required to file for a birth certificate is the date, time, and place of the birth, as well as parental information. Once documented, a record of a live birth, called the *Certificate of Live Birth* (Fig. 10.1), is signed by the physician, healthcare provider, or any other person in attendance at the birth, including a midwife, who can certify that the infant was born alive at the place and time on the record. The **Certificate of Live Birth** includes the baby's name, parent's names, healthcare provider's name, hospital, sex, race, date of birth, and person completing the record. The certificate is filed with the registrar of the local county, usually within a year of the birth, and is considered an unofficial birth certificate. The certificate is then sent to the Office of Vital Statistics or state registrar and will be verified before a *birth certificate* is issued. Although the Certificate of Live Birth shows that the baby was born medically alive, the **birth certificate** is the official record declaring a live birth.

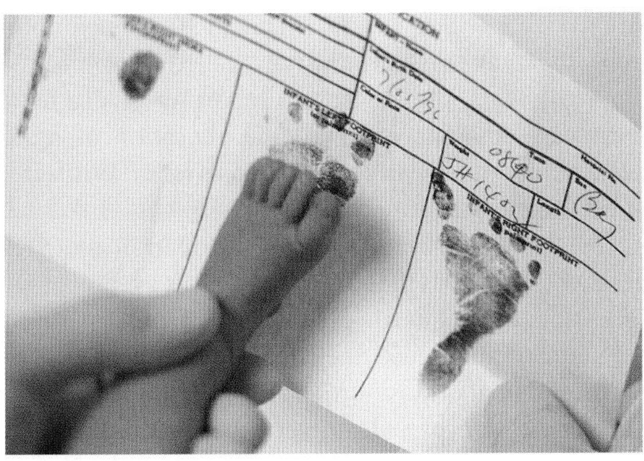

Fig. 10.1 The attending physician or midwife completes the initial birth certificate and then submits it to the local (usually county) agency for recording. From there the government's official certificate of birth is released. (Copyright © Comstock/Stockbyte/Thinkstock.com.)

As with all legal documentation, it is important that a birth certificate be accurate, legible, and complete when submitted to the local authorities. Some states and local authorities can impose severe penalties against individuals for incorrectly, improperly, or knowingly reporting false information on birth certificates.

Deaths

Just as important as it is to report live births, it is equally important to report deaths and the cause of death. As with a birth certificate, a death certificate is a legal record of an individual's death. A death certificate is needed for proof of death for many other reasons: banking purposes, insurance and pension benefits, transfer of real and personal property, and for Internal Revenue Service and Social Security notification. As it is a legal document, a death certificate may be introduced in court as evidence when a question about the death arises.

A death certificate also plays a very important role in medical and health research efforts. For example, during the 1980s, physicians were reporting causes of death for many patients with acquired immunodeficiency syndrome (AIDS) as pneumonia. However, the actual underlying causes of death were from opportunistic infections associated with the human immunodeficiency virus (HIV), which causes AIDS, such as pneumonia from *Pneumocystis carinii* (now called *Pneumocystis jirovecii*). Thus, the inaccurate reporting of deaths in these cases may have slowed the allocation of much needed funds and healthcare resources for HIV-infected individuals and treatment.

The death certificate provides information about the decedent, or deceased individual, such as age; sex; race; education; date of death; his or her parents; if married, the name of the spouse; the circumstances and cause of death; and final disposition, such as burial or cremation. The registration of a death certificate is submitted to the state government, and the reporting follows individual state laws and regulations. Death certificate data from each state are also reported to the CDC's National Center for Health Statistics, which allows the federal government to use information to produce national vital statistics.

Although most death certificates follow similar standards, there are some mandatory regulations that differ among individual states. For example, in the case of fetal death, state laws may differ about the gestational age at which fetal deaths must be reported. Some states require the reporting of all fetal deaths regardless of the length of gestation, whereas other states require reporting of deaths for fetuses weighing 350 g or more or after 20 weeks of gestation. Thus, if an infant was stillborn at 22 weeks of gestation and the state requirement was 20 weeks, both a birth certificate and a death certificate would need to be issued.

Depending on the situation and the state law, a primary physician, an attending physician, a nonattending physician, a medical examiner, a nurse practitioner, a forensic pathologist, or a coroner can sign a death certificate. A **coroner** is an elected or appointed position. Some coroners may be physicians, whereas others may be sheriffs or funeral home directors. **Medical examiners** are also appointed to their positions, although almost all of them are physicians with training in forensic pathology. A coroner or a medical examiner would complete the death certificate in the following cases: a criminal act, such as a homicide; a lack of attendance at death; a patient found dead at home; accidental deaths; suicides; the cause of death is unknown; and when a postmortem needs to be performed (Fig. 10.2).

A **postmortem**, also called an *autopsy*, is an examination that is performed on an individual after death to determine time and cause of death. Often, an autopsy will be requested if an individual dies under suspicious circumstances; however, in the absence of suspicious circumstances, an autopsy is not performed without the consent or request of the surviving next of kin.

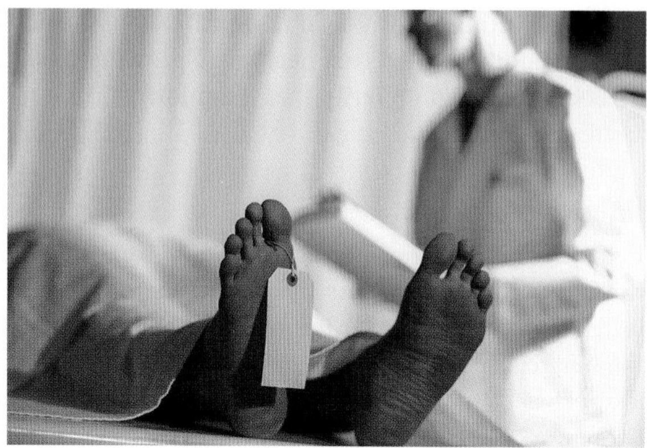

Fig. 10.2 A coroner or a medical examiner would complete the death certificate in cases, such as, a criminal act, a patient found dead at home, accidental deaths, suicides, or if the cause of death is unknown. (iStock.com/Fstop123.)

When an individual dies at home or while using in-home hospice services, a coroner is called to determine whether there were any factors that might warrant an **inquest**, even without suspicious circumstances. In some states, a coroner or medical examiner would not be contacted if the individual is older than 90 years of age and there is no evidence of foul play.

APPLY THIS

The cause of death is unknown for an individual found dead on his living room sofa. Neighbors have called the police, who find that the individual is an 80-year-old man and appears to have died of natural causes.

1. Who should be called to determine death and sign the death certificate?
2. Would an autopsy be performed?
3. Would the family be under investigation?

Communicable Diseases

If a disease that can be quickly transmitted to many individuals may endanger the general population and may create an epidemic, it is the responsibility of healthcare professionals to notify the proper authorities to prepare and, hopefully, prevent or limit the spread of that disease or illness. In fact, it is a legal and ethical mandate that these cases are reported to the local department of health, which may then be reported to the CDC. In addition, the information gained from reporting allows the local, state, and federal government to make informed decisions on laws and policies about specific activities, such as food handling, insect control, sexually transmitted infections and disease tracking, and immunization programs.

Although this may vary by state, in general, physicians; veterinarians; podiatrists; nurse practitioners; physician assistants; nurses; nurse midwives; infection control practitioners; medical examiners; coroners; dentists; and administrators of health facilities and clinics, dispensaries, correctional facilities, or any other institution that diagnoses or treats a communicable disease are required to report communicable diseases to their local health department. Most local and state health departments have specific forms for reporting and, at a minimum, require the submission of the patient's full name, date of birth, race, sex, marital status, address, telephone number, place of employment, stage of disease, medication and amount given, and the date of onset. The local or state health department will then notify the CDC and will conduct an investigation to determine who else might be in danger of possible exposure and to arrange for testing and treatment of those individuals.

Although not all contagious illnesses are reported as communicable diseases, there are more than 120 "nationally notifiable diseases," according to the CDC, or diseases required by law to be reported to government authorities, which include:

- Tuberculosis
- Rubeola
- Rubella
- Tetanus
- Diphtheria
- Cholera
- Rheumatic fever
- Poliomyelitis (polio)
- Acquired immunodeficiency syndrome (AIDS)
- Meningitis
- Certain strains of the influenza virus, such as swine flu
- Sexually transmitted diseases
- Zika virus

A complete list of nationally notifiable diseases may be found at https://wwwn.cdc.gov/nndss/conditions/notifiable/2017/.

Sexually transmitted infections. Some of the most commonly reported communicable diseases are sexually transmitted infections (STIs), sometimes referred to as *sexually transmitted diseases (STDs).* The term STIs is broader and more accurate than STDs because a patient may be diagnosed with an infection but has not presented with any symptoms, which would constitute a disease. This is an important point when contacting the sexual partners of an infected individual: the sexual partner may not have presented with any symptoms and is unaware he or she is infected with an STI.

STIs are reportable to the local health department. Most states require all cases of communicable diseases, including STIs, to be reported within a specific timeframe as mandated by the local health department, usually not to exceed 2 weeks. Once confirmed, the local health department will try to locate sexual contacts of infected people to make sure they get tested and then treated if they are infected. In addition, if a healthcare provider notifies a patient that he or she has an STI, the provider must also counsel the patient regarding the risks of transmission.

APPLY THIS

An HIV-positive patient has an appointment at your office. Several of the medical staff are hesitant to assist the physician during this patient's examinations.

1. Does a nurse or medical assistant have the right to refuse to assist the physician with the patient?
2. What precautions should be taken in preparation for the patient?

Case Investigation and Contact Tracing

Once a communicable disease has been diagnosed in a patient, the process of case investigation and contact tracing begins. They are an essential disease control measure employed by local and state health department personnel to prevent further spread of diseases.

Case investigation is part of the process of supporting patients with suspected or confirmed infection. In case investigation, public health staff work with patients to help them recall everyone with whom they have had close contact during the timeframe while they may have been infectious. For example, a patient who is diagnosed with a sexually transmitted infection is asked about his sexual partners.

Contact tracing follows case investigation and is the process to identify, monitor, and support individuals who may have been exposed to a person with a communicable disease. Public health staff may then warn those exposed individuals (or contacts) of their potential exposure as rapidly and confidentially as possible. To protect patient privacy, contacts are only informed that they may have been exposed to a patient with the infection. They are not told the identity of the patient who may have exposed them. Contacts are provided with education, information, and support to understand their risk, what they should do to protect themselves and others, and what other tests and treatments may be necessary. Health departments are responsible for leading case investigations, contact tracing, and outbreak investigations.

In most situations, a patient's medical information cannot be released without the patient's authorization, based on the Health Insurance Portability and Accountability Act (HIPAA) Privacy Rule. However, HIPAA recognizes the legitimate need for public health authorities and others responsible for ensuring public health and safety to have access to protected patient information to carry out their public health mission and to protect the health and safety of the public at large. As a result, HIPAA permits covered entities and their authorized business associates to disclose protected health information without the patient's authorization for specified public health purposes, such as preventing or controlling diseases, injuries, or disabilities.

ABUSE

Abuse is defined as a misuse or maltreatment. In relationships, abuse may be emotional, physical, psychological, economic, and/or sexual trauma inflicted on another individual to satisfy a desire to control and have power over that individual. An abusive person uses physical force, mental degradation, intimidation, and other manipulative means to gain power over another individual. Abuse may take many forms but includes the following types and actions:

- *Physical*—pushing, hitting, shoving, punching, biting, choking, and physically trapping or impeding movement
- *Verbal/emotional*—criticizing, degrading, swearing, blaming, attacks that harm self-esteem
- *Psychological*—isolating you from your family and friends, controlling actions and decisions, stalking, invading privacy or space
- *Sexual*—forcing or demanding sex, forcing you to have unwanted sex with another person, forcing engagement into prostitution or pornography, refusing to use safe sex practices
- *Economic*—forbidding you from working, controlling access to money, exploiting your citizenship or lack of citizenship to work or to prevent you from working

Statutes in each state provide more specific details describing the behaviors that are considered grounds

DISCUSSION

Case Study: Kimberly Ann Bergalis

Kimberly Ann Bergalis was one of six patients infected with HIV after undergoing a dental procedure from David J. Acer, a Florida dentist who was HIV positive, in December 1987. Bergalis was diagnosed with HIV in January 1990 and died of AIDS at the age of 23 in December 1991. It was one of the first known cases of clinical transmission of HIV. Dr. Acer had been diagnosed with HIV several years earlier and continued to practice dentistry without disclosing his status to his patients, which was not required by law.

As a result of this case, the CDC proposed barring HIV-infected healthcare professionals from procedures in which the virus might be transmitted. However, opponents of the proposed regulations argued that this case was an anomaly and that testing all healthcare professionals would be inefficient and ineffective and would unfairly discriminate against them. Thus, the legislations did not pass.

1. Should it be mandated that HIV-positive healthcare professionals inform their patients of their status?
2. What can be done to prevent exposure of HIV and other infectious diseases in a healthcare setting?
3. What should the consequences be if an HIV-positive healthcare professional infected his or her patients today?

From Lambert, B. (1991). Kimberly Bergalis is dead at 23; symbol of debate over AIDS tests. *The New York Times*. Available from: htttps://www.nytimes.com/1991/12/09/obituaries/kimberly-bergalis-is-dead-at-23-symbol-of-debate-over-aids-tests.html; Ciesielski, C. A., Marianos, D. W., Schochetman, G., et al. (1994) Division of HIV/AIDS, Centers for Disease Control and Prevention. *Annals of Internal Medicine, 121*(11), 886–888; The 1990 Florida dental investigation: the press and the science. Available from: https://www.ncbi.nlm.nih.gov/pubmed/7978703.

for abuse or neglect, and the penalties and proof needed to sustain the cases. In addition, every state has mandatory reporting laws for abuse, specifically child abuse and elder abuse, and many states have requirements for reporting domestic violence.

Child Abuse

Child abuse is a leading cause of death among children younger than 5 years of age. In a report published by the Children's Bureau of the U.S. Department of Health and Human Services, more than 7.8 million referrals of alleged mistreatment involving children were reported. Every state has statutes that require specific professionals and persons to report suspected child abuse and neglect to appropriate agencies. In fact, 48 states and the District of Columbia require that specific professions are designated as mandatory reporters of child abuse. The other two states—New Jersey and Wyoming—require that all persons report incidences of child abuse, regardless of their profession. In fact, most cases of child abuse are reported by professionals. Although these mandatory reporters may vary by state, they often include the following:

- Social workers
- Teachers, principals, and other school personnel
- Physicians, nurses, and other healthcare professionals
- Counselors, therapists, and other mental health professionals
- Childcare providers
- Medical examiners or coroners
- Law enforcement officers

Other states may require commercial film and photographic processors, animal control officers, and public and private college administrators to report child abuse. In addition, many healthcare facilities and clinics have internal policies and procedures for handling reports of abuse, and these usually require the person who suspects abuse to notify the supervisor of the facility that abuse has been discovered or is suspected, which then needs to be reported to child protective services or other appropriate authorities.

Anyone in the healthcare profession is required to report incidents or suspicion of abuse to the appropriate authorities (Fig. 10.3). Although the circumstances under which a mandatory reporter must make a report vary based on the state, a report generally must be made when the healthcare professional suspects or has reason to believe that a child has been abused or neglected. Other states may require the standard that the healthcare professional has knowledge of or has observed a child being subjected to abuse. When reporting an incident, the healthcare professional does not have to provide proof that abuse or neglect has occurred. There are a number of signs of child abuse, such as the following:

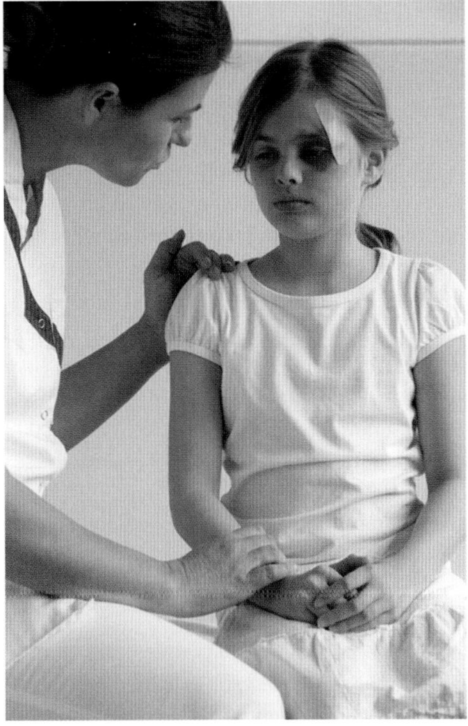

Fig. 10.3 Everyone in the healthcare profession is required to report incidents, or suspicion, of child abuse to the appropriate authorities. In addition, as with other cases, the child should be asked—while alone—whether he or she feels safe. (Copyright © Creatas Images/Creatas/Thinkstock.com.)

- Previously filed reports of physical or sexual abuse of the child
- Documented abuse of other family members
- Different stories between parents and child on how an accident happened
- Stories of incidents and injuries that are suspicious
- Injuries blamed on other family members
- Repeated visits to the emergency department for injuries
- Discolorations/bruising on the buttocks, back, and abdomen
- Elbow, wrist, and shoulder dislocations
- Delays in the normal growth and development patterns
- Erratic school attendance
- Poor hygiene

- Malnutrition
- Obvious dental neglect
- Neglected well-baby procedures (e.g., immunizations)

In most states, a confidential report can be filed and even anonymously in some states so that there is no fear of liability or reprisal from filing a report. In fact, nearly every state imposes penalties, such as a fine or imprisonment, on mandatory reporters who fail to report suspected child abuse or neglect as required by law. For example, there have been several lawsuits against physicians alleging medical malpractice when they failed to report cases in which child abuse was suspected (see *Landeros v. Flood*, 551 P.22d [Calif. 1976]; *Becker v. Mayo Foundation*, 737 NW2d 200 [Minn. 2007]). In the case of a child with signs of injury and abuse being brought to the emergency department, the healthcare professional may be required to immediately contact the appropriate authorities.

Elder Abuse

It is projected that 1 out of 10 people older than the age of 60 years has experienced some form of abuse, neglect, and exploitation, although this is likely an underestimate because of underreporting. The most common types of abuse among persons older than the age of 60 are physical abuse, sexual abuse, emotional abuse, neglect, abandonment, and financial abuse. Elder abuse can also include inappropriate use of medications or physical restraints; force-feeding; failure to provide food, clothing, shelter, or other essentials, such as medical care or medications; and forging an older person's signature in order to steal money or possessions. Neglect, abandonment, and desertion can also include failing to pay nursing home or assisted-living facility costs if there is a legal responsibility to do so.

As a result, legislation has been passed to protect adults older than age 60 from abuse, neglect, abandonment, and exploitation, called the **Older Americans Act of 1987 (OAA)**. In addition to providing training, research, and community services, the OAA provides public education services and protection against elder abuse, neglect, and exploitation. In many states, elder abuse may be a criminal offense.

As in child abuse, 48 states, the District of Columbia, and several territories require mandatory reporting of elder abuse, especially reporting by healthcare professionals. A failure to report elder abuse may result in fines, imprisonment, and civil lawsuits for medical malpractice, depending on the state. In some states, reporting of the elder abuse must be made to the appropriate authorities within 5 calendar days.

APPLY THIS

A patient is brought into the emergency department by her son. She is suffering from Alzheimer's dementia and is disoriented by her surroundings and family member. Her son gives a history that indicates his mother fell down the stairs. On examination, a number of bruises are observed on the patient's body in various stages of healing, and the patient exhibits general apprehension and apparent fear when many of the male staff speak to her or try to touch her.

1. What should be done to establish if this is a case of elder abuse?
2. Because the patient cannot provide her history, what evidence should be gathered in this case?

Domestic Violence and Abuse

Domestic violence is any abusive act between family members, ex-spouses, intimate cohabitants, former intimate cohabitants, dating couples and former dating couples in which one party seeks to gain/maintain power and control over the other partner. One form of domestic violence is **intimate partner violence (IPV)** and is a more inclusive term to include relationships between two people, with or without a marital or sexual relationship. IPV describes physical, sexual, or psychological harm by a current or former partner or spouse and can occur between heterosexual or same-sex couples and does not require sexual intimacy. Another form of domestic violence **nonintimate partner violence**, which is violence between individuals who are not intimate partners, but have a familial relationship, such as mother/adult son, or brother/sister.

There are many forms of abuse in domestic violence, although two or more types are commonly present in the same relationship. Emotional abuse often occurs with or before physical or sexual abuse in the relationship. Domestic violence tends to occur in cycles, often escalating in severity over time, with the abuse not stopping without intervention. Some signs of domestic violence include the following:

- Repeated injuries or bruises
- Unusual marks, scars, or rashes
- Bite marks

- Swelling or pain anywhere on the body, including the genital area
- Venereal disease and genital abrasions or injuries
- Unexplained fractures
- Repeated accidental injuries
- Black eyes or wearing dark glasses
- Makeup worn to hide bruising

According to the National Intimate Partner and Sexual Violence Survey conducted by the CDC, more than one in three women have experienced physical violence at the hands of an intimate partner, which included being slapped, pushed or shoved, beaten, burned, or choked. In addition, more than 27% of women and 11% of men in the United States have experienced IPV, including sexual violence, physical violence, and/or stalking by an intimate partner in their lifetime, and nearly 1 in 10 women (9.4%) have been raped by an intimate partner in her lifetime. However, these statistics are believed to be much higher because of underreporting.

As a result, many major medical associations and advocacy organizations have recommended universal screening for IPV by healthcare professionals in hopes of reducing its incidence and severity. In 1992, the Joint Commission on the Accreditation of Hospitals and Health Care Organizations mandated that emergency departments develop written protocols for identifying and treating survivors of domestic violence to receive hospital accreditation. Since then, the American Medical Association, American Congress of Obstetrician Gynecologists, and the American Nurses Association (ANA) have all recommended routine universal screening for domestic violence, regardless of the healthcare setting.

Although the prevalence of screening for intimate partner violence differs across healthcare specialties, only 3%–41% of healthcare providers reported routine screening for domestic violence. Furthermore, 10% of healthcare providers had never screened a patient for partner abuse. The reasons for the low percentage of universal screening for domestic violence by healthcare providers were time constraints; lack of knowledge, education, or training on the issue; and inadequate follow-up resources and support staff. In addition, healthcare providers reported feeling uncomfortable discussing domestic violence, as well as fearing for their personal safety and misdiagnosing patients.

Most states have enacted mandatory reporting laws, which require the reporting of specified injuries and wounds, and suspected abuse or domestic violence for individuals being treated by a healthcare professional. However, the laws vary from state to state, but generally fall into four categories:

- States that require reporting of injuries caused by weapons
- States that mandate reporting for injuries caused in violation of criminal laws, as a result of violence, or through nonaccidental means
- States that specifically address reporting in domestic violence cases
- States that have no general mandatory reporting laws

The U.S. Department of Health and Human Services provides a list of state statutes and policies on reporting domestic violence by state at https://www.acf.hhs.gov/sites/default/files/fysb/state_compendium.pdf.

When screening for domestic violence, it is important to ask questions when the patient is alone to determine whether the patient feels safe or fears for his or her safety. Often, the abusive partner may insist on speaking for the patient and may be resistant to leaving the patient alone. The healthcare professional should observe the demeanor of the patient, such as acting apprehensive or fearful or having an exaggerated concern for the partner.

SUBSTANCE ABUSE

Addiction is a compulsive behavior in which a person engages in a habit or action despite its negative consequences and effects. Healthcare professionals have an important role to play in screening patients for drug use, providing brief interventions, referring them to substance abuse treatment if necessary, and providing ongoing monitoring and follow-up. Specific groups need to be particularly screened for substance abuse, such as adolescents and pregnant women.

Although illicit drugs, such as cocaine and heroin, continue to be substances for abuse, a growing trend has been the abuse of prescription drugs. Results from the 2017 National Survey on Drug Use and Health report an estimated 18 million people (more than 6% of those aged 12 and older) have misused such medications at least once in the past year. This issue is a growing national problem in the United States. Prescription drugs are misused and abused more often than any other drug, except marijuana and alcohol. This growth is fueled by misperceptions about prescription drug safety and increasing availability. Furthermore, abuse of prescription drugs now ranks second, after marijuana, among illicit drug users. A patient who becomes dependent on a prescription drug may visit several different healthcare providers to obtain an oversupply of that drug. Many go to emergency departments to try to get prescriptions or injections of that same drug.

There are many reasons for this alarming trend of prescription drug abuse, including a significant increase in the prescribing of medications and the misperceptions of their safety when used nonmedically or by someone other than the prescription recipient. The number of prescriptions for many of these commonly abused prescription medications has increased dramatically since the early 1990s—more than eight times for stimulants and four times for opioids. In addition, there is the perception that abuse of prescription drugs is less harmful than that of illicit ones. This is not the case, however, because prescription drugs act similarly on the body system as illicit drugs do and may result in abuse, addiction, and a variety of other adverse health effects.

As with the other kinds of abuse discussed in this chapter, anyone can intervene to help people with addictions. Locally, there are many agencies and community service departments that can be contacted to aid individuals in obtaining treatment. In addition, many employers have **employee assistance programs (EAPs)** that will provide resources to help people overcome their addictions. As a healthcare provider, an important role is to counsel the patient and recommend professional counseling to assist the patient with his or her addiction.

Federal Drug Agencies

The U.S. Drug Enforcement Administration (DEA) and the U.S. Food and Drug Administration (FDA) oversee all providers who are licensed to prescribe drugs and regulate the use of drugs to patients, respectively. Depending on the type of drug and its potential for addiction, a healthcare provider is restricted in what kind, how much, and how often prescriptions can be written and filled. In addition, any healthcare provider licensed and authorized to prescribe medication must have a registered DEA number, which is used for authenticating and tracking prescriptions for controlled substances. The DEA enforces strict protocols for prescribing and distribution that include requiring certain prescriptions to be written using a triplicate copy prescription pad that is then submitted to the authorities to be monitored and tracked. Other categories of drugs require a written prescription and cannot be phoned or transmitted electronically to the pharmacy. In both categories, refills may not be allowed or are limited in number. For example, if a healthcare provider is writing excessive prescriptions for a certain medication, this will alert the DEA to the possibility of a problem with that provider's prescribing habits, which may result in a federal investigation.

In 1971, the U.S. Congress passed the **Controlled Substances Act**, which established federal drug policies under which the manufacture, importation, possession, use, and distribution of certain substances are regulated. As a result of the Act, prescribed medications and controlled substances are classified based on their medical use in treatment and potential for abuse. Table 10.1 shows the DEA's classification of controlled substances, which divides drugs into five classes or "schedules." Schedule I drugs have the highest potential for abuse or addiction, and Schedule V drugs have the lowest potential for abuse or addiction. Since its passage, the Act has been amended several times. Table 10.2 shows these updates.

DISCUSSION

More than half of adults in the United States, over 128 million people, have tried marijuana, despite it being an illegal drug under federal law. Nearly 600,000 Americans are arrested for marijuana possession annually, yet public support has grown in favor of legalizing marijuana from 12% in 1969 to 66% today. In 1996, California became the first state to legalize marijuana for medical purposes when voters passed Proposition 215. By the end of 2000, eight states had legalized medical marijuana. By 2017, 29 states and Washington, DC, had legalized it.

1. Despite its legalization in many states, marijuana is still a Schedule I substance. Why do you think the designation has not changed yet?
2. Do you think the federal government should legalize it? Why or why not?
3. What are some legal implications with marijuana's legalization in some states but not at the federal level?

TABLE 10.1 Drug Classifications According to the Controlled Substances Act of 1970

Drug Schedule	Characteristics	Prescription Regulations	Examples
Schedule I	High potential for abuse, severe physical or psychological dependence For research use only	No accepted use in United States Marijuana may be used for cancer and glaucoma research and may be obtained for patients in research situations	Narcotics: heroin Hallucinogens: peyote mescaline, PCP, hashish, amphetamine variants, LSD, cannabis (marijuana, THC) Designer drugs: ecstasy, crack, crystal meth
Schedule II	High potential for abuse, severe physical or psychological dependence Accepted medicinal use with specific restrictions	Dispensed by prescription only Oral emergency orders for Schedule II drugs may be given, but physician must supply written prescription within 72 h Refills require new written prescription from physician	Narcotics: opium, codeine, morphine, methadone, hydromorphone (Dilaudid), meperidine (Demerol), oxycodone (OxyContin), fentanyl (Duragesic), pentobarbital (Nembutal) Stimulants: amphetamines, amphetamine salts (Adderall), methylphenidate (Ritalin) Depressants: pentobarbital (Nembutal)
Schedule III	Moderate potential for abuse, high psychological dependence, low physical dependence Accepted medicinal uses	Dispensed by prescription only May be refilled five times in 6 months with prescription authorization by physician Prescription may be phoned to pharmacy	Narcotics: paregoric (opium derivative), certain codeine combinations (with acetaminophen) Depressants: pentobarbital (Nembutal) (rectal route) Stimulants: benzphetamine (Didrex)
Schedule IV	Lower potential for abuse than Schedule III drugs Limited psychological and physical dependence Accepted medicinal uses	Dispensed by prescription only May be refilled five times in 6 months with physician authorization Prescription may be phoned to pharmacy	Narcotics: pentazocine (Talwin) Depressants: chloral hydrate (Noctec), phenobarbital, diazepam (Valium), chlordiazepoxide (Librium), alprazolam (Xanax), clorazepate (Tranxene), benzodiazepines (lorazepam [Ativan], flurazepam [Dalmane]), midazolam (Versed), meprobamate (Equanil), temazepam (Restoril) Stimulants: phentermine (Adipex-P)
Schedule V	Low potential for abuse Abuse may lead to limited physical or psychological dependence Accepted medicinal uses	OTC narcotic drugs may be sold by registered pharmacist depending on state laws Buyer must be 18 years of age, show identification, and sign for medications	Preparations containing limited quantities of narcotics, generally cough and antidiarrheal preparations: cough syrups with codeine, diphenoxylate hydrochloride with atropine sulfate (Lomotil) and attapulgite (Parepectolin)

LSD, Lysergic acid diethylamide; *OTC*, over the counter; *PCP*, phencyclidine hydrochloride; *THC*, tetrahydrocannabinol.
From Drug Enforcement Administration (DEA), *Local DEA offices can provide current lists of medications on these schedules.* Washington, DC: U.S. Department of Justice.

TABLE 10.2 **Amendments to the Controlled Substances Act of 1970**

Amendment	Effect
Psychotropic Substances Act of 1978	Enabled federal government to add substances under schedules of controlled substances to the Convention of Controlled Substances (UN treaty designed to control illegal trade in psychoactive substances)
Controlled Substances Penalties Amendments Act of 1984	Strengthened penalties and removed ambiguity for both state and foreign drug felony convictions, particularly for recidivists; doubled penalties for distribution of controlled substances within 1000 ft. of school property
Chemical Diversion and Trafficking Act of 1988	Implemented new provisions required by *United Nations Convention Against Illicit Traffic in Narcotic Drugs and Psychotropic Substances of 1988;* regulated chemicals and drug manufacturing equipment (effectively diminished US criminal export of raw materials to cocaine manufacturers in South America)
Domestic Chemical Diversion and Control Act of 1993	Initiated registration of distributors of single-entity ephedrine products (a methamphetamine precursor); enabled DEA to revoke a company's registration without proof of criminal intent
Federal Analog Act	Enabled DEA to treat any substance intended for human consumption that is "substantially similar" to an illegal drug as if it was a Schedule I drug; designed to combat "designer drugs"

CONCLUSION

Healthcare professionals play a pivotal role in protecting public health and safety. All healthcare professionals must be aware of any mandatory reporting laws for their local, state, and the federal governments, as well as their profession, especially with regard to births and deaths, communicable diseases, and abuse. This should be not only a legal mandate but also an ethical standard to uphold.

CHAPTER REVIEW QUESTIONS

1. The acronym DEA means
   A. Drug and Ethics Administration.
   B. Drug Enforcement Administration.
   C. Drug Evaluation Agency.
   D. Drug Ethical Administration.
2. Which of the following would NOT be a possible sign of abuse?
   A. Black eyes
   B. Repeated fractures
   C. Chickenpox
   D. Unusual bruises
3. All the following health professionals may sign a death certificate except a
   A. nurse practitioner.
   B. physician.
   C. physician assistant.
   D. coroner.
4. Which of the following is not an example of a vital statistic that must be reported?
   A. Death certificates
   B. Divorce records
   C. Birth records
   D. Negative case in contract tracing
5. EAP means
   A. employer assistance program.
   B. employee assistance program.
   C. equal assistance program.
   D. employee aid program.
6. A characteristic that might be observed in an abused patient could be
   A. poor eye contact.
   B. guarding or guarded behavior.
   C. wearing sunglasses or makeup to hide bruises.
   D. All the above

7. A patient is found deceased in her home. Which of the following health professionals is likely to complete the death certificate?
   A. Nurse practitioner
   B. Physician
   C. Sheriff
   D. Coroner
8. According to the CDC, which of the following is not considered a communicable disease that must be reported?
   A. AIDS
   B. Cholera
   C. Diabetes
   D. Tetanus
9. A drug that has high potential for abuse and must be prescribed would be classified as a
   A. Schedule I.
   B. Schedule II.
   C. Schedule III.
   D. Schedule IV.
10. The process of identifying and monitoring people who may have been exposed to a person with a communicable disease is called
   A. case investigation.
   B. contact tracing.
   C. employee assistance program.
   D. mandatory reporting.

SELF-REFLECTION QUESTIONS

1. If you suspected a neighbor of child abuse or neglect, how would you respond?
2. As discussed, a low rate of healthcare professionals report screening patients about their risk of domestic violence. Why do you think that is?
3. What types of evidence would you report for a case of elder abuse?

INTERNET ACTIVITIES

1. Determine the laws in your state for reporting HIV/AIDS by accessing the CDC website: https://www.cdc.gov.
2. Read the article posted on the following website: https://www.ncbi.nlm.nih.gov/pmc/articles/PMC1403376/pdf/pubhealthrep00067-0011.pdf. It describes the investigation into the case of the dentist in Florida who was HIV positive. What recommendations for prevention would be most important, and what is the reality of the risk for patients now to be exposed from a healthcare provider who is HIV positive?
3. Research and investigate the role of case investigation and contact tracing in the COVID-19 epidemic. What type of questions were asked to identify contacts?
4. Research the CDC's Violence Prevention website: https://www.cdc.gov/violenceprevention/intimatepartnerviolence/fastfact.html. As a healthcare professional, what role can you have in identifying domestic violence in your patients?

ADDITIONAL RESOURCES

https://americanspcc.org/child-abuse-statistics/
http://emedicine.medscape.com/article/805727-treatment
https://www.aidshealth.org
https://www.cdc.gov/hiv/statistics/overview/geographicdistribution.html
https://www.apnews.com/bff06292e84e47d324af-9ca9314c0423

BIBLIOGRAPHY

Chu, S. Y., Buehler, J. W., Lieb, L., et al. *Causes of death among persons reported with AIDS*. Available from: https://www.ncbi.nlm.nih.gov/pmc/articles/PMC1694865/.

https://americanspcc.org/child-abuse-statistics/.

https://americanspcc.org/wp-content/uploads/2014/03/2015-Child-Maltreatment.pdf.

https://www.samhsa.gov/data/sites/default/files/NSDUH-FRR1-2014/NSDUH-FRR1-2014.pdf.

https://www.samhsa.gov/topics/prescription-drug-misuse-abuse.

National Center for Health Statistics. *State definitions and reporting requirements: for live births, fetal death, and induced terminations of pregnancy. 1997 version*. Available from: https://www.cdc.gov/nchs/data/misc/itop97.pdf.

National Center for Injury Prevention and Control. *Child maltreatment*. Available from: https://www.cdc.gov/violenceprevention/pdf/childmaltreatment-facts-at-a-glance.pdf.

Office of the Assistant Secretary for Planning and Evaluation. *Screening for domestic violence in health care settings*. Available from: https://aspe.hhs.gov/report/screening-domestic-violence-health-care-settings.

11

Conflict Management

CHAPTER OBJECTIVES

1. Define conflict, differentiating between positive and negative conflict.
2. Identify various conflict behavioral styles.
3. Identify the emotional, cognitive, and physical responses to conflict.
4. Define characteristics of disruptive behavior.
5. Compare and contrast the different types of conflict management and conflict resolution.
6. Define alternative dispute resolution.
7. Identify the components of alternative dispute resolution.

KEY TERMS

Accommodating Conflict behavior style in which an individual allows the needs of a group or team to supersede the individual's own needs, also known as "smoothing."

Alternative Dispute Resolution (ADR) The procedure for settling disputes by means other than litigation.

Arbitration A process using a mediator to resolve a dispute between two parties without using a judge and/or a trial process.

Avoiding Conflict behavior style in which the issue is not addressed at all or is ignored.

Collaborating Conflict behavior style in which the needs and goals of the individuals are combined to meet a common goal.

Competing Conflict behavior style in which an individual's own needs are advocated over the needs of others.

Compromising Conflict behavior style in which people give and receive in a series of tradeoffs.

Conflict The mental struggle resulting from incompatible or opposing needs, drives, wishes, or external or internal demands.

Conflict management The long-term management of disputes and conflicts, which may or may not lead to resolution.

Conflict resolution The process of ending a disagreement between two or more people in a constructive fashion for all parties involved.

Disruptive behavior Personal conduct, whether verbal or physical, that affects or that potentially may affect patient care negatively.

Facilitation The process by which a third party (facilitator) assists in the resolution of a dispute.

Mediation The process by which a neutral third party who is trained in mediation techniques facilitates and assists in resolving a dispute.

Negative conflict A conflict that has devolved into disruptive behaviors or violence.

Negotiation Any communication used in an attempt to achieve a goal, approval, or action by another.

Positive conflict The idea that healthy discussion can happen in the face of a disagreement, regardless of differing personalities, education levels, or responsibilities.

INTRODUCTION

Conflict is an unavoidable part of almost any profession and workplace. However, the healthcare industry is subject to higher incidences of conflict and severity owing to the increasing demand for broader access to care, greater accountability, and improved quality of care. This is further compounded by healthcare professionals and industry facing more demanding work, staffing shortages, stricter regulatory enforcement, a more litigious society, and decreased reimbursement. The healthcare professional's typical day involves a race to coordinate resources, provide care, perform procedures, gather data, respond to emergencies, and interact with diverse groups of people with a variety of different expectations and needs. Thus, healthcare professionals face more conflict and greater obstacles than many other fields or professions. And yet very few have been provided the necessary training and skills to manage and negotiate the various hurdles of their profession and workplace, particularly in cases of conflict management and resolution.

Although some level of friction is inevitable in any group setting, it is especially likely in the healthcare setting, where there are differences in authority and the constant pressure of patient care. In most cases, minor conflicts can highlight problems and inconsistencies in an organization or process and serve as a catalyst for necessary changes and improvements. However, chronic conflict and unacceptable behavior at any level can breed fear and distrust, making teamwork impossible, which may affect patient care and outcomes. Thus, it is critical for healthcare professionals to have proper conflict resolution training to better understand how to diffuse difficult situations and reach an agreement that satisfies all parties.

WHAT IS CONFLICT?

Conflict is the internal struggle resulting from incompatible or opposing needs, drives, wishes, or external or internal demands. It is often the result of differences from varying perspectives. As opposed to a disagreement, which is simply a failure to agree, a conflict involves a perceived threat to an individual's needs, interests, or concerns because of a disagreement.

Conflict is, in fact, a natural and normal part of human interactions. Conflict generally can have two forms: *positive* and *negative.*

Positive vs. Negative Conflict

Conflict can appear in a positive, or functional, way that can result in improvements. Positive conflict is the idea that healthy discussion can occur in the face of a disagreement, regardless of different personalities, education levels, or responsibilities. Positive conflict can be utilized in many ways. When conflict arises, diverse attitudes and backgrounds can produce creative approaches to solve problems and reach goals in an organization (Fig. 11.1). Employees who feel free to disagree or offer different viewpoints are more likely to engage in workplace problem-solving and discussions. In addition, conflict can trigger critical thinking in a team in an effort to seek resolution, as well as improve team effectiveness and cohesiveness. When a team learns to resolve conflict, it often helps them to better understand their goals, both individually and as a team.

Negative conflict is when conflict devolves into disruptive behaviors or violence, usually attributable to the lack of trust, communication, and discussion. There is a natural tendency to avoid conflict because it can be uncomfortable and unpleasant. However, it is important to understand that conflict does not have to be a bad or unproductive situation. In fact, although conflict is difficult, it can bring growth and change if handled appropriately. Conflict can be an indicator that change may be coming or necessary. The important thing to note is that if conflict is identified and managed early and properly, it can lead to a positive result.

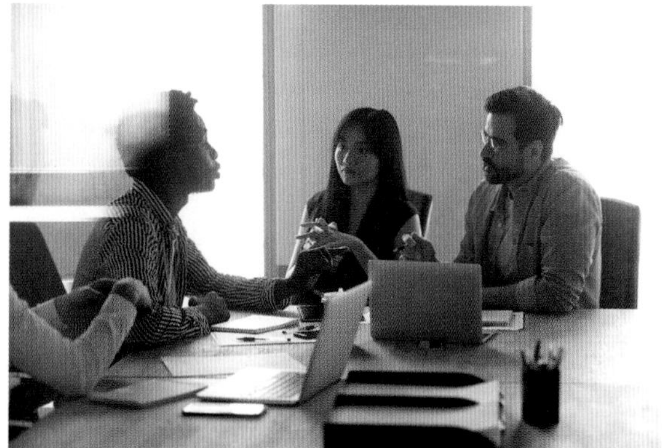

Fig. 11.1 Positive conflict allows people with diverse attitudes and backgrounds to produce creative approaches to solve problems and reach goals in an organization. (iStock.com/Fizkes.)

DISCUSSION

Susan attended a departmental meeting to discuss new attendance policies and clinical guidelines. The discussion became quite heated, with the department dividing into two groups arguing different sides of the policy issues. By the end of the meeting, a consensus had been reached with both sides satisfied with the resolution. In fact, there was some good-natured joking between several team members afterward.

However, later that day during lunch, one of Susan's coworkers started talking about the meeting and how uncomfortable and upset it made her feel. The coworker stated that she does not like it when people argue and did not know why "we all just can't get along."

1. What could Susan say to her coworker about conflict?
2. Would you consider this a positive or negative conflict?

Contributing Factors in Conflicts

Patients and healthcare professionals understand that healthcare delivery is a complex environment. Some of the key characteristics and contributing factors that may create misunderstandings, disputes, and conflicts in the healthcare setting are:

- The healthcare system involves a wide variety of knowledge, power, and control held by the various parties. Although it is normal for most conflicts to involve some level of differences between parties, what is unusual are the institutionalized differences brought about by differing levels of responsibility and education, as is the case in health care (Fig. 11.2).
- The ethnic and socioeconomic diversity of both patients and providers of healthcare services in many communities may be significant and can create potential barriers to helping participants determine solutions.
- Strong gender inequities remain in health care in terms of the services offered to patients, the opportunities for staff, and the diversity within groups of healthcare professionals.
- Health care involves people interacting with other people to repair and preserve the health and personal integrity of patients. Often, this involves people's strongly held personal or religious values that may be irreconcilable.

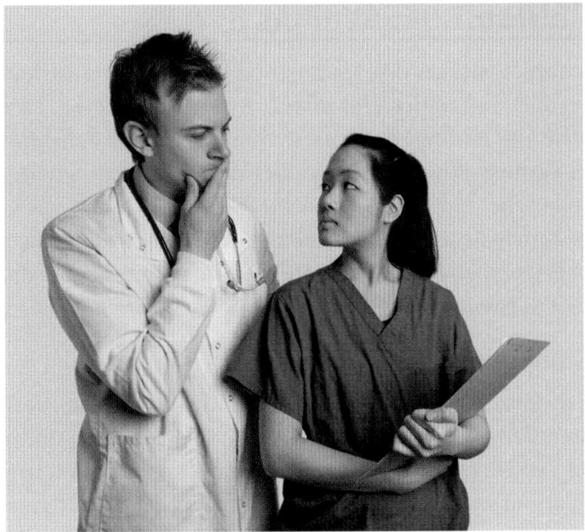

Fig. 11.2 The wide variety of knowledge, power, and control held by the various participants in health care introduces institutionalized differences in how to handle some situations. (Copyright © moodboard/moodboard/Thinkstock.com.)

All these factors contribute to make healthcare environments particularly prone to conflict. It is therefore important for all healthcare professionals to understand the origins of conflict and to develop strategies to manage the conflicts they experience.

APPLY THIS

Judy was recently hired as a certified medical assistant in a new pediatrician's office. After working several months, she noticed that another medical assistant, Debbie, was arriving late every day. It was Debbie's job to arrive early to turn on the computers, restock the examination rooms, and make sure the messages from the answering service were given to the physicians. Judy was upset because she was doing Debbie's job because of her constant tardiness at work.

One day Debbie was more than an hour late, and the waiting room was full of waiting patients. Judy muttered under her breath how unfair it was that she was left doing both Debbie's job and her job. Debbie overheard her and started yelling at Judy that it was not her fault that traffic was bad.

1. How should Judy have handled the situation?
2. What could Judy do to have prevented Debbie's outburst?

CONFLICT BEHAVIORAL STYLES

Conflict is often best understood by examining various conflict behaviors and styles. By understanding each style and its consequences, we may adjust our behaviors in various situations. This does not mean that any one style is better or worse than another, but it does allow us to anticipate and understand the expected consequences of each type. In general, there are five main types of conflict behavioral styles.

Competing

Competing is a style in which an individual's own needs are advocated over the needs of others. It relies on an aggressive style of communication, low regard for future relationships, and the exercise of coercive power. Those using a competitive style tend to seek control over a discussion. They fear that loss of such control will result in solutions that fail to meet their needs. In general, this type of conflict behavioral style may offer short-term rewards, but it may be detrimental to an organization in the long term.

Accommodating

Accommodating, also known as "smoothing" or "giving in," is the opposite of competing. People using this style allow the group's needs to take priority over their own in an effort to preserve the relationship. Although this style can lead to maintaining peace and a quick resolution, it can also lead to feeling of resentment from the accommodator toward the other party.

Avoiding

Avoiding, or withdrawing, is a common response to the negative perception of conflict. Some examples include pretending there is nothing wrong or completely shutting down. What generally occurs is that feelings are repressed, views remain unexpressed, and the conflict does not go away but grows until it becomes too big to ignore. Because individual needs and concerns remain unexpressed, people are often left feeling confused, wondering what went wrong in a discussion or relationship.

Compromising

Compromising is an approach to conflict in which people gain and give in based on a series of tradeoffs. For example, one person may agree to negotiate larger points and let go of the smaller points, which expedites the resolution process. Although seemingly satisfactory, compromise is generally not satisfying. Although there is a resolution, each party does not ultimately get what it wants and does not necessarily make efforts to understand the other party.

Collaborating

Collaborating is the pooling of individual needs and goals toward a common goal. Often called "win–win problem-solving," collaboration requires assertive communication and cooperation in order to achieve the best solution. It offers the chance for agreement, the integration of needs, and the potential to exceed the expectations of the conflict resolution. Collaboration requires thinking creatively to resolve the problem without concessions.

EMOTIONAL, COGNITIVE, AND PHYSICAL RESPONSES TO CONFLICT

In addition to the behavioral responses summarized by the various conflict styles, we have emotional, cognitive, and physical responses to conflict as well. These are important aspects of our experience during conflict, and they frequently tell us more about what the true source of our perception of a threat is. Also, by understanding our thoughts, feelings, and physical responses to conflict, we may get better insights into the best potential solutions to the situation.

In emotional responses, these are the feelings we experience in conflict, ranging from anger and fear to despair and confusion. Emotional responses are often misunderstood because people tend to believe that others feel the same as they do. Thus, differing emotional responses are confusing and, at times, threatening.

Cognitive responses are our ideas and thoughts about a conflict, often present as our inner voice or internal observer during a situation. For example, we might think any of the following things in response to someone taking a parking spot just as we are ready to park:

"That jerk! Who does he think he is?"

or

"He sure seems distracted. I wonder if he is okay."

or

"What am I supposed to do now? I'm going to be late for my meeting. I should give him a piece of my mind! But what if he gets mad at me?"

Such different thoughts contribute to emotional and behavioral responses, where self-talk can promote either a positive or a negative feedback loop in the situation.

Physical responses can play an important role in our ability to meet our needs in the conflict. They include increased physical tension, increased perspiration, tunnel vision, shallow or accelerated breathing, nausea, and rapid heartbeat. These "fight or flight" responses are those we experience in high-anxiety situations, and they may be managed through stress management techniques. Establishing a calmer environment in which emotions can be managed is more likely if the physical responses are effectively addressed as well.

Disruptive Behavior

Disruptive behavior has been defined by the American Medical Association as "personal conduct, whether verbal or physical, that affects or that potentially may affect patient care negatively." It specifically includes "conduct that interferes with one's ability to work with other members of the healthcare team." Whether the disruptive behavior comes from patients or another healthcare professional, the challenge is to find a way of addressing any disruptive behavior before it impedes patient care. The following can be examples of potentially disruptive behaviors among healthcare professionals:

- Profane or disrespectful language
- Demeaning behavior, such as name calling
- Sexual comments or innuendo
- Inappropriate touching, sexual or otherwise
- Racial or ethnic jokes
- Outbursts of anger
- Throwing instruments, charts, or other objects
- Criticizing other caregivers in front of patients or other staff
- Comments that undermine a patient's trust in other caregivers or the hospital
- Failure to adequately address safety concerns or patient care needs expressed by another caregiver
- Intimidating behavior that can suppress input by other members of the healthcare team
- Deliberate failure to adhere to organizational policies without adequate reason

When behavior goes against an expectation or if there is the perception that it does, then conflict may exist. Whether it is surgical technologists filing complaints about having instruments thrown at them or medical assistants humiliated by their supervisors, victims of disruptive or abusive behavior may come to view litigation as the only way to protect their safety and dignity. To combat this risk, an increasing number of healthcare organizations are adopting a zero-tolerance policy for the more severe offenses, such as sexual harassment and physical violence, and offering counseling, education, and training for more minor offenses. By responding swiftly and decisively to observed incidents and complaints, healthcare organizations can protect themselves against liability for condoning a hostile or discriminatory work environment.

RELATE TO PRACTICE

A surgical technologist is walking past a scrub sink where she sees a coworker washing her hands and crying. The coworker tells her that during a just-completed procedure, the surgical saw stopped working for some reason. The surgeon "lost it" and threw the saw against the wall while yelling for a replacement saw. The coworker said she was scared and was afraid the surgeon was going to throw the saw at her. She is upset and does not know what she can do about it.

1. What can the surgical technologist advise her coworker to do?
2. What kind of behavior(s) did the surgeon display?

CONFLICT MANAGEMENT

Conflict management is the long-term management of disputes and conflicts, which may or may not lead to resolution. For decades, healthcare organizations and professionals have recognized the need for managing conflict within the healthcare workplace to ensure that conflict does not affect the quality of care and patient safety.

In 2009, The Joint Commission, the organization that accredits hospitals and other healthcare organizations, began requiring that healthcare organizations establish policies and procedures for conflict management among their leadership and management staff (Standard LD.02.04.01). Based on The Joint Commission's recommendations, the standards and their elements of performance refer to:

(1) "a system for resolving conflicts among individuals working in the hospital" (Standard LD.01.03.01),
(2) "an ongoing process for managing conflict among leadership groups" (Standard LD.02.04.01),
(3) "a process for managing disruptive and inappropriate behavior" (Standard LD.03.01.01, Element of Performance 5).

In addition, The Joint Commission issued a Sentinel Event Alert titled "Behaviors That Undermine a Culture of Safety." It urged healthcare organizations to address unprofessional behaviors through formal policies, and it identified the lack of conflict management skills as a root cause of disruptive behavior. The Joint Commission recommended interventions such as educating team members, encouraging interprofessional dialogue, and developing an organizational process for responding to intimidating and disruptive behavior.

Any conflict management an organization implements must create and maintain a culture of safety that, in turn, promotes and protects the quality of patient care. The challenge for healthcare organizations is to assess their current problem-solving techniques and responses to conflict. How a particular healthcare organization implements policies and procedures to meet the standards of The Joint Commission will be unique and specific to that organization.

Conflict Resolution

Conflict resolution is the process of resolving a disagreement between two or more parties in a constructive way that all parties involved feel that their needs have been met. Most conflicts are interpersonal or occur when a person or group of people frustrates or interferes with another person's efforts at achieving a goal. Interpersonal conflict should be managed and resolved before it degenerates into a verbal assault, which may cause irreparable damage to a team. Dealing with interpersonal conflict can be a difficult and uncomfortable process. Healthcare professionals need to use carefully worded statements to avoid adding friction and tension to a situation and to deescalate a situation in which each party feels able to openly communicate and express his or her frustration and needs. So how do we start?

The first step in resolving interpersonal conflict is to acknowledge its existence. Recognizing a conflict allows team members to build common ground by putting the conflict within the context of the larger goal of the team and the organization. Moreover, the larger goal can help by giving team members a motive for resolving the conflict.

In addition, when it comes to conflict, communication is both the cause and the resolution. Open and supportive communication is vital to a high-performing team. A conflict-friendly team environment must encourage effective listening. This means listening to one another without interruption and not having side conversations, doodling, or staring vacantly. The fundamentals to resolving team conflict include the following elements:

1. Before stating one's view, the speaker should try to understand what others have said.
2. Try to find common ground—seek what the opposing sides have in common. This helps to reinforce what is shared between the disputants.
3. Whether or not an agreement is reached, team members should thank the other team members for having expressed their views and feelings. Thanking the other recognizes the personal risk the individual took in expressing themselves and should be viewed as an expression of trust and commitment.

When interpersonal conflict occurs, all sides of the issue should be recognized without finger-pointing or blaming. When one team member is yelled at or blamed for something, it has the effect of silencing the rest of the team. It communicates to everyone that dissent is not allowed, and, as discussed earlier, dissent may be one of the most fertile resources for new ideas.

Alternative Dispute Resolution

There may be occasions when conflict can progress beyond interpersonal conflict techniques and require a third party to assist with the resolution, which may be especially true in a professional setting. Alternative dispute resolution (ADR) is the procedure for settling disputes by means other than litigation, which may be costly and time consuming.

ADRs are increasingly being utilized in disputes that would otherwise result in litigation, such as labor disputes, divorce actions, and personal injury claims. Many people prefer ADR because they view it as a more creative process focused on problem-solving, unlike litigation, which is viewed more as a "win–lose" scenario and can be very adversarial. Some of the more common ADR techniques are negotiation, mediation, facilitation, and arbitration to resolve conflict.

Negotiation

Negotiation is any communication used in an attempt to achieve a goal, approval, or action by another. Negotiating takes place every time two or more individuals resolve a disagreement, an area of contention, or an area that requires some compromises on one or both sides. It may be formal or informal. Those in healthcare use negotiation skills daily when interacting with patients, families, coworkers, and employers. In fact, we learn the process of negotiating at a young age. When you were a child and asked your parents for four cookies and they said one, you may have finally settled on two cookies. This is negotiating.

Negotiation is similar to compromising, in that there is a back-and-forth dialogue with a series of tradeoffs. However, there is a difference between the two. The objective of any negotiation process is to get a "win–win" result, in which both parties gain or lose together. In contrast, the process of compromise has one party lose something; the loss can be big or small. Thus, negotiation can be done without compromise, but compromise cannot be done without negotiation.

Mediation

Mediation is the process by which a neutral third party, such as an attorney, judge, or other person trained in mediation techniques, facilitates and assists the parties in resolving a dispute. The fundamental principle of mediation is self-determination. Mediation relies on the ability of the parties to reach a voluntary, uncoerced agreement. The mediator may offer a possible resolution for discussion, help parties explore options, identify issues, and provide information (Fig. 11.3).

The mediation process is commonly used to resolve medical malpractice claims, personal injury claims, and employee disputes. It is the least adversarial method of ADR and can assist the parties to identify the real issues and options for settlement. Ultimately, the parties are able to maintain control of the outcome.

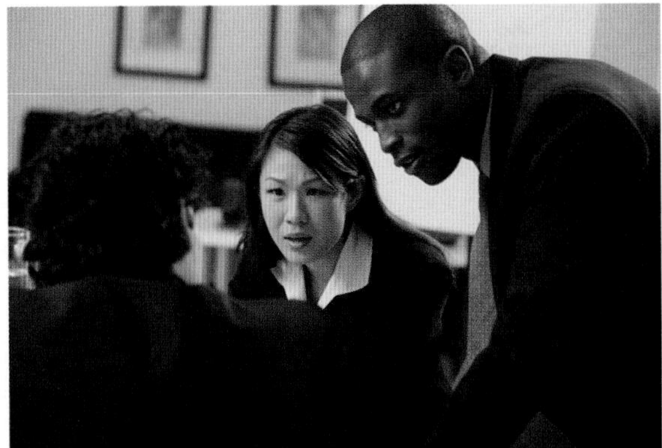

Fig. 11.3 A mediator may offer a possible resolution for discussion, help parties explore options, identify issues, and provide information. (Copyright © Comstock Images/Stockbyte/Thinkstock.com.)

Facilitation

Facilitation is the process by which a third party, a facilitator, assists in the resolution of the dispute. The following are some types of processes and techniques that a facilitator may use to resolve issues:

- Guided dialogue
- Consensus building
- Action planning
- Strategic planning
- Vision planning
- Focused conversation
- Systems-change dynamics of human transformation

A trained facilitator uses these processes to guide and aid the group to reach its goals. Every participant is treated as equal and influences the processes used.

Arbitration

Arbitration is the process of resolving issues in a conflict in a more structured setting, similar to formal litigation. There can be one arbitrator or a panel of arbitrators that can award damages, interest, attorney's fees, and punitive damages, if allowed by law. Arbitration is usually voluntary, but the law can mandate it for specific disputes, such as labor disputes and civil litigation.

Arbitration may be either "binding" or "nonbinding." Binding arbitration means that the parties waive their right to a trial and agree to accept the arbitrator's decision as final. Generally, there is no right to appeal an arbitrator's decision. However, nonbinding arbitration means that the parties are free to request a trial if they do not accept the arbitrator's decision.

APPLY THIS

Nadia is a newly hired patient care technician at the hospital. During her first 2 weeks on the job, she made several errors, including not taking a patient's vital sign on time and incorrectly documenting in a patient's medical record. On a particular day, Barbara, a nurse on the unit, begins yelling at Nadia and throws a package of gloves at her. Nadia is embarrassed and humiliated over the situation.

1. What kind of disciplinary actions should hospitals and other healthcare organizations have for disruptive behavior?
2. What kind of action or resolution should be taken in this situation?

CONCLUSION

Members of a healthcare team work in stressful environments that can bring about conflict. Conflict arises when individuals or parties disagree and perceive a threat to their needs, interests, or concerns. However, conflict is a normal part of human behavior. It may seem unpleasant, but it does have a purpose. If conflict is managed correctly, it can produce positive results where respective parties are satisfied with the outcome and change can occur. The key to successful conflict resolution is communication, being aware of your conflict behavioral style, and responses to conflict. However, if conflict is not effectively addressed, it can result in disruptive behavior and potential litigation.

CHAPTER REVIEW QUESTIONS

1. Conflict occurs when one individual perceives a threat to his or her
   A. needs.
   B. interests.
   C. concerns.
   D. All the above
2. Disruptive behavior is an example of
   A. positive conflict.
   B. negative conflict.
   C. disagreement.
   D. None of the above
3. What is the key point in dealing with conflict to enable a positive outcome?
   A. Communication
   B. Speaking loudly
   C. Waiting to discuss the event
   D. Physical gestures to communicate a point
4. The ADR process that is similar to compromising is
   A. mediation.
   B. arbitration.
   C. negotiation.
   D. facilitation.
5. The conflict behavior style that is also known as "smoothing" is
   A. avoiding.
   B. collaborating.
   C. compromising.
   D. accommodating.
6. All the following are reasons that conflicts may arise in the healthcare setting except
   A. demand for healthcare services has increased.
   B. shortage of staffing has led to a more stressful work environment.
   C. healthcare professionals are often equally trained and educated but will have conflicting opinions.
   D. a stricter and more litigious work environment.
7. During a staff meeting, a disagreement occurs between two of your coworkers. One of them starts raising her voice and makes a rude comment to the other coworker about her performance. She demands that everyone should agree with her suggestion. This is an example of
   A. accommodating.
   B. avoiding.
   C. collaborating.
   D. competing.
8. A new policy for staffing needs to be created. However, several staff members have differing opinions on what should be included in the policy. The office manager recommends that members from each department form a committee. This is an example of
   A. accommodating.
   B. avoiding.
   C. collaborating.
   D. compromising.
9. All the following are physical responses to conflict except
   A. increased peripheral vision.
   B. increased perspiration.
   C. increased breathing.
   D. increased heart.
10. Negotiation is an attempt to achieve a goal or approval by another. A similar conflict behavior style to negotiation is
   A. avoiding.
   B. collaborating.
   C. compromising.
   D. accommodating.

SELF-REFLECTION QUESTIONS

1. How do I personally feel about conflict? How do I manage it at home and at work?
2. How would I handle disruptive behavior from a coworker?
3. Is it possible for conflict to be healthy?
4. Does your workplace have a conflict management policy? If so, do you know what it is?
5. Think about a conflict that you have experienced in the past. What was the outcome? Positive or negative? What are the steps that led to that outcome? Could it have been handled differently?

INTERNET ACTIVITIES

1. Go to the website of the International Association for Conflict Management at https://www.iacm-conflict.com. When were they founded and what is their mission statement?
2. Go to the website of University of Maryland Francis King Carey School of Law at https://www.law.umaryland.edu/programs/cdrum/documents/md_school_conflict_brochure.pdf. Why is it important to teach children in K–12 about conflict resolution? What other conflict-related skills do they teach?

ADDITIONAL RESOURCES

http://www.courts.ca.gov/3074.htm
https://hbr.org/2013/10/four-steps-to-resolving-conflicts-in-health-care
https://www.jointcommission.org/
http://www.cspsteam.org
https://www.ama-assn.org/
https://www.iacm-conflict.org/

BIBLIOGRAPHY

Academic Leadership Support. *About conflict.* Available from: https://www.ohrd.wisc.edu/onlinetraining/resolution/aboutwhatisit.htm.

Donner, D. *Description of positive conflict.* Available from: https://www.ehow.com/about_6802533_description-positive-conflict.html.

Free Dictionary. *Captain of the ship doctrine.* Available from: http://medical-dictionary.thefreedictionary.com/Captain+of+the+Ship+Doctrine.

Greenhalgh, L. (2006). Managing conflict. *MIT Sloan Management Review*, (Summer), 45–51.

Harvard Law School, Program on Negotiation. *Conflict resolution.* Available from: https://www.pon.harvard.edu/category/daily/conflict-management/.

John Ford & Associates. *Contextualizing disruptive behavior in health care as a conflict management challenge.* Available from: http://johnford.blogs.com/jfa/2009/03/contextualizing-disruptive-behavior-in-health-care-as-a-conflict-management-challenge.html.

Lafasto, F., & Larson, C. (2001). *When teams work best.* Thousand Oaks, CA: SAGE.

Learn about the law. Available from http://public.findlaw.com.

Leonard, K. *Positive & negative conflicts in the workplace.* Available from http://smallbusiness.chron.com/positive-negative-conflicts-workplace-11422.html.

Locke, E. Handbook of principles of organizational behavior, 2nd ed. Available from: http://dmcodyssey.org/wp-content/uploads/2014/02/Organization-Behavior-Textbook-2009.pdf.

Managing groups and teams/conflict. Available from: http://en.wikibooks.org/wiki/Managing_Groups_and_Teams/Conflict.

Overton, A., & Lowry, A. (December 2013). *Conflict management: Difficult conversations with difficult people.* Available from: https://www.ncbi.nlm.nih.gov/pmc/articles/PMC3835442/.

Porto, G., & Lauve, R. (2006). *Disruptive clinician behavior: A persistent threat to safety, patient safety quality healthcare.* PSNet Patient Safety Network. Available from: https://www.psqh.com/julaug06/disruptive.html.

Ramsay, M. A. E. *Conflict in the healthcare workplace.* Available from: https://www.ncbi.nlm.nih.gov/pmc/articles/PMC1291328/.

Shah, M. *Impact of interpersonal conflict in healthcare setting on patient care; the role of nursing leadership style on resolving the conflict.* Available from: http://medcraveonline.com/NCOAJ/NCOAJ-02-00031.pdf.

Siegel, M. (1998). The perils of culture conflict. *Fortune*, (Nov), 257–262.

Simons, T. L., & Peterson, R. S. (2000). Task conflict and relationship conflict in top management teams: The pivotal role of intragroup trust. *Journal of Applied Psychology*, *85*(1), 102–111.

Simpson, A. *The role of law in conflict management.* Available from: https://www.mediate.com/articles/simpson.cfm.

Stack, L. *Conflict in the workplace: Conflict can be positive and productive.* Available from: http://www.aviationpros.com/article/10385718/conflict-in-the-workplace-conflict-can-be-positive-and-productive.

Taylor, S. M. (2003). Manage conflict through negotiation and mediation. In E. A. Locke (Ed.), *Handbook of principles of organizational behavior: Indispensable knowledge for evidence-based management* (2nd ed.). John Wiley & Sons, Ltd.

The Joint Commission. Available from: https://www.jointcommission.org/.

U.S. Equal Employment Opportunity Commission. *Federal sector alternative dispute resolution.* Available from: https://www.eeoc.gov/federal/adr/federal-adr.cfm.

VanBuren, V. *Applying conflict resolution skills in health care. Part I: Principled negotiation method.* Available from: http://www.karlbayer.com/blog/applying-conflict-resolution-skills-in-health-care-part-i-principled-negotiation-method/.

12

Birth and Life

CHAPTER OBJECTIVES

1. Discuss the history of involuntary sterilization and eugenics in the United States.
2. Discuss the legal cases related to contraception.
3. Discuss the legal cases related to abortion rights and access and *Roe v. Wade*.
4. Discuss the legal issues surrounding adoption.
5. Discuss bioethical issues related to assisted reproductive technology (ART).
6. Define what an emancipated minor is and their rights in healthcare.
7. Describe ethical issues associated with organ donation and transplantation.

KEY TERMS

Abortion A procedure to end a pregnancy by a medical or surgical procedure to remove the embryo or fetus and placenta from the uterus.

Adoption The legal action that bestows parental rights on a person who was not the child's legal parent before the proceeding.

Artificial insemination (AI) Injection of seminal fluid into the female vagina, which contains male sperm from a husband, partner, or other donor, to aid in conception.

Contraception The intentional prevention of conception through the use of various devices, sexual practices, chemicals, drugs, or surgical procedures, also commonly called birth control methods.

Emancipation The legal process of a minor achieving independence from his or her parents.

Eugenics The study of all agencies under human control which can improve or impair the racial quality of future generations.

Fertilization Assistance in conception, most commonly performed either as artificial insemination or as in vitro fertilization to produce pregnancy.

In vitro fertilization Process to assist in conception by harvesting an ovum from a woman and combining it with the man's sperm outside of the uterus and then implanting the fertilized embryo back into the uterus.

Minor A person who does not have the legal rights of an adult and has not yet reached the age of majority.

Sterilization Any procedure performed to permanently prevent reproduction.

Surrogacy A method of assisted reproduction that helps a party start a family when that party otherwise could not.

INTRODUCTION

Throughout our lives, ethics and laws continue to play critical roles. This becomes more complex with significant advancements in technology, science, and health care, such as how do we determine life, how and should we sustain that life, and who should have authority over their or someone else's life? Some of these questions are not new controversies and have been issues that society and our government have been trying to address for decades, while others are new and challenge our society as it evolves in our laws, ethics, and morality.

In this chapter, we will cover some of the current and often controversial ethical and bioethical areas of concern and debate regarding birth and life. These issues include family planning, reproductive health, abortion rights, organ donations, and autonomy and the rights of specific populations, such as pediatrics and those with mental health and disabilities. As medicine and society continue to advance and evolve, so will the ethical and bioethical issues and our need to address them.

ETHICAL ISSUES IN REPRODUCTIVE HEALTH

There are many ethical aspects which derive from the application of reproduction control in women's health. The main issues that raise ethical dilemmas are the development of assisted reproduction techniques, including the process of in vitro fertilization; surrogacy; the right to procreate or reproduce; and abortion, women's right to body autonomy, and the moral status of the embryo.

Religious beliefs are major contributors to the ethical and legal questions surrounding the issues of contraception and abortion. The controversy includes everything from the many different types of contraception to the "morning-after pill" to the options of abortion vs. adoption for pregnancies conceived outside a parent's willingness or ability to keep a child.

Currently, a spouse has no legal right veto or to be informed of his wife's decisions on contraception, sterilization, or abortion. However, a spouse has the right to veto care that will result in the conception of a child under the circumstances of artificial insemination (AI) or embryo transplants. Unless the state or federal government has passed a law governing consent or access to the care in question, the decision rests primarily with the woman with consultation from her healthcare provider.

Healthcare providers should encourage women to discuss reproductive choices with their spouses or partners, but it is inappropriate to require their consent. In fact, healthcare providers who obtain a spouse's consent rather than the woman's can be sued for breaching the confidential relationship and even liable for battery to the woman, unless the spouse is the legal guardian or has been delegated the right to consent in a durable power of attorney. If a patient does not want a spouse or family member to be informed about medical care, this wish must be honored.

Sterilization

Some patients seek surgical procedures voluntarily to alter their ability to reproduce, called **sterilization**. Female sterilization methods aim to prevent the ovum from leaving the fallopian tubes or sperm from fertilizing the ovum. Males may opt to undergo a vasectomy, where the vas deferens is severed and then tied or sealed to prevent sperm from entering the seminal fluid.

Patients may choose these procedures for many reasons. It may be economical (e.g., the patient cannot afford children), therapeutic (e.g., the patient is at risk because of conditions such as cancer), or some patients simply do not wish to reproduce. Regardless of the reason, healthcare professionals must use careful screening and ensure that patients fully understand the procedures they will be undergoing.

Some physicians will not perform these procedures on anyone younger than 30 years of age and prefer that the patient has already had children before making this choice. In most states, the law forbids the sterilization of any minor, except in extremely rare cases involving a court order.

Involuntary Sterilization

The United States has a long history of involuntary or coerced sterilization. In fact, the United States was an international leader in **eugenics** or discouraging reproduction by people with "undesirable" qualities. Eugenic applied theories of biology and genetics to human breeding and determined who was "fit" vs. "unfit." This often resulted in eugenic policies against immigrants, people of color, poor people, unmarried mothers, the disabled, and the mentally ill.

In 1849, Gordon Lincecum, a Texas biologist and physician, proposed a bill mandating the eugenic sterilization of the mentally handicapped and others whose genes he deemed undesirable. Although the legislation was never sponsored or brought up for a vote, it represented the first serious attempt in U.S. history to use forced sterilization for eugenic purposes.

Between 1890 and 1920, the United States was the first country to perform compulsory sterilization programs for the purpose of eugenics. Federally funded sterilization programs took place in 33 states throughout the 20th century, with more than 65,000 individuals being forcibly sterilized, most of them members of ethnic minorities. A third of the sterilizations were done on girls under 18, even as young as 9. Approximately 20,000 sterilizations took place in state institutions, comprising one-third of the total number performed in the 32 states where such actions were legal.

Although Michigan and Pennsylvania were the first to propose forced sterilization laws, Indiana was the first state to pass the world's first sterilization law in 1907 (Fig. 12.1). By the 1930s and 1940s, involuntary sterilization programs were common practices and were even mandated in many states.

Beginning in 1909 and continuing for 70 years, California had one of the largest involuntary sterilization programs that mostly targeted Asians and Mexicans. Even more recently, between 2006 and 2010, California prisons were reported to have authorized forced sterilizations of nearly 150 female inmates. Many other states, particularly Southern states, also employed sterilization as a means of controlling African American populations. "Mississippi appendectomies" was another name for unnecessary hysterectomies or tubal ligations performed on predominantly poor Black women without their knowledge at teaching hospitals in the South for medical students. Between 1970 and 1976, young Native American women underwent sterilization by tubal ligations without their knowledge when they believed they were getting appendectomies. It is estimated that as many as 25%–50% of Native American women were forcibly sterilized. Box 12.1 list landmark cases that brought awareness to involuntary sterilization programs and forced changes to the laws.

In December 2015, the United States Senate voted unanimously to pass the Eugenics Compensation Act that provided compensation for living eugenics victims. Currently, only two states have implemented a Eugenics Compensation Program as part of the Act. North Carolina was considered to have one of the most egregious eugenics programs, which operated between

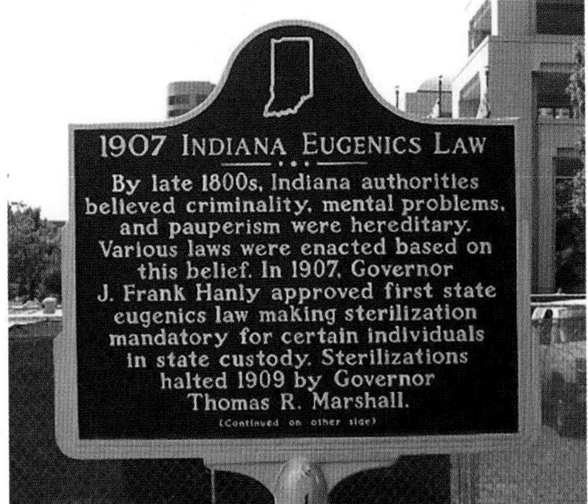

Fig. 12.1 Indiana was the first state to pass the first sterilization law in 1907 that permitted sterilization mandatory for certain individuals in state custody. Involuntary sterilizations halted in 1909 (https://www.in.gov/history/images/eugenics2.jpg). (Indiana Historical Bureau, Indiana State Library.)

BOX 12.1 Landmark Cases in Involuntary Sterilization in the United States

- *Buck v. Bell*: In 1927, Carrie Buck, a poor white woman, was the first person to be sterilized in Virginia under a new law. Carrie's mother had been involuntarily institutionalized for being "feebleminded" and "promiscuous." Carrie was assumed to have inherited these traits and was sterilized after giving birth. The Supreme Court case led to the sterilization of 65,000 Americans with mental illness or developmental disabilities from the 1920s to the 1970s.
- *Madrigal v. Quilligan*: A small group of Mexican immigrant women sued county physicians, the state, and the U.S. government after they were sterilized while giving birth at Los Angeles County-USC Medical Center during the late 1960s and early 1970s. They argued that a woman's right to bear a child is guaranteed under the Supreme Court decision in *Roe v. Wade*.
- *Relf v. Weinberger*: Mary Alice and Minnie Relf were poor Black sisters from Alabama and were sterilized at the ages of 14 and 12. Their mother, who was illiterate, had signed an "X" on a piece of paper she believed gave permission for her daughters, who were both mentally disabled, to receive birth control shots. In 1974, the Southern Poverty Law Center filed a lawsuit on behalf of the Relf sisters, revealing that 100,000–150,000 poor people were being sterilized each year under federally funded programs.

1929 to 1974, and paid $35,000 to 220 surviving victims of its eugenics program. Virginia agreed to give surviving victims $25,000 each.

Contraceptives

With few exceptions, a competent adult woman has the autonomy and authority to consent to her health care, including the use of contraceptives. **Contraception**, commonly called birth control methods, is defined as the intentional prevention of conception using various devices, sexual practices, chemicals, drugs, or surgical procedures. Thus, any device or act whose purpose is to prevent a woman from becoming pregnant can be considered as a contraceptive.

To get contraceptive medication, or birth control pills, a prescription is necessary from a healthcare provider and, in some states, a pharmacist. One of the important changes that came with the passage of the Affordable Care Act in 2011 was in reproductive health, which ensured more than 63 million women had access to birth control. Many states also explicitly permit all or some people younger than 18 to obtain contraceptive.

However, since its passage, several lawsuits against the contraceptive mandate were filed. In *Hobby Lobby v. Burwell* in 2014, the Supreme Court agreed that employers that object to the coverage of contraceptives for religious or moral reasons can decline to cover contraceptives for employees or students. In another case, *Zubik v. Burwell* in 2016, was the accommodation process—which enabled employees and students of objecting employers to access contraceptives without cost-sharing—is now optional, meaning many women will have to look elsewhere for contraceptive coverage and potentially pay out-of-pocket for this medical care.

APPLY THIS

A patient does not want more children and talks to her physician about taking oral contraceptives. She asks her physician to not inform her husband since he still wants to more children and has told her not to take contraceptives. A few months later, the physician gets a phone call from the patient's husband. He asks the physician why the couple had not conceived since they have been trying.

1. What should the physician tell the patient's husband?
2. What if the physician informs the husband that the patient is taking oral contraceptives? What would the physician be liable for?

Abortion

Abortion continues to be one of the most polarizing issues in the United States. An **abortion** is a procedure to end a pregnancy by a medical or surgical procedure to remove the embryo or fetus and placenta from the uterus. In September 2000, the United States Food and Drug Administration approved mifepristone, also known as RU 486, to be marketed as a method of medical abortion. Currently, medication abortion is provided up to 10 weeks' gestation.

Abortion raises many ethical, moral, and legal issues related to the rights of the woman vs. the rights of the fetus. Some believe that life begins the moment that the sperm and ovum are joined, and the **fertilization** process begins. For those who consider life to begin at conception, abortion always equals murder and is therefore forbidden. Others argue that life begins once the fertilized egg becomes an embryo at 8–14 days, while still others contend that life does not begin until the embryo becomes a fetus at the eighth and ninth weeks and organs are developed. Then, there are some other groups who argue that a life does not begin until the child is born. Those who believe in the absolute autonomy of the woman over her body take the other approach. A woman should have supreme rights and authority over her own body as a premise of freedom and that nobody—legal, moral, or otherwise—should force a person to bear in her womb and give birth to an unwanted child if she does not want to. The discussion surrounding abortion usually centers on whether it should be legal or illegal.

Before abortion was legal, many women were desperate for this service and subjected themselves to illegal, unsterile, and dangerous procedures to end the pregnancy. It was not unusual for both the woman and her fetus to die because of the procedure. With the passage of *Roe v. Wade* that legalized abortion rights in 1973, more than 59 million abortions were performed in the United States between 1973 and 2014, although total abortions dropped by almost 25% from 1998 to 2013. Approximately 862,320 abortions were performed in 2017, down 7% from 926,190 in 2014.

Roe v. Wade is the central court decision that created current abortion laws in the United States. In this 1973 decision, the Supreme Court ruled that women had a constitutional and fundamental right to choose whether or not to have abortions without excessive government restriction, and that this right was based on an implied right to personal privacy based on the Constitution. In *Roe v. Wade*, the Supreme Court said that a fetus is not a person but "potential life," and, thus, does not have constitutional rights of its own. The Supreme Court also set up a framework in which the woman's right to abortion and the state's right to protect potential life shifts:

- during the first trimester of pregnancy, a woman's privacy right is strongest, and the state may not regulate abortion for any reason
- during the second trimester, the state may regulate abortion only to protect the health of the woman
- during the third trimester, the state may regulate or prohibit abortion to promote its interest in the potential life of the fetus, except where abortion is necessary to preserve the woman's life or health

State laws vary on abortion rights and what is considered the legal life of an unborn child. Individual states have a variety of regulations and laws the limit whether, when, and under what circumstances a woman may obtain an abortion. For example, most states require an abortion be performed by a licensed physician with some requiring that they be done in a hospital after a specific point in the pregnancy. Majority of states prohibit abortion after a specific point in the pregnancy, usually 20–24 weeks, with the generally allowable exceptions when an abortion is necessary to protect the patient's life or health. Some states require mandatory counseling and/or a waiting period before seeking an abortion, usually 24 h. Almost every state allows healthcare providers to refuse to participate in an abortion as part of the conscience protection laws.

Because of their own religious and moral standards, some healthcare professionals may refuse to perform voluntary abortions. This brings up important ethical questions. Does a healthcare professional have the right to refuse medical services based on religious or moral standards? In terms of the physician–patient relationship, once a patient and a physician have voluntarily entered into a treatment or care relationship, the relationship may be terminated by mutual consent. A patient may unilaterally terminate a physician–patient relationship for any reason. Physicians do not have the same flexibility and are duty bound to continue to treat a patient once treatment has begun. However, both federal and state laws do allow termination of patient treatment based on a few reasons, most commonly as a result of religious reasons or based on the *conscience clause* or *objection*.

ADOPTION

Adoption is the legal action that bestows parental rights on a person who was not the child's legal parent before the proceeding. Adoption involves the termination of the existing legal parent's parental rights and the determination that the potential adoptive parent is fit. All conflicting parental rights must be terminated before an adoption is final.

If a parent marries a person who is not the child's legal parent, this stepparent does not have full parental rights unless he or she formally adopts the child. Such an adoption will require the rights of the previous parent, if known and still living, to be terminated. If a married couple, neither of the parents of the child, or a single adult seeks to adopt a child, the rights of both of the child's existing parents must be terminated.

Parents may voluntarily relinquish their parental rights in an adoption proceeding, but most states protect the parent (usually the mother) from precipitous decisions concerning termination of parental rights. These protections may include a ban on agreements signed before the baby is born and a waiting period after birth during which the parent may revoke the decision to give up parental rights.

In most states, it is illegal to pay parents to induce them to terminate their parental rights. It would be legal to give the mother almost anything as long as she did not give up her baby. It is acceptable to pay for the mother's medical expenses and support during the pregnancy, but this cannot be conditioned on a waiver of parental rights.

In addition to bans on paying parents, the courts are sensitive to efforts to coerce parents into relinquishing their parental rights. For example, it is improper for healthcare providers to participate in obtaining a waiver of parental rights from the patients. Although it is acceptable for healthcare providers to receive their routine fees from an agency or prospective parent, any payment in excess of the fees charged in other situations could subject the healthcare provider to prosecution for receiving money in connection with an adoption.

The healthcare provider's legal and ethical duty is to protect the patient's best interests, consistent with public health and safety. If the healthcare provider has doubts about the mother's fitness to care for the baby, they should be reported to the child welfare department.

Adoption Agencies and Guidelines

Federal legislation sets the framework for adoption in the United States, and individual states pass laws to comply with federal requirements and in order to become eligible for federal funding. Thus, adoption is primarily regulated by state laws, and these laws vary from state to state.

Because adoption laws are primarily governed by states, who may adopt varies and what are the requirements to adopt. For example, currently, 11 states permit state-licensed child welfare and adoption agencies to refuse to place and provide services to children and families to certain people and families if doing so conflicts with their religious beliefs. This includes same-sex couples and people who identify as lesbian, gay, bisexual, trans, or queer (LGBTQ). Additionally, there was a strong bias against single parent adoption. However, that bias is lessening and, in the last several decades, there has been a steady, sizable increase in the number of single parent adoptions. According to a 2013 report based on 2009 U.S. Census figures, approximately one-third of all adoptions from foster care are by single people.

Each state's adoption statutes may be found at: https://www.childwelfare.gov/topics/adoption/laws/laws-state/domestic/.

ASSISTED CONCEPTION ISSUES

Bioethical issues are also raised when addressing assisted or artificial conception, often referred to as *assisted reproductive technology (ART)*. These can take several forms, ranging from AI, in vitro fertilization, and surrogate motherhood. With new advancements in ART come new challenges to bioethics legislation regarding marriage, sex, and reproduction.

These issues are often further complicated by the fact that many states have not yet established laws concerning ART. Healthcare professionals who perform or participate in ART should ensure that informed consent is received from both the patient, the partner, and anyone involved with the ART to protect against any legal repercussions.

Artificial Insemination (AI)

Artificial insemination (AI) has been widely practiced for decades, so many there are already many legal protections and regulations in place. AI is commonly used for patients who are unable to conceive a child by natural methods and involves implanting male sperm into the woman's vagina to aid in conception. The sperm may originate from the woman's partner or husband or from a known or unknown donor. This is rarely an issue when the procedure is performed for a husband and wife or for a couple and the donor is known.

Ethical and legal issues may arise when the procedure involves unknown donors, which then requires an individual's consent. For example, some cases have involved women using frozen sperm collected from a husband before his death to conceive a child. Is the deceased husband's sperm the property of the wife and does she still have his consent even after death? In addition, in many states, this raises legal questions regarding the rights that the child has to the father's estate, pension, or social security benefits.

In Vitro Fertilization

Another procedure in ART to assist couples in conception involves the harvesting of the woman's ova that are combined with sperm cells to then be fertilized outside of the womb. The now fertilized ova are then implanted into the uterus. This procedure—**in vitro fertilization**—was first successfully performed in 1977 and is now commonly carried out. In fact, many insurance companies currently reimburse the costs for this procedure (Fig. 12.2).

However, ethical issues still arise. First, the patient and partner must be completely informed, and each party must provide informed consent of the procedures.

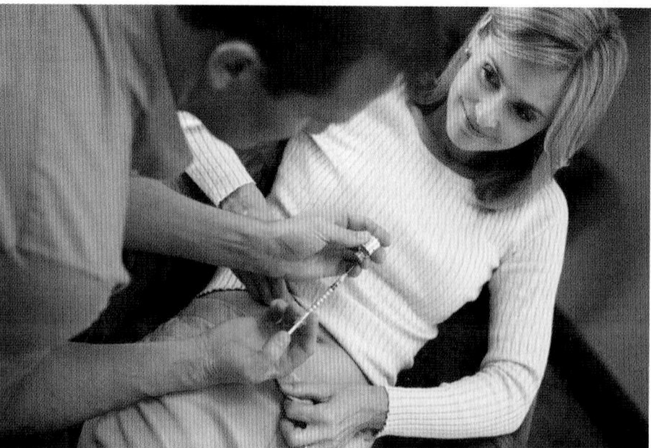

Fig. 12.2 Man helping woman inject drugs in preparation for in vitro fertilization. (Copyright © Monkey Business Images/Monkey Business/Thinkstock.com.)

Each party must also make his or her wishes known on what should be done with any unused ovum and sperm, as well as unused fertilized eggs. Should they be disposed of? Or does one party have the right to any of the unused specimens for future use?

RELATE TO PRACTICE

Maria, a nurse in a psychiatric facility, is 12 weeks pregnant. She has just arrived at work and has been on the floor making medication rounds for 20 min when a patient attacks her. The patient punches her, knocks her to the floor, and kicks her in an attempt to leave the facility. Maria was injured and hospitalized, and her unborn child was killed in utero during the assault. Can the patient be charged with murder? Why or why not?

Surrogacy

Surrogacy is a method of assisted reproduction that helps a party start a family when that party otherwise could not. The most common case of surrogacy is when a woman, a gestational surrogate, agrees to have a child for another party, which could be a single man or woman or a couple. The surrogacy may be by carrying the fertilized embryo of a married couple for a woman unable to carry the child. In other cases, in which the woman is unable to produce ova, the in vitro method may be used to impregnate the surrogate, using the surrogate's or another donor's ovum. In each of these types of surrogacy methods, the sperm may or may not be obtained from the male partner or spouse. This has led to a number of legal and ethical issues, especially in regard to custody.

In one of the most controversial surrogacy custody cases, *Baby M*, William and Elizabeth Stern contracted with Mary Beth Whitehead to be their gestational surrogate in 1984. Whitehead would be inseminated with Stern's sperm and carry the pregnancy to term, and she would relinquish her parental rights to Elizabeth Stern. However, once the baby was born, Whitehead decided she wanted to keep the child. The Sterns then sued to be recognized as the child's legal parents. After the case was heard by the Superior Court and Supreme Court of New Jersey, the case was remanded to family court, which awarded custody to the Sterns and Whitehead was given visitation rights (*New York Times*, 1988, in re Baby M., 537 A.2d 1227, 109 NJ 396, 1988).

DISCUSSION

In the case of *Baby M*, the original case was heard by the Superior Court of New Jersey in 1987, which formally validated the surrogacy contract and awarded custody of the baby to the Sterns under a "best interest of the child analysis." However, in, 1988, the Supreme Court of New Jersey invalidated the surrogacy contract as against public policy but affirmed the court's use of a "best interest of the child" analysis and remanded the case to family court, with the lower court again awarding custody to the Sterns and giving Whitehead visitation rights.

1. Should a surrogate mother be allowed to change her mind once a child is born? If so, under what circumstances?
2. Would your answer be different depending on whose ovum and sperm were used?

Consent in ART

This is a rare area of medical care in which the consent of the patient is not sufficient. The consent of the husband should be obtained before a married woman is impregnated by AI. Legal questions can arise when a married woman is artificially inseminated with donor sperm. In most states, this child is legally defined as legitimate to the husband. This presumption can be defeated if the healthcare provider fails to follow the statutory requirements. If the statute requires the permission of husband and wife, failing to obtain the husband's permission could allow him to deny paternity.

Unconsented AI may have the same legal consequences as adultery. Although the courts might view this as strictly between the husband and wife, they might honor a suit against the healthcare provider for any mental pain and suffering the unconsented insemination caused the husband.

Choosing a sperm donor can be fraught with legal risks, especially if the proper procedures, forms, and consent are not in place. If the husband is the source of the sperm, there are few legal problems. Custody and paternity are not at issue because the biologic father and the legal father are the same man.

In the case a sperm donor is used and if the laws of the state cut off parental rights for a sperm donor, the donor might make a legal challenge if he knows who his biologic child is. Many states have specific laws on AI that specify that the donor father has no legal rights.

However, if a couple wants to choose their own donor or to arrange a contract pregnancy, the laws are not as clear. Custody fights and criminal charges of baby selling are known problems with these arrangements.

ETHICAL ISSUES IN MINORS

Healthcare providers and professionals are generally expected to keep patient information confidential and obtain informed consent from patients before treating them. However, when the patient is a minor, questions arise about whether the healthcare provider has the same moral obligations of confidentiality and respect for patient choice (autonomy). Although the definition of a minor may differ based on the state or circumstance, a **minor** is a person who does not have the legal rights of an adult and has not yet reached the age of majority. In most states, a person reaches majority and acquires all the rights and responsibilities of an adult when he or she turns 18 years of age. Until a minor reaches the legal age of adulthood, he or she may not be responsible for his or her own actions. This includes the capacity to enter into a contract for damages for negligence or intentional wrongs without a parent being liable, nor for punishment as an adult for a crime.

In health care, many ethical and legal situations with managing the minor's rights and privacy as a patient and not having the full authority of an adult. For example, is it morally acceptable for minor patients to keep health information private from their parents? Do they have a legal right to keep this information from their parents? Do they have the right to make their own healthcare decisions? What happens when the parents' decision conflicts with the minor patient and the healthcare provider?

Minors' Access to Contraception

In general, minors are constrained in their ability to consent to medical care. Ideally, minors and their parents will agree on the need for medical care, including contraception, and the parent will authorize it. However, many parents do not want their children to use contraceptives because they believe that their availability will encourage sexual activity. Minors may purchase nonprescription contraceptives in all states (i.e., condoms, spermicides), and many states explicitly allow some minors to consent to prescription contraceptives without parental consent. Healthcare provider also may counsel minors about contraception without parental consent.

BOX 12.2 Provisions of 2021 Title X Final Rule on Family Planning

- Discussion with clients about their reproductive life plan
- A broad range of acceptable and effective family planning methods and services for delaying or preventing pregnancy
- The broad range of family planning services does not include abortion as a method of family planning
- Pregnancy testing, and counseling
- Services centered around preconception health and achieving pregnancy, which should include basic infertility services, sexually transmitted infection prevention education, screening, and treatment, HIV testing and referral, and screening for substance use disorders.

Some states do not explicitly allow minors to consent to prescription contraceptives, but no state prohibits minors from receiving prescription contraceptives. As a part of Title X Service Grants, the U.S. Department of Health and Human Services' Office of Population Affairs provides family planning services for all Americans, including services achieving pregnancy, preventing pregnancy, and assisting women, men, and couples with achieving their desired number and spacing of children. Box 12.2 lists core family planning services provided by Title X.

This federal legislation encourages healthcare providers to make contraceptives available to minors. Although this legislation has a provision requiring the parents of minor patients to be notified after the minors receive care, the enforcement of this provision has been prohibited by the courts. Healthcare providers have an ethical duty to respect the privacy of minors. However, many states legally allow healthcare providers to breach the provider–patient relationship and notify parents of medical care provided to their minor children. Currently, no state requires parents to be notified when a minor is prescribed contraception.

Healthcare providers prescribing contraceptives should provide the minor with all the information that would normally be provided to adult patients. If the contraceptives are prescribed without parental permission, it is advised that for the following to be considered:

- Inquiry should always be made as to the feasibility of parental consent.
- A full case history, including preexisting sexual activity, should be obtained and maintained.

- Documentation in the medical record should be of the benefit of contraception or the more serious consequence of pregnancy.
- The minor should be clearly aware of the issues and consequences and that full consent is given or to the extent a minor can give it. This includes being aware of the side effects of contraceptive pills to be prescribed. The minor patient should be required to sign a consent form acknowledging this information.
- Where follow-up care is indicated, it should be insisted on.

DISCUSSION

Most healthcare providers worry about the risks of giving minors prescription contraceptives without parental consent. However, a more problematic issue is when the parent forces contraceptives on an unwilling minor. For example, the parent may be worried about the minor's ability to care for a child.

1. What ethical and legal issues may arise for the healthcare provider in this situation?
2. What are the issues regarding consent for the minor?
3. What if the minor suffers from a stroke or other side effect as a result of the contraceptive? Who would be liable?

Minors' Consent to Abortion

In 1992, in *Planned Parenthood v. Casey*, the Supreme Court affirmed that a woman of adult years and sound mind has the same exclusive right to consent to an abortion as to any other medical care. Biological fathers and husbands have no right to be informed or consulted about the woman's decision to have an abortion. However, the rights of minors are more limited. Although the U.S. Supreme Court has not allowed states to prevent minors from having abortions, states can require minors who do not have parental consent for an abortion to seek consent from a court and to demonstrate that the abortion is in their best interest.

Currently, 37 states require some type of parental involvement in a minor's decision to have an abortion. Twenty-seven states require one or both parents to consent to the procedure, while 10 require that one or both parents be notified.

EMANCIPATED MINORS

Emancipation is the legal process or action of when a minor has achieved independence from his or her parents. Generally, this has been on the condition of a person reaching the age of 18, in most situations, and is free from the custody of his or her parents. They are now expected to support and care for themselves.

A minor may be emancipated by either express emancipation or implicit emancipation. *Express emancipation* occurs in a court order, such as voluntary emancipation by the minor's parents, an orphan turning 18 years of age, and constructive emancipation, which is a release from abusive or irresponsible parents. *Implicit emancipation* occurs when a minor reaches the age of majority, usually 18 years of age; gets married; leaves school or home; enlists in the military; is convicted as an adult; or cohabitates without parental consent.

Though emancipated minors are now able to participate in society as adults, many states have laws that limit their ability to engage in certain activities, such as labor contracts. In fact, violation of contractual law can result in minors having their emancipation revoked.

ETHICAL ISSUES IN ORGAN DONATION AND TRANSPLANTATION

Since the first successful organ transplant in 1954, the transplantation of organs and tissues has enabled thousands of individuals increased longevity by replacing diseased or damaged organs and tissues. The great need for organ transplants—with demand far exceeding available organs for the over 100,000 on the U.S. national transplant waiting list—has introduced issues surrounding the allocation of organs, and the meeting of this great need through issues of consent, dead donor determination, for-profit models of organ transplantation, organ trafficking and medical tourism, synthetic and artificial organs, xenotransplantation, the possibility of bioengineered and/or three-dimensional printed organs, and even the potential for fetal organ farming.

According to the United States Government Information on Organ Donation and Transplantation, as of 2021, more than 106,000 people are awaiting an organ transplant. **Organ transplantation** is the surgical process of removing an organ or tissue from one person and placing it in another. Organs that can be donated include the liver, kidney, pancreas, heart, and many others, with kidneys being the most transplanted and in the greatest need.

Currently, organ donation may come either from a deceased or living donor. Living donors are those individuals who are alive at the beginning of organ donation and are expected to be alive at the end. In most situations, living donors donate one organ, whereas one deceased donor can donate more than eight organs. However, even the number of cadaveric organs (from deceased donors) is currently unable to meet the demands that exist today.

Use of Deceased Donors

Individual may declare themselves an organ and tissue donor, for example, in a living will or driver's license, in the event of their death (Fig. 12.3). The decision to become a donor can be revoked at any time.

If a deceased individual is a potential donor candidate, an organ procurement organization (OPO) will usually be immediately contacted. If there was no instruction or refusal to donate organs or tissue, such as in a living will, the OPO may approach the family to discuss their wishes for making the deceased family member a potential donor. The family may specify which organ(s) may be donated.

Use of Living Donors

Although living organ donors are selected because they are healthy and alive after the donation, some have stated that living organ donation violates one of the prime tenets of medicine: *primer non nocere* or "first, do no harm." Although living donors are not physically better off after the donation, they can receive a psychological benefit from having helped a loved one or another person. However, living organ donation has the potential to do great harm. For example, the living donor is taking a risk of death from the operation, and, even if the donor survives the operation, long-term health outcomes may result from the operation or the loss of the organ in the future.

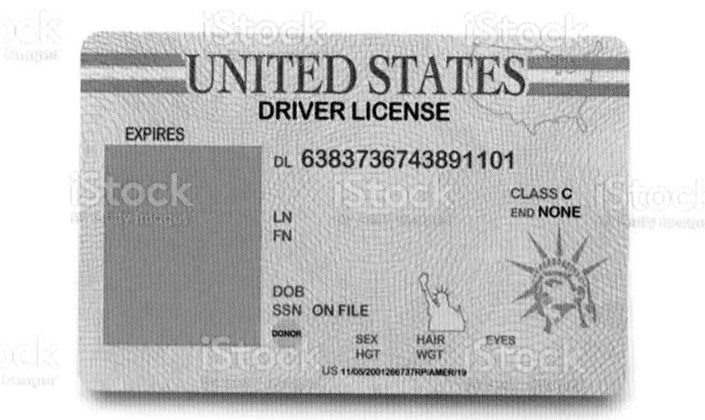

Fig. 12.3 Individuals may declare themselves an organ and tissue donor on their driver's license in the event of their death (https://www.governor.pa.gov/newsroom/wolf-administration-reminds-license-id-card-holders-that-organ-donation-can-save-lives/). (iStock.com/Michael Burrell.)

Financial Incentives

One of the most controversial issues is whether incentives—financial or otherwise—should be used to increase organ donation. Financial incentives in organ donation are any material gain or valuables obtained by those directly consenting to or involved in the organ donation process.

The field of organ donation and transplantation is well regulated. Both state and federal laws and regulations provide a safe and fair system for allocation, distribution, and transplantation of donated organs. In the United States, Congress passed the National Organ Transplant Act in 1984 and made offering organs for "valuable consideration" illegal despite several surveys finding that a majority of people are in favor of some sort of reimbursement. Opponents of incentives stress the possible risk to donors and the effect incentives might have on society's moral outlook. They cite harms such as coercion, misuse, and undermining dignity. Some individuals believe that providing financial incentives for organs causes the human body to be seen as a commodity, which contradicts some people's religious teachings and may be ethical and moral challenges.

However, those in favor of incentives point out that the current system is not functioning adequately, as demonstrated by the long waitlist for an organ and the increasing number of deaths because of the lack of supply of organs. Currently, more than 8000 people die each year from the lack of available organs for transplant. Some individuals favor regulated markets and maintain that a government-regulated system would prevent the concerns voiced by opponents. Those in favor of incentives claim those who are against having at least a trial of incentives are willing to see people on the waiting list die to preserve their own moral purity. Recently, the National Living Donor Assistance Center began providing assistance to individuals for travel and lodging but not for lost wages.

Organ Allocation

While a shortage of organs for transplantation exists, there will be a requirement that those organs be offered to patients on the waiting list. In 2015, the Organ

Procurement and Transplant Network/United Network for Organ Sharing provided a framework for regulating organ allocation policies. The three ethical principles that govern organ allocations policies are "utility (doing good and avoiding harm); justice; and respect for persons."

Utility refers to the maximization of the benefit to the community, which takes into consideration the amount of benefit that would be provided and the possible harm. In addition, it takes into consideration the probability of such benefit and harm. Justice refers to equity in the pattern of distribution of the benefits and burdens of an organ procurement and allocation program. Justice does not refer to treating all patients the same but does "require giving equal respect and concern to each patient." Factors to be considered in the application of justice include medical urgency, likelihood of finding an organ for transplant in the future, waiting list time, first vs. repeat transplant, age, and geography. Autonomy requires treating people with respect and recognition that they are "ends in themselves," not merely means.

Waiting Lists

Since 1984, the nonprofit United Network for Organ Sharing (UNOS) has operated under the National Organ Transplant Act, which established the Organ Procurement and Transplant Network, under a contract with the Division of Transplantation in the U.S. Department of Health and Human Services. UNOS maintains a central computer network containing the names of all patients waiting for kidney, heart, liver, lung, intestine, pancreas, and multiple-organ transplants.

Patients on the waiting list are in end-stage organ failure and have been evaluated by a transplant physician at hospitals where organ transplants are performed. In addition, policies are created and revised by committees composed of transplant physicians, government officials, donor families, transplant recipients, and members of the general public. Any proposed changes to the organ allocation rules are openly debated and published for public comment before being implemented.

Waiting list rules and guidelines vary by organ. General principles that guide the allocation of organs include a patient's medical urgency; blood, tissue, and size match with the donor; time on the waiting list; and proximity to the donor. Under certain circumstances, special allowances are made for children. For example, children younger than age 11 who need kidneys are automatically assigned preference. Factors such as a patient's income, celebrity status, gender, and race or ethnic background play no role in determining allocation of organs.

CONCLUSION

Healthcare professionals work with a variety of patients of different ages and needing different medical services. As part of providing patient care, there are many ethical aspects and legalities that must be managed. This includes providing and counseling patients on reproductive health, including family planning, contraception, and the need for an abortion. In many of these clinical situations, the healthcare professional may have to provide care to minors and it will be important to understand the ethical and legal responsibilities of confidentiality, consent, and when the rights of the minor patient or parents must be considered and followed.

CHAPTER REVIEW QUESTIONS

1. In vitro fertilization involves
   - **A.** use of a surrogate.
   - **B.** harvesting ova to mix with sperm and grow outside the uterus.
   - **C.** artificial insemination.
   - **D.** implantation of embryonic stem cells.
2. Which of the following allows a pharmacist to refuse to dispense oral contraceptives to a patient with a prescription based upon religious beliefs?
   - **A.** Conflict of interest
   - **B.** Conscience clause
   - **C.** Informed consent
   - **D.** *Primer non nocere*

3. All the following are ethical principles used in organ donation except
   A. confidentiality.
   B. justice.
   C. respect for the person.
   D. utility.
4. Which of the following factors is *not* taken into consideration when allocating organs?
   A. Patient's blood, tissue, and size match with the donor
   B. Patient's medical urgency
   C. Patient's time on the waiting list
   D. Patient's age and gender
5. Which of the following legal right does a husband have regarding the reproductive health services his wife receives from her healthcare provider?
   A. He has a legal right to know she is taking birth control pills.
   B. He has a legal right to know that she is seeking an abortion.
   C. He has a legal right to know she is using his sperm for in vitro fertilization.
   D. He has the legal right to know she is seeking a tubal ligation to prevent further pregnancies.
6. Which country had the first sterilization program?
   A. Germany
   B. United States
   C. China
   D. United Kingdom
7. Which legal case resulted in the legalization of abortion rights in 1973?
   A. *Planned Parenthood v. Casey*
   B. *Hobby Lobby v. Burwell*
   C. *Zubik v. Burwell*
   D. *Roe v. Wade*
8. An emancipated minor is all the following except
   A. a person who gets a job and helps pays bills while living with the parent.
   B. a person who enlists in the military
   C. a person who gets married.
   D. a person reaching the age of 18.
9. Which organ is the most transplanted and has the greatest need?
   A. Heart
   B. Kidney
   C. Liver
   D. Pancreas
10. Which of the following is *not* a type of assisted reproductive technology?
   A. Artificial insemination
   B. Surrogacy
   C. In vitro fertilization
   D. Mifepristone

SELF-REFLECTION QUESTIONS

1. What other factors do you think should be considered when allocating organs?
2. Do you think there are certain traits or genes that should be removed from the populations, such as those for diseases? What are some examples?
3. As a healthcare professional, should you be permitted to refuse to perform a medical procedure or service, such as an abortion or providing a teenager with contraceptives, if it is against your religious beliefs?
4. Should the donor's medical information be available to a child conceived through ART so that he or she knows his or her genetic background and any history of diseases?
5. Should the child be informed of any siblings to prevent marrying and conceiving with an unknown sibling?
6. Should genetic parents have visitation rights in the case of surrogacy?

INTERNET ACTIVITY

1. Research the controversy surrounding Nadya Suleman, who underwent fertility treatment and gave birth to octuplets. Did her medical team violate guidelines by implanting more than the generally accepted number of embryos?
2. Research compulsory sterilization programs in the 50 states at the following site: https://www.uvm.edu/~lkaelber/eugenics/. What programs existed in your state?
3. Research the history of women's reproductive rights and the passage of *Roe v. Wade*. What was Norma (Jane Roe) McCorvey's reason for filing a lawsuit?

BIBLIOGRAPHY

Abortion statistics. *United States data and trends*. Available from: http://www.nrlc.org/uploads/factsheets/FS01AbortionintheUS.pdf.

http://optn.transplant.hrsa.gov/policiesAndBylaws/nota.asp.

http://www.pbs.org/independentlens/blog/unwanted-sterilization-and-eugenics-programs-in-the-united-states/.

https://cdn.intechopen.com/pdfs-wm/52101.pdf.

https://law.justia.com/cases/new-jersey/supreme-court/1988/109-n-j-396-1.html.

https://www.organdonor.gov/legislation/index.html.

New York Times. (1988). *Opinion: "Justice for all in the baby M case,"*. New York Times. Available from: www.nytimes.com/1988/02/04/opinion/justice-for-all-in-the-baby-m-case.html.

Social Security Administration. *SI 01130.736 Payments to Victims from a State Eugenics Compensation Program*. https://secure.ssa.gov/POMS.NSF/lnx/0501130736.

The Center for Investigative Reporting. *Female inmates sterilized in California without approval. Available from.* https://www.revealnews.org/article/female-inmates-sterilized-in-california-prisons-without-approval/.

13

Death and Dying

CHAPTER OBJECTIVES

1. Define death and relate the process of dying.
2. Describe the stages of grief.
3. Discuss the different laws regarding end-of-life planning.
4. Define and differentiate the various types of advance directives.
5. Identify the functions of hospice.
6. Discuss the different types of euthanasia and the legal and ethical issues surrounding this issue.
7. Describe the criteria for determining death.

KEY TERMS

Active euthanasia The active acceleration of death by the use of drugs, whether by oneself or with the aid of a physician.

Advance directive The treatment preferences and designation of an alternate decision maker in the event that a person should become unable to make medical decisions on his or her own behalf.

Brain death The irreversible loss of function of the brain, including the brainstem.

Death The permanent cessation of all biological functions that sustain a living organism.

Do-not-resuscitate order (DNR order) Sometimes called a "No Code," it is a legal order written either in the hospital or on a legal form to communicate the wishes of a patient to not undergo CPR or advanced cardiac life support if the patient's heart stops or the patient stops breathing.

Durable power of attorney A type of advance medical directive in which legal documents provide the power of attorney to another person in the case of an incapacitating medical condition.

Euthanasia Termination of a life to eliminate pain and suffering related to a terminal illness, usually performed by giving a drug or agent to induce cessation of body functions. Also known as *assisted suicide*.

Healthcare proxy A legal document in which an individual designates another person to make healthcare decisions if he or she is rendered incapable of making his or her wishes known.

Hospice Organization or program involving a multidisciplinary group of medical professionals available to aid in support of the terminally ill and their families.

Involuntary euthanasia The active effort to end the life of a patient who has not explicitly requested aid in dying. This term is most often used with respect to patients who are in a persistent vegetative state and who probably will never recover consciousness.

Living will A document in which the patient states his or her wishes regarding medical treatment, especially treatment that sustains or prolongs life by extraordinary means, in the event that the patient becomes mentally incompetent or unable to communicate.

Nonvoluntary euthanasia Euthanasia conducted when the consent of the patient is unavailable, such as the patient is in a coma, is a young child or infant, has dementia, is severely mentally retarded, or has severe brain damage.

Passive euthanasia The act of allowing a patient to die without medical intervention.

Patient Self-Determination Act Federal law that requires all healthcare institutions receiving Medicare or Medicaid funds to provide patients with written information about their right under state law to execute advance directives. The written information must clearly state the institution's policies on withholding or withdrawing life-sustaining treatment.

Persistent vegetative state (PVS) Condition characterized by the irreversible cessation of higher brain functions, usually as a result of damage to the cerebral cortex.

Physician-assisted suicide The practice whereby a physician provides a potentially lethal medication to a terminally ill patient at his or her request to end life.

Physician orders for life-sustaining treatment (POLST) An approach to encourage healthcare providers to speak with patients to help create specific medical orders to be honored by healthcare professionals during a medical crisis.

Terminally ill Relating to an illness where regardless of the medical treatment, to a reasonable degree of certainty, will not lead to a restoration of health or will prolong the dying process.

Thanatology The study of the effects of death and dying, especially the investigation of ways to lessen the suffering and address the needs of the terminally ill and their survivors.

Uniform Determination of Death Act (UDDA) Model state legislation that has since been adopted by most U.S. states and is intended "to provide a comprehensive and medically sound basis for determining death in all situations."

Uniform Rights of the Terminally Ill Act Legislation that allows a person to declare a living will specifying that he or she does not wish to be kept alive through life support if terminally ill or in a coma.

Voluntary euthanasia Conscious medical act that results in the death of a patient who has given consent.

INTRODUCTION

Death and dying are an evitable part of life and, until recently, there were few options on how and when to die. End-of-life decisions were often limited to choosing for or against cardiopulmonary resuscitation (CPR) or other medical interventions to sustain life. In the last several decades, however, advances in medical knowledge and technology have provided and forced many more end-of-life decisions. With these decisions concerning the dying patient, many complex ethical and legal dilemmas arise that must be addressed.

This chapter discusses the various issues dying persons, their families, and healthcare professionals must consider regarding what kind of caregiver help and medical intervention a dying person wants or needs. Dying persons may have to make decisions about how much family involvement they want and who will be making decisions for them once they are unable to.

PROCESS OF DYING

The nature of death has for centuries been a topic within religious traditions, as well as of philosophical and scientific study. These approaches may include a belief in resurrection or reincarnation or the idea that consciousness simply ceases to exist. In fact, scientific interest has led to the development of the field of **thanatology**, which is devoted to the study of effects of death and dying. Thanatology examines the mechanisms of death and the psychological aspects of the grieving process and provides those studying thanatology with advanced and practical skills needed to provide compassionate care to those dealing with dying, death, and grief. It helps us answer such questions as: Why do we die? What happens after we die? How can we prolong life? How can we have a "good" death?

The definition and process of death and dying has changed over time. For example, death was once defined as the absence of a heartbeat and breathing. But the development of CPR and defibrillators have rendered that definition obsolete because breathing and heartbeat can sometimes be restarted and continue. Even without a functioning heart or lungs, life can sometimes be sustained with a combination of life-support devices, organ transplants, and artificial pacemakers.

Our understanding of the brain raises questions of what makes us human and alive. For example, patients who sustain damage to the cerebrum, which is the largest region of the brain, and are unconscious for at least 4 weeks are considered to be in a persistent vegetative state (PVS). It sometimes is confused with a coma, but comatose patients are never conscious. Patients in PVS may exhibit limited wakefulness, breathe on their own, have spontaneous body movements, blink and track objects with their eyes, and smile. Although these responses are reflexes and largely physical responses to stimuli, PVS is associated with varying degrees of consciousness.

The chances of recovery from a PVS to have some brain functions are possible but limited and, unfortunately, uncommon, particularly the longer the patient is in a PVS. At this point, the physician may recommend to the patient's family removing the patient from life support, unless a "do-not-resuscitate" (DNR) order is already in place, which will be discussed later in this chapter. Family members viewing a loved one in a PVS and in the process of dying can raise conflicting feelings regarding whether or not the person is truly "there" and "alive" and produce feelings of grief and emotional suffering.

COMMON CAUSES OF DEATH

According to the Centers for Disease Control and Prevention, in 2019, the 10 leading causes of death in the United States were:

- heart disease
- cancer
- unintentional injuries and accidents
- chronic lower respiratory disease
- stroke (cerebrovascular disease)
- Alzheimer's disease
- diabetes
- nephritis, nephrotic syndrome, and nephrosis
- influenza and pneumonia
- intentional self-harm (suicide).

With 7 of the top 10 causes of death being from chronic diseases, most patients diagnosed with a terminal illness are dying from and/or with one or more chronic disease and the associated symptoms for months to years before dying. In many chronic and progressive conditions, such as cancer, heart disease, or dementia, the symptoms become more intolerable and difficult to control as the disease progresses to an advanced stage. As a result, an end-stage illness can significantly impair a person's function.

In addition, aggressive treatments may offer little benefit while posing significant risk and jeopardizing the patient's quality of life and well-being. Thus, when there is no further cure or only limited treatment options to control the progression of the disease, hospice can offer support for patients and families.

GRIEF

An important aspect of thanatology is related to understanding how people respond to a terminal illness and grief. Grief is a natural response to any significant loss. It is the emotional suffering one feels when something or someone is taken away. Loss can be categorized as either physical or abstract. Physical loss is related to something that the individual can touch or measure, whereas other types of loss are abstract and relate to aspects of a person's social interactions.

One of the most cited models of grief is by psychologist Elisabeth Kübler-Ross in her book, *On Death and Dying*. Kübler-Ross proposed that both the individual, or patient, facing the reality of impending death and those who care about the person tend to experience a series of predictable emotions, often referred to as the "five stages of grief" (Fig. 13.1):

- **Denial**—Denial is often the first of the five stages of grief and is usually only a temporary defense for the patient. The patient may initially be unable to accept that his or her condition is terminal, and that death is inevitable. Denial assists an individual in coping and making survival possible. Denial allows an individual to measure feelings of grief. These feelings are generally replaced with heightened awareness of possessions and individuals who will be left behind after death.
- **Anger**—In the second stage, the patient recognizes that denial cannot continue. Anger can manifest itself in different ways. People can be angry with themselves or with others, especially those who are close to them. During the anger stage, the individual may feel deserted and abandoned.
- **Bargaining**—In the third stage, the patient hopes to somehow postpone or delay death. The patient may try to "negotiate" with a higher power for an extended life in exchange for a reformed lifestyle. During this stage, a patient wants life to return to its previous form.

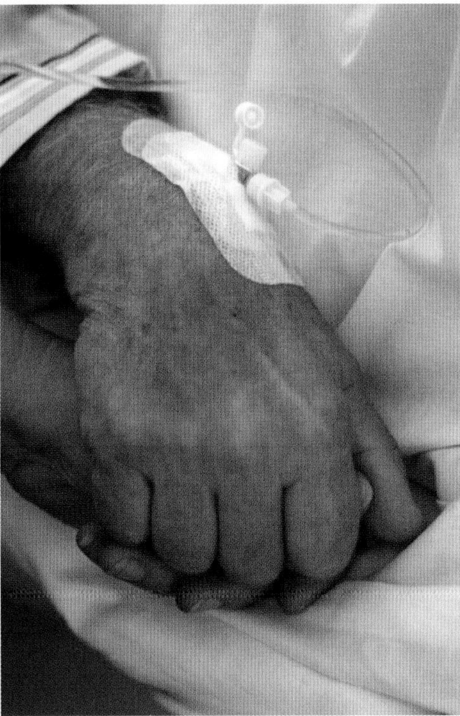

Fig. 13.1 Both the individual facing the reality of impending death, as well as those who care about the individual, tend to experience a series of predictable emotional "stages" of grief. (Copyright © Nina/Malyna/iStock/Thinkstock.com.)

- **Depression**—During the fourth stage, the patient begins to understand that death is imminent. As a result, the patient may become more isolated, refuse visitors, and spend more time crying and grieving. It is natural to feel sadness, regret, fear, and uncertainty when going through this stage. Although this stage is the most difficult for people, it is an essential and helpful process that allows the dying person to disconnect and make way for a sense of acceptance.
- **Acceptance**—In this last stage, the patient may begin to come to terms with his or her mortality. This stage varies according to the person's situation. The patient can enter this stage well before his or her family members.

Because reactions to personal losses of any kind are as unique as the person experiencing them, Kübler-Ross noted that these stages may occur in any order, the person may not experience all five stages of grief or may experience other emotions.

END-OF-LIFE PLANNING

Advancements in technology and medicine have enabled healthcare professionals to resuscitate patients in cardiac or respiratory arrest and maintain their life indefinitely with life-sustaining support measures. Not all patients wish for these measures to be taken, however. In 1985 the **Uniform Rights of the Terminally Ill Act** was enacted and authorized all adult patients the right to make decisions regarding life-sustaining treatment by executing a declaration instructing a physician to withhold or withdraw life-sustaining treatment in the event the person is in a terminal condition and is unable to participate in medical treatment decisions.

In addition, the Uniform Rights of the Terminally Ill Act authorizes the physician to withhold or withdraw life-sustaining treatment in the absence of a declaration on the consent of a close family member if the action would not conflict with the known intentions of the patient. In 1993 owing to state law variations, the Uniform Rights of the Terminally Ill Act was replaced with the Uniform Health-Care Decisions Act (UHCDA). The UHCDA allows an adult with capacity or an emancipated minor to give an oral or written instruction to a healthcare provider, which remains in force even after the individual loses capacity.

In 1990, the federal government passed the **Patient Self-Determination Act (PSDA)**, which mandates that hospitals, nursing homes, hospice providers, and other healthcare agencies that receive Medicare or Medicaid funds provide written information to patients regarding their rights to make medical decisions and execute advance directives. Patients are given written notice on admission to the healthcare facility of their decision-making rights, and policies regarding advance directives in their state and in the facility where they have been admitted. The PSDA also requires healthcare facilities to maintain written policies and procedures with respect to advance directives; document in the patient's medical record whether or not the patient has executed an advance healthcare directive; and educate their staff and the communities they serve about state law governing advance directives. According to the PSDA, patient rights include the following:

- The right to facilitate their own healthcare decisions
- The right to accept or refuse medical treatment
- The right to make an advance healthcare directive

Advance Directives

Advance directives, also commonly referred to as *advance medical directives* or *advance healthcare directives,* are usually written documents detailing the treatment preferences and designation of an alternate decision maker in the event that a person should become unable to make medical decisions on his or her own behalf. Advance directives are designed to outline a person's wishes and preferences in regard to medical treatments and interventions, and to identify a potential **healthcare proxy**—that is, an individual the person authorizes to act on the patient's behalf to make decisions consistent with and based on the patient's stated will, in case the person becomes incapacitated or unable to communicate. Often, drafting a proper advance directive form may require assistance from a physician and/or an attorney, especially because advance directive policies may differ from one state to another.

An individual with an advance directive should keep the original copies of his or her advance directives where they can be easily found. The individual should also provide a copy of the advance directive to his or her healthcare proxy, healthcare providers, hospital, nursing home, and family and friends. It is recommended that the advance directive be reviewed annually. Healthcare providers and facilities are not allowed to discriminate based on whether patients have an advance directive or not. It is also important to note that an individual's wishes expressed in an advance directive supersede those of the family or significant other.

Advance directives generally fall into two main categories: a living will and a durable power of attorney.

Living Will

A **living will** is a written document that specifies what types of medical treatment are desired should the individual become incapacitated, permanently unconscious, or cannot make your own decisions about emergency treatment. A living will can be general or very specific. For example, a statement in a living will may include: "If I suffer an incurable, irreversible illness, disease, or condition and my attending physician determines that my condition is terminal, I direct that life-sustaining measures that would serve only to prolong my death be withheld or discontinued."

More specific living wills may include information regarding an individual's desire for services, such as the following:

- Analgesia (pain relief)
- Antibiotics and antivirals
- Artificial hydration (intravenous or IV)
- Artificial feeding (feeding tube)
- Cardiopulmonary resuscitation (CPR)
- Life-support equipment and procedures, including ventilators and dialysis
- Organ donations
- Do-not-resuscitate (DNR) order

Durable Power of Attorney

A **durable power of attorney (DPOA)** is a type of advance directive that provides the power of attorney to others in the case of an incapacitating medical condition. A DPOA can also specifically designate different individuals to act on a person's behalf for specific affairs. For example, one individual can be designated the DPOA of healthcare or medical power of attorney, similar to a healthcare proxy, whereas another individual can be made the DPOA for finance.

For example, the DPOA for finance is the one who needs to pay for the healthcare services. The DPOA for finance allows an individual who has been appointed to act in a person's place for financial purposes when and if the person becomes incapacitated by allowing the individual to make bank transactions, sign Social Security checks, apply for disability, or write checks to pay bills.

Healthcare Proxy

A **healthcare proxy**, sometimes called a durable power of attorney for health care, is a legal document in which an individual designates another person to make healthcare decisions, if he or she is rendered incapable of making his or her wishes known. An individual does not have to be terminally ill for a healthcare proxy to go into effect. The healthcare proxy communicates the same rights to request or refuse treatment that the individual would have if capable of making and communicating these decisions. The healthcare proxy is legally authorized to make a wide range of healthcare decisions, such as:

- admitting or discharging the person from a hospital or nursing home,
- determining treatments or medicines the person does or does not want to receive, and
- who has accessibility to the person's medical records.

If an individual does not designate a healthcare proxy and cannot make healthcare decisions, state law often appoints an individual who can make decisions on the individual's behalf, including (in order of priority):

- court-appointed guardian or conservator,
- spouse or domestic partner,
- adult child,
- adult sibling,
- close friend, and
- nearest living relative.

Do Not Resuscitate

Another common type of advance directive is a do-not-resuscitate order (DNR order), sometimes called a "No Code," is a legal order written either in the hospital or on a legal form to communicate the wishes of a patient to not undergo CPR or advanced cardiac life support if the patient's heart stops or the patient stops breathing.

This introduces an important distinction. How does a DNR order differ from a living will or other types of advance directives? It is a matter of authorization. Advance directives and living wills are documents written by individuals themselves to state their wishes for care if they are no longer able to communicate their wishes. In contrast, it is a physician or hospital staff member who is authorized to write a DNR order based on the wishes previously expressed by the patient in his or her advance directive or living will. Likewise, if the patient is unable to express his or her wishes but has previously used a healthcare proxy, the physician can write such a DNR order at the request of the alternate decision maker. Furthermore, a DNR order does not affect any treatment other than that which would require intubation or CPR. Patients who have a DNR order can continue to get chemotherapy, antibiotics, dialysis, or any other life-sustaining treatments.

Physician Orders for Life-Sustaining Treatment

Many states offer programs that address a range of emergency life-sustaining treatments, including CPR, for people with advanced illness. These programs are commonly called Physician Orders for Life-Sustaining Treatment (POLST) and are used in many healthcare settings. POLST, sometimes called Medical Orders for Life-Sustaining treatment (MOLST) depending on the state, involves a physician-initiated discussion and shared decision-making process with patient with advanced or terminal illnesses. It results in a set of medical orders written by the physician that adheres to a patient's goal of care and wishes in regard to the use of CPR, artificial nutrition, hydration, hospitalizing, ventilation, intensive care, and other medical interventions.

POLST began in 1991 in Oregon and is now currently used in 42 states. POLST encourages healthcare providers to speak with patients to help create specific medical orders to be honored by healthcare professionals during a medical crisis. Thus, in a medical crisis, emergency medical technicians and other healthcare professionals should first follow POLST.

APPLY THIS

You witness a comatose patient's family member tell the attending physician that the family wishes the patient to be a "DNR." You do not know if the patient has a living will on file or if the patient has a healthcare proxy naming this family member his or her decision maker.

1. What should you do?
2. How would you explain what a DNR and a healthcare proxy are?

Hospice Care

Another end-of-life decision may be the use of hospice care. Some people have the mistaken notion that hospice is used to hasten or prolong death. But, in fact, hospice is an organization or program involving a multidisciplinary group of medical professionals available to aid in support of the terminally ill patient and their families. Hospice is, more accurately, a service that provides palliative care for patients in the late stages of a terminal illness (Fig. 13.2). Patients and families who transfer into hospice find themselves served by a healthcare team who focuses on providing a peaceful, symptom-free, and dignified transition to death for patients whose diseases are advanced beyond a cure or treatment. The focus of hospice care is then on improving the quality of life and one free of pain and suffering rather than on its length.

A hospice team often consists of physicians; nurses; social workers; clerics; volunteers; and speech, physical, and occupational therapists, who work together with the common goal to provide comfort, reduce suffering, and preserve patient dignity to terminally ill patients and

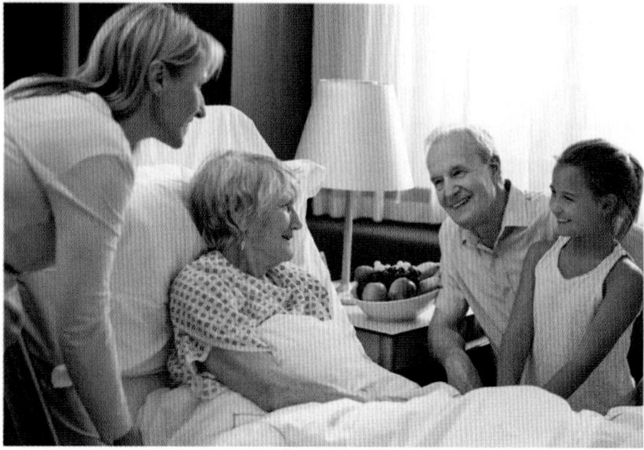

Fig. 13.2 Hospice care provides support for both patients and their loved ones. (Copyright © monkeybusinessimages/iStock/Thinkstock.com.)

their families and caregivers. The complex care of hospice patients may include the following:

- Managing evolving medical issues (e.g., infections, medication management, pressure ulcers, hydration, nutrition, physical stages of dying)
- Treating physical symptoms (e.g., pain, shortness of breath, anxiety, nausea, vomiting, constipation, confusion)
- Counseling about the anxiety, uncertainty, grief, and fear associated with end of life and dying
- Dietary counseling
- Rendering support to patients, their families, and caregivers with the overwhelming physical and psychological stresses of a terminal illness
- Guiding patients and families through the difficult interpersonal and psychosocial issues and helping them with finding closure
- Paying attention to personal, religious, spiritual, and cultural values
- Assisting patients and families reaching financial closures (living will, trust, advance directive, funeral arrangements)
- Providing bereavement counseling to the mourning loved ones after the death of the patient
- More and more patients and their families are choosing hospice as an end-of-life care, especially with Medicare, Medicaid, and most private insurance carriers providing hospice benefits. Medicare hospice benefits also include pharmaceuticals, medical equipment, social services, chaplain visits, 24/7 access to nursing care, and grief support after a death.

APPLY THIS

An important role of medical assistants in health care is to provide patient education. Jeanette has been a medical assistant at an internal medicine clinic for 7 years with Dr. Willet. The medical office serves mainly older high-risk patients; therefore, it is customary practice to discuss and educate patients on the importance of advance directives, living will, and power of attorney.

At the request of Dr. Willet, Jeanette is asked to temporarily assist at Glendale Summit Medical Clinic, where the patient population is different from that at Jeanette's current medical clinic. Here, many of the patients are much younger, and a significant number are from lower socioeconomic backgrounds. Jeanette relishes this change and is enthusiastic about expanding her experience working with this new patient population. At the request of the office manager, Jeanette assists in auditing patient charts. She notices many patients do not have advance directives on file.

1. Should Jeanette be concerned about this? Why or why not?
2. How should Jeanette approach this concern? And with whom?
3. What should Jeanette include as part of the advance directive?

EUTHANASIA

As we discuss the ability of having a "good death," **euthanasia** is the Greek term meaning "good death" and refers to the practice of intentionally ending a life in order to relieve pain and suffering through medical means. It is important to note that the word "intentionally" is key to the definition of euthanasia. Although this definition may seem similar to premeditated murder—the ending of a life—the important difference lies in the reasoning behind the intent: to relieve pain and suffering.

Euthanasia may be classified according to whether a person gives informed consent as: voluntary, nonvoluntary, or involuntary.

- **Voluntary euthanasia**: Euthanasia conducted with the consent and participation of the patient. In cases of voluntary euthanasia, the patient may ask for assistance in dying, may refuse treatment or medication, ask for medical treatment or life support machines to be switched off, or refuse to eat in order to hasten death. Voluntary euthanasia is legal in some countries and several states in the United States.

- **Nonvoluntary euthanasia**: Euthanasia conducted when the consent of the patient is unavailable, such as the patient is in a coma, is a young child or infant, has dementia, is severely intellectually disabled, or has severe brain damage. This term is most often used with respect to patients who are in a PVS and who probably will never recover consciousness.
- **Involuntary euthanasia**: Euthanasia conducted against the wishes of the patient or the patient's surrogate decision maker. Involuntary euthanasia would be performed on a person who would be able to provide informed consent, but does not, because he or she does not want to die or because he or she was not asked. Involuntary euthanasia is widely opposed and is regarded as a crime in all legal jurisdictions.

Passive and Active Euthanasia

Voluntary, nonvoluntary, and involuntary euthanasia can all be further divided into passive or active. **Passive euthanasia** entails the withholding of common life-sustaining treatments. Examples of passive euthanasia include discontinuing life-support machines, disconnecting a feeding tube, or not carrying out a life-extending operation. Passive euthanasia ensures that the patient dies "naturally." **Active euthanasia** is much more controversial and entails the conscious use of lethal substances or forces, such as administering a lethal injection, to end a patient's life, whether by the patient or someone else. Whereas passive euthanasia results in the omission of an act, active euthanasia is brought about by commission of an act.

Death With Dignity Acts and Physician-Assisted Suicide

Euthanasia that is conducted in the presence of or with the cooperation of a physician is termed ***physician-assisted suicide***. Physician-assisted suicide refers to the practice whereby a physician provides a potentially lethal medication to a terminally ill patient at his or her request to end life. Unlike euthanasia, which is the act of ending a life in order to end a person's suffering, physician-assisted suicide has legal authorization.

Death with Dignity laws, also known as *physician-assisted dying* or *aid-in-dying laws*, stem from the basic idea that it is the terminally ill people who should be the sole decision makers in end-of-life decisions and determine how much pain and suffering they should endure, not governments, politicians, or religious leaders. Death with Dignity statutes allow mentally competent adult state residents who have a terminal illness with a confirmed prognosis of having 6 or fewer months to live to voluntarily request and receive a prescription medication to hasten their imminent deaths.

Currently, Death with Dignity laws exist in 10 states or jurisdictions (Box 13.1). In these states with Death with Dignity laws, physicians cannot be prosecuted for

DISCUSSION

In 1973, Donald "Dax" Cowart was severely burned by an accidental propane explosion while trying to start his car. He was unaware that a propane pipeline ran beneath the dry riverbed where he was parked and that it was leaking. Coward was able to pull himself from the car and ran for help. He ran for a half-mile before encountering a farmer and the farmer's nephew, who ran to call an ambulance.

Cowart lost both of his hands and most of his face, suffered significant hearing loss, and had significant scarring over most of his body due to burns. After 14 months of hospitalization, he was released into his mother's care. The burns disabled Cowart and he plead to be allowed to die. Physicians did not honor his request and forced treatment on him. Cowart's mother wanted him to continue treatment, believing he would change his mind with time and treatment. He endured years of depression and severe sleep problems. He twice attempted suicide.

Though he went on to marry, graduated from Texas Tech University in 1986 with a law degree, and practiced personal injury law, he still believed he should have been allowed to refuse treatment and be allowed to die. Cowart became a fierce advocate for patients' rights and autonomy and against medical paternalism. He died in 2019 from complication from leukemia and liver cancer.

1. What legal and ethical issues that are involved in this case?
2. Should the physicians feel justified in not honoring Cowart's request to die since he was later able to live a fairly fulfilling life? Even considering Coward suffered from depression and attempted suicide twice?
3. What is medical paternalism? Are there current examples of this?

Source: Gerrek, M. L. (2018). Getting past Dax. *AMA Journal of Ethics, 20*(6), 581–588. https://doi.org/10.1001/journalofethics.2018.20.6.mhst1-1806.

BOX 13.1 Current Death with Dignity Laws

- California (End of Life Option Act; approved in 2015, in effect from 2016)
- Colorado (End of Life Options Act; 2016)
- District of Columbia (D.C. Death with Dignity Act; 2016/2017)
- Hawaii (Our Care, Our Choice Act; 2018/2019)
- Maine (Death with Dignity Act; 2019)
- New Jersey (Aid in Dying for the Terminally Ill Act; 2019)
- New Mexico (Elizabeth Whitefield End of Life Options Act; 2021)
- Oregon (Death with Dignity Act; 1994/1997)
- Vermont (Patient Choice and Control at the End of Life Act; 2013)
- Washington (Death with Dignity Act; 2008)

prescribing medications to hasten an individual's death as long as the individual resides in the state.

Ethical and Legal Considerations in Euthanasia

The topic of euthanasia is extremely controversial, and there are numerous arguments on both sides of the issue. Over the years, there have been a number of political and social movements, organizations, studies, articles, campaigns, books, speeches, and even films dedicated to this issue, and yet it remains controversial and unresolved.

There have been many legal cases for and against euthanasia. The next section will discuss the most pivotal and landmark court decisions that have had a significant effect on the issues of euthanasia, right to die, and advance directives. These court decisions continue to be controversial and are still the subject of much debate. However, they have laid much of the legal framework courts and lawmakers use in making many end-of-life decisions.

Karen Ann Quinlan

In 1976, the court case of Karen Ann Quinlan was an important precedent in the history of the right-to-die issue in the United States. At the age of 21, Quinlan became unconscious after arriving home after a party. After she collapsed and stopped breathing twice for more than 15 min, she was rushed to the hospital, where she lapsed into a PVS. She was kept alive on a ventilator for several months but showed no improvement. Her parents requested that her physicians and the hospital discontinue active care and allow her to die. Quinlan's physicians refused because they thought removing life-sustaining treatment was the equivalent of murder. They felt they had an inherent duty to protect life and specifically to keep Ms. Quinlan alive.

The court case eventually made it to the New Jersey Supreme Court, which ruled in her parents' favor and request to discontinue the ventilator. The court found that families are adequate surrogates for incapacitated patients who did not and could not make their wishes known. Although Quinlan was removed from a ventilator in 1976, she continued to survive in a PVS and on a feeding tube for almost a decade until her death from pneumonia in 1985.

Quinlan's case continues to raise important questions in bioethics, euthanasia, and legal guardianship. Specifically, two significant outcomes arose from her case: (1) the development of formal ethics committees in hospitals, nursing homes, and hospices; and (2) the development of advance directives.

Nancy Cruzan

In 1983, Nancy Cruzan lost control of her car and was thrown 35 ft. from her car, where she landed face down in a water-filled ditch. Paramedics found her with no vital signs but were able to resuscitate her. Although Cruzan was able to breathe without the aid of a ventilator, she remained in a coma for several weeks and was diagnosed as being in a PVS. After 4 years, her parents requested to have her feeding tube removed so that she might be allowed to die. However, Cruzan's physicians refused the request, with the Missouri Governor and Missouri Supreme Court siding with the physicians.

Cruzan's parents' petition went before the U.S. Supreme Court, which allowed the parents to authorize the withdrawal of the feeding tube and allow their daughter to die. Cruzan died 11 days later on December 26, 1990, at the age of 25 years.

Terri Schiavo

One of the most recent and controversial "right-to-die" cases is that of Terri Schiavo. In 1990 at the age of 27 years old, Schiavo had a cardiac arrest. Schiavo's husband found her unconscious, and she was not breathing and had no pulse. She had suffered massive brain damage due to a lack of oxygen and remained in a coma for more than 2 months before her diagnosis was changed to PVS. The court appointed Schiavo's husband, Michael, as her legal guardian, with no objections from Schiavo's parents.

After several years of unsuccessful rehabilitation and experimental therapies, in 1998, Schiavo's husband petitioned the courts to remove her feeding tube. Without a living will, he believed Schiavo would not want to be kept alive in a PVS, which her parents opposed. The Schiavo case involved 14 appeals and numerous motions, petitions, and hearings in the Florida courts, and 5 suits in federal district court. In 2005 a judge ordered the removal of Schiavo's feeding tube, and she died 2 weeks later at the age of 41 years.

DISCUSSION

Jack Kevorkian was a retired pathologist and an advocate for physician-assisted suicide. Between 1990 and 1998, Kevorkian assisted in the suicide of a reported 130 people; most were terminally ill and diagnosed as having less than 6 months to live or were disabled or chronically ill. Despite being arrested and tried multiple times, Kevorkian was acquitted, usually because of the absence of existing laws against assisted suicide. However, in 1998 the Michigan legislature enacted a law making assisted suicide a felony punishable by a maximum 5-year prison sentence or a $10,000 fine. Yet Kevorkian continued to provide assisted suicide for patients. In 1999 a jury in Oakland County, Michigan, convicted Kevorkian of second-degree murder and the illegal delivery of a controlled substance, and he was sentenced to 10–25 years in prison with the possibility of parole.

During the next 3 years, Kevorkian attempted to appeal, including to the U.S. Supreme Court, but his request was refused. In 2007 after serving a little more than 8 years of his sentence, Kevorkian was released from prison on good behavior and, on the condition, he would not assist in any more suicides. Kevorkian once said of his work: "My aim in helping the patient was not to cause death. My aim was to end suffering. It's got to be decriminalized." Kevorkian died in 2011 at the age of 83.

1. Were Kevorkian's actions ethically or legally wrong? Or both?
2. Did Kevorkian commit a crime even if there were no laws against assisted suicide?

DETERMINATION OF DEATH

Healthcare professionals will often use the terms "brain death" or "biological death" to define when a person is dead. However, as mentioned earlier, what constitutes life and death has changed as a result of medical advances, changing legal and ethical boundaries and societal norms. So, with such increasing complexity and a changing environment, how does a physician determine the moment of death? How is brain death determined? In general, **death** is defined as the permanent ending of all biological functions that sustain a living organism. But the determination of **brain death** can be complicated. For example, in the past, it was presumed that, if there was no electrical activity in the brain, it indicated the end of consciousness and death. Electroencephalogram (EEG) studies, however, have shown spurious electrical impulses in unconscious patients, including those in certain sleep stages, coma, hypoxia, hyperthermia, hypoglycemia, and with certain drugs. As a result, what constitutes death must be in accordance with accepted medical standards.

To provide physicians and other healthcare professionals with a more consistent definition and guideline for the determination of death, the **Uniform Determination of Death Act (UDDA)** was approved in 1981. The UDDA is a draft state law created by the Uniform Law Commission, also known as the *National Conference of Commissioners on Uniform State Law*, which provides nonpartisan, draft legislation to state statutory laws to promote uniformity among the states. The UDDA has been approved by both the American Medical Association and the American Bar Association and has been adopted by all states and the District of Columbia, with several states having additional regulations in the determination of death.

The UDDA provides a more legal definition and determination of death based on (1) irreversible cessation of circulatory and respiratory functions or (2) irreversible cessation of all functions of the entire brain, including the brainstem.

Unlike PVS, brain death is the irreversible loss of all functions of the brain; this includes the brainstem, which controls breathing and other vital functions. The diagnosis of brain death is based on three main components:

- Coma: The patient should be completely unresponsive and unconscious, usually tested with painful stimuli.
- Absence of brainstem reflexes: The patient should be unresponsive to stimuli that otherwise would trigger an involuntary response, such as dilation of the pupils in the presence of a bright light.
- Apnea test: The patient, when disconnected from a respirator, should not have respiratory movements and will show other measurable signs supporting the diagnosis of brain death, such as no coughing or gagging reflexes, blinking reflexes, or grimace reflexes.

Based on the UDDA guidelines, if the patient is diagnosed as brain dead, he or she will be declared clinically and legally dead. Being able to define death as outlined by the UDDA is pertinent for many different legal situations, such as the following:

- Organ donation: The declaration of brain death is necessary before an individual's organs can be removed and donated to another individual.
- Criminal cases: The law requires a legal declaration of death before prosecutors may indict a defendant with homicide.
- Tort action: A wrongful death malpractice lawsuit cannot be brought without a declaration of an individual's death.
- Estate law: An individual may not inherit an individual's estate without a declaration of death.
- Life insurance: Determination of death allows the disbursement of life insurance funds to the beneficiaries.

CONCLUSION

Issues surrounding death and dying are numerous and complex. Although some of the more controversial aspects of responding medically to the dying are likely never to be completely resolved completely, the increasing dialogue on such issues is helping us all to think more consciously about and become more sensitive to the rights and needs of both dying patients and those who will care for and grieve for them.

CHAPTER REVIEW QUESTIONS

1. DNR stands for
   A. Do Not Revive.
   B. Do Not Repeat.
   C. Do Not Restrict.
   D. Do Not Resuscitate.
2. Which advance directive allows a person to designate another person to make healthcare decisions if he or she is rendered incapable of making his or her wishes known?
   A. Living will
   B. Durable power of attorney
   C. Healthcare proxy
   D. DNR
3. The law mandating that hospitals, nursing homes, hospice providers, and other healthcare agencies provide written information to patients regarding their rights to make medical decisions and execute advance directives is called the
   A. Uniform Determination of Death Act.
   B. Durable Power of Attorney.
   C. Patient Self-Determination Act.
   D. Uniform Rights of the Terminally Ill Act.
4. The __________ states that all patients have the right to create a living will to make their wishes known in the event they are incapacitated, as well as to designate alternate decision makers through a healthcare proxy or durable power of attorney.
   A. Uniform Determination of Death Act
   B. Durable Power of Attorney
   C. Patient Self-Determination Act
   D. Uniform Rights of the Terminally Ill Act
5. Which piece of legislation precipitated the enactment of the Uniform Health-Care Decisions Act (UHCDA)?
   A. Uniform Determination of Death Act
   B. Durable Power of Attorney
   C. Patient Self-Determination Act
   D. Uniform Rights of the Terminally Ill Act
6. An individual who has executed a DNR order typically would not receive
   A. chemotherapy.
   B. antibiotics.
   C. IV fluids.
   D. CPR.
7. A __________ is a form of advance directive that specifies what types of medical treatment are desired should the individual become incapacitated.
   A. living will
   B. healthcare proxy
   C. durable power of attorney
   D. DNR
8. Turning off a life-support machine is an example of
   A. active euthanasia.
   B. involuntary euthanasia.
   C. passive euthanasia.
   D. All the above

9. The advance directive used to designate an individual(s) to act on a person's behalf to make medical decisions and carry out the patient's wishes is the:
   A. POLST.
   B. living will.
   C. DPOA.
   D. DNR order.

10. Which of the following is not true of the Uniform Determination of Death Act (UDDA)?
    A. It is recognized by all states and the District of Columbia.
    B. It provides the legal definition and determination of death.
    C. It determines death based only on the irreversible cessation of brain activity.
    D. It determines death based on the patient being in a persistent vegetative state (PVS) for more than 4 weeks.

SELF-REFLECTION QUESTIONS

1. Should a patient who is suicidal be allowed to refuse treatments to artificially sustain life (e.g., inserting a feeding tube)?
2. Think about a time that you experienced a loss. Looking back, did you go through all five stages of grief? Describe how you handled each stage.
3. Do you or any of your family members have advance directives? If so, do you know what they are or what your family's wishes would be?
4. As a part of your role in patient education, what information would you supply the patient regarding advance directives?

INTERNET ACTIVITIES

1. Visit https://www.medicare.gov/what-medicare-covers/part-a/how-hospice-works.html. List three questions you should ask when deciding which hospice program is right for you or a family member.
2. Go to https://www.helpguide.org/mental/grief_loss.htm. What are three tips to help someone cope with grief?
3. Research a state with a Death with Dignity Law. What conditions must be met in order to allow for a physician-assisted suicide?

ADDITIONAL RESOURCES

https://www.medicare.gov/manage-your-health/advance-directives/advance-directives-and-long-term-care.html.

https://www.medicareinteractive.org/get-answers/caring-for-yourself-or-a-loved-one-with-medicare/preparing-for-your-future-health-care-needs/health-care-proxies.

https://www.cms.gov/Outreach-and-Education/Medicare-Learning-Network-MLN/MLNProducts/Downloads/AdvanceCarePlanning.pdf.

https://www.gpo.gov/fdsys/pkg/GAOREPORTS-HEHS-95-135/pdf/GAOREPORTS-HEHS-95-135.pdf.

BIBLIOGRAPHY

U.S. Department of Health and Human Services. (2016). *Health, United States*. Available from https://www.cdc.gov/nchs/data/hus/hus16.pdf#019.

Centers for Disease Control and Prevention, Leading Causes of Death. (2019). https://www.cdc.gov/nchs/fastats/leading-causes-of-death.htm.

Cruzan V., Missouri Dept. of Health, 497 U.S. 261 (Mo. 1990).

'Jacob Jack' Kevorkian dies; death with dignity proponent remembered. (2011). Available from medicalnewstoday.com (last update).

Kübler-Ross, E. (1968). *On death and dying*. New York: Routledge.

Kübler-Ross, E. (2005). *On grief and grieving: finding the meaning of grief through the five stages of loss*. New York: Simon & Schuster.

In re Quinlan, 70 N.J. 10, 355 A.2d 647 (N.J. 1976).

14

Key Trends in Healthcare Law and Ethics

CHAPTER OBJECTIVES

1. Discuss the role of public health in the United States
2. Describe the history of vaccine mandates in the United States
3. Discuss the different legal cases supporting and against vaccine mandates
4. Describe the different exemption laws for vaccine mandates
5. Explain the difference between sex, gender identity, and gender expression
6. Discuss the obstacles to healthcare access for transgender and gender nonconforming people

KEY TERMS

Epidemic An outbreak that affects many people at one time and can spread through one or several communities.

Gender Refers to the various socially constructed roles, behaviors, expressions and identities of girls, women, boys, men, and gender-diverse people.

Gender expression Refers to how people present their gender on the outside, often through behavior, clothing, hairstyle, voice, or body characteristics.

Gender ID data Information that includes gender identification, birth-assigned sex, legal sex, preferred name, and legal name.

Gender identity Refers to one's internal knowledge of one's gender, such as being a man, a woman, or another gender.

Gender nonconforming (GNC) Refers to a gender identity—one's personal and subjective sense of gender—that is neither male nor female. It can also refer to a gender expression characterized by mannerisms and behaviors that are not conventionally associated with an assigned gender.

Mandate An order or requirement an executive body given by the legislature in a state of emergency.

Medical exemptions A request to not receive a state mandated vaccine due to believing that the vaccine would not be safe for themselves or their child.

Pandemic An outbreak that affects many people at one time and the spread is global.

Parens patriae The doctrine in which the state exerts authority over child welfare.

Philosophical exemptions Also called personal exemptions, an exemption based on individuals or parents' personal beliefs about vaccines, such as vaccine safety.

Public health The science of protecting and improving the health of people and their communities, achieved by promoting healthy lifestyles; researching disease and injury prevention; and detecting, preventing, and responding to infectious diseases.

Quarantine A state, period, or place of isolation in which people or animals that have arrived from elsewhere or been exposed to infectious or contagious disease are placed.

Religious exemption laws Also called "Religious Freedom Restoration Acts" or RFRAs, permit people, churches, non-profit organizations, and sometimes corporations to seek exemptions from state laws that burden their religious beliefs.

Transgender A broad term that can be used to describe people whose gender identity is different from the gender they were thought to be when they were born; "trans" is often used as shorthand for transgender.

INTRODUCTION

Few industries face as much change and fluctuations as the healthcare industry. As we have discussed throughout this book, there are various laws, standards, codes, and ethics that help to regulate the practice of health care and healthcare professionals. However, these laws, standards, and codes are not static but are ever changing and reflect the health care needs of the population and the evolving political, social, and economic environment.

The healthcare industry must adapt to these internal and external forces and influences. In some cases, they may be controversial for both healthcare professionals and the public. Regardless, they are occurring, and the laws and ethics must adapt and be prepared to address and meet these changes. Some of the issues the healthcare industry is currently facing are the legal duty and authorization of governments to manage public health and health mandates. COVID-19 has dominated much of the news in the last few years. It has impacted almost every industry, especially health care, and the economy worldwide, and it has resulted in many deaths since the first documented case in Wuhan, China.

Another topic for the legal and healthcare community is the expanding awareness of people who are transgender or gender nonconforming and how this affects their health care. What are the existing laws to protect them from discrimination? What role does the healthcare community have and what actions need to be taken to provide equitable and appropriate patient care?

PUBLIC HEALTH AND VACCINE MANDATES

It would be difficult to discuss the impact on the healthcare system and, in fact, the world in the last few years without discussing the COVID-19 pandemic (Box 14.1). The coronavirus disease 2019 (COVID-19), is a disease caused by a novel (or new) coronavirus that had not previously been seen in humans. The first documented cases of COVID were in Wuhan, China, with as many as 59 cases at this point, and additional cases being reported in Thailand and Japan. The first confirmed case of COVID-19 in the United States was on January 21, 2020, in Washington State in a patient who had recently returned from Wuhan, China. On January 31, 2020, with a worldwide death toll of more than 200 and an exponential jump to more than 9800 cases, the World Health Organization (WHO), an international public health agency of the United Nations, declared a public health emergency, for just the sixth time in its history. Three days later, the United States declares a public health emergency due to the coronavirus outbreak.

BOX 14.1 Disease Occurrence

- **Endemic**—describes a disease that is present permanently in a region or population
- **Epidemic**—is an outbreak that affects many people at one time and can spread through one or several communities
- **Pandemic**—is the term used to describe an epidemic when the spread is global.

As the scientific and medical community learned more about the virus and its mode of transmission, several public health measures and initiatives were put into place to combat the spread of the disease. This included travel restrictions and bans on non-essential travel and on countries with high rates of COVID infections. States issued stay-at-home orders and mandates; ordered business closures; limited large gathering and close contact with people who they did not live with or with anyone who is sick; mask mandates or face covering over the nose and mouth in public settings mandates; and vaccine mandates.

With development of effective vaccines against the coronavirus, President Joe Biden announced two sweeping vaccine mandates to control the spread of the disease. These mandates would apply to more than 100 million Americans.

Despite these broad measures, as of December 2021, the cases of COVID continue to rise with more than 51.3 million cases and 808,000 deaths due to COVID. These mixed results and the United States' struggle with controlling the COVID pandemic has been largely due to conflicting responses and the legal battle between federal and state governments over who has authority to enforce public health mandates and their role in protecting their citizens. There have been protests, objections, and legal lawsuits against these mandates and the different measures to control disease transmission saying that the federal government is overreaching and that these measures are unconstitutional and even unethical. In some cases, these protests and objections have led states to grant religious and philosophical exemptions from such mandates.

Public backlash against vaccine requirements is not a new phenomenon and has a long history in this country. However, governments have a long history of mandating vaccines to curb transmission of infectious diseases with several landmark Supreme Court cases upholding this authority and that public health takes precedence.

PUBLIC HEALTH'S ROLE IN DISEASE CONTROL

Public health has long played a critical role in ensuring and maintaining the health of communities and populations. Public health is the science of protecting and improving the health of people and their communities. This is achieved by promoting healthy lifestyles; researching disease and injury prevention; and detecting, preventing, and responding to infectious diseases. The growth of a public health system for protecting community health depended both on scientific discovery and social action. Two factors have shaped the modern public health system: the growth of scientific knowledge about sources and means of controlling disease, and the growth of public acceptance of disease control as both a possibility and a public responsibility.

When little was known about the causes of disease, society tended to regard illness with a degree of resignation and few actions were taken. As understanding of sources of contagion and means of controlling disease became more refined, more effective interventions against health threats were developed. Public organizations and agencies were formed to employ newly developed interventions and strategies against these health threats. As scientific knowledge grew, public health authorities expanded to take on new actions, including sanitation, immunization, health education, and creating new laws and regulations.

Before the 18th century, epidemics such as the plague, cholera, and smallpox evoked sporadic public efforts to protect citizens in the face of a dread disease. Although epidemic diseases were often considered a sign of poor moral and spiritual condition, some public effort was made to contain the epidemic spread of specific disease through isolation of the ill and quarantining of travelers. Several European cities appointed public authorities to adopt and enforce isolation and quarantine measures (Fig. 14.1).

By the 18th century, isolation of the ill and quarantining of the exposed became common measures for containing and controlling contagious diseases. Several American port cities adopted rules for trade quarantine and isolation of the sick. In 1701, Massachusetts was the first state to pass laws for isolation of smallpox patients and for ship quarantine as needed.

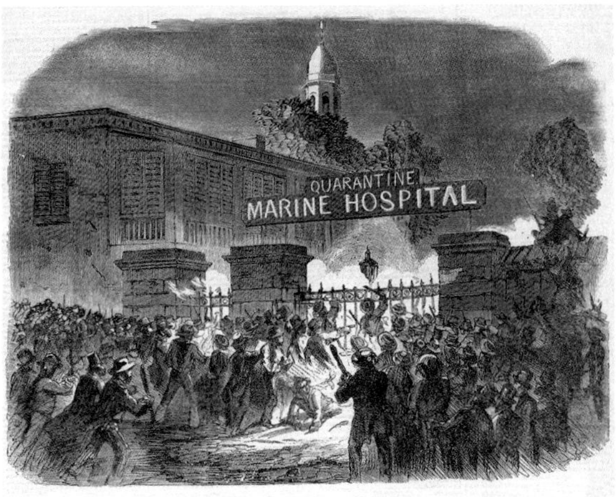

Fig. 14.1 By the 19th century, quarantine facilities were built to care for patients showing symptoms of highly infectious diseases, such as smallpox and yellow fever. This one was built in 1799 on Staten Island. (iStock.com/Keith Lance.)

By the end of the 18th century, several cities, including Boston, Philadelphia, New York, and Baltimore, had established permanent councils to enforce quarantine and isolation rules. These initiatives reflected new ideas about both the cause and meaning of disease. Diseases were seen less as natural effects of the human condition and more as potentially controllable through public action.

From the 1930s through the 1970s, local, state, and federal responsibilities in health continued to increase. The federal role in health also became more prominent with the passage of several legislative acts and laws (Box 14.2). A strong federal government and a more prominent government role in ensuring social welfare were publicly supported social values of this era. The federal and state government with local health agencies took on greater roles in providing and planning health services, in health promotion and health education, and in financing health services.

Vaccine Mandates

Federal and state governments have long recognized the importance of vaccines for protecting the public's health by passing legislation and establishing agencies

BOX 14.2 United States' Public Health Milestones

- The Social Security Act was passed in 1935. One title of the act established a federal grant-in-aid program to the states for establishing and maintaining public health services and for training public health personnel. Another title increased the responsibilities of the Children's Bureau in maternal and child health and capabilities of state maternal and child health programs.
- The National Mental Health Act, establishing the National Institute of Mental Health as a part of NIH, was passed in 1946. This institute was also authorized to finance training programs for mental health professionals and to finance development of community mental health services in local areas, as well as to conduct and support research.
- The Medicare and Medicaid programs, titles 18 and 19 of the Social Security Act, were passed in 1966.

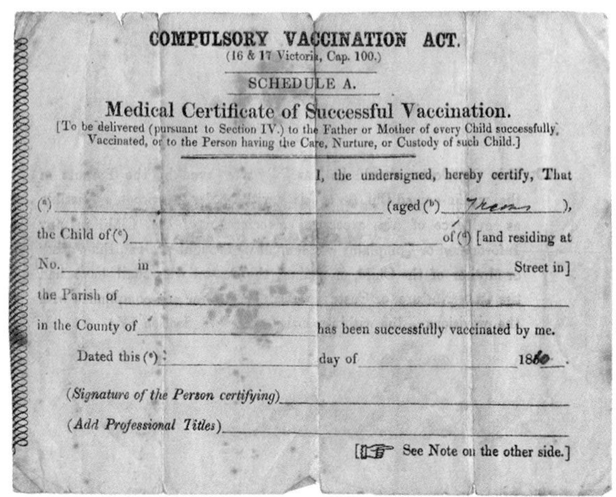

COMPULSORY VACCINATION ACT.
(16 & 17 Victoria, Cap. 100.)

SCHEDULE A.

Medical Certificate of Successful Vaccination.
[To be delivered (pursuant to Section IV.) to the Father or Mother of every Child successfully Vaccinated, or to the Person having the Care, Nurture, or Custody of such Child.]

I, the undersigned, hereby certify, That
(a) ______ (aged (b) ______),
the Child of (c) ______ of (d) [and residing at
No. ______ in ______ Street in]
the Parish of ______
in the County of ______ has been successfully vaccinated by me.
Dated this (e) ______ day of ______ 1860.
(*Signature of the Person certifying*) ______
(*Add Professional Titles*) ______
[☞ See Note on the other side.]

Fig. 14.2 Governments have a long history of requiring vaccines, usually for children. This is a certificate of compulsory vaccination, dated 1860 for a child aged 7 weeks against smallpox, which was widespread during the 19th century. (iStock.com/Whitemay.)

to oversee their safe manufacture and distribution. Additionally, governments have a history of mandating vaccines for a population. The first state law mandating vaccination was enacted in Massachusetts in 1809 and authorized local boards of health to require smallpox vaccinations for those over 21 years of age (Fig. 14.2). Other states subsequently passed similar legislation. However, opposition to mandatory vaccinations increased as states began to enforce these laws, with vaccine mandates being repealed in California, Illinois, Indiana, Minnesota, Utah, West Virginia, and Wisconsin during this time.

In 1905, the U.S. Supreme Court issued its landmark ruling in *Jacobson v. Massachusetts* upholding the right of states to compel vaccination. The Supreme Court held that a health regulation requiring smallpox vaccination was a reasonable exercise of the state's power and that did not violate the liberty and rights of individuals under the Constitution.

Despite the ruling, opposition continued for vaccine mandates. In most cases, vaccine mandates have been for school-age children. In another court case, *Zucht v. King* in 1922, the Supreme Court decided in the case that unvaccinated students could be constitutionally excluded from attending schools in the district of San Antonio, Texas. The decision upheld the right of local governments to require vaccinations as a condition for attending public schools, ruling that unvaccinated individuals could be denied access to education. The Court argued that public health supersedes an individual's right to education.

Additionally, in 1944, the Supreme Court ruled that mandating childhood vaccines comes under the doctrine of **parens patriae**, in which the state exerts authority over child welfare. In this decision, the Court wrote that parental authority is not absolute and can be restricted if doing so is in the child's best interest. They went on to say freedom of religion does not give parents the right to expose their community or their child to a communicable disease, or the child to the possibility of illness or death.

Although the Centers for Disease Control and Prevention (CDC) has a recommended schedule for child and adolescent immunization, it does not set vaccination requirements for schools. The CDC points out that each state makes its own decisions about which vaccines are required for school attendance in that state. Today, all 50 states have vaccine mandates for children attending school.

Exemption Laws

Some states allow for religious and medical exemptions, and these laws can vary from state to state. **Religious exemption laws**, sometimes called "Religious Freedom Restoration Acts" or RFRAs, permit people, churches, non-profit organizations, and sometimes corporations to seek exemptions from state laws that burden their religious beliefs. The individual or organization must seek out an exemption, such as through court proceedings. Medical exemptions may be requested if individuals or parents believes that the vaccine would not be safe for themselves or their child due to having a disease or taking a medication that would weaken their or their child's immune system, have severe allergy to the vaccine or an ingredient in the vaccine, or have a serious reaction to the vaccine or an ingredient in the vaccine in the past. To get a medical exemption, individuals must have their or their child's healthcare provider sign a medical exemption form. Many states ask whether the exemption is temporary or permanent, and almost half of states require healthcare providers to sign a new form every year. Less recognized are personal or philosophical exemptions. This exemption is based on individuals or parents' personal beliefs about vaccines. Some parents are concerned about vaccine safety. Others believe that getting sick is good for the child because it strengthens the immune system. Many of these concerns have been debunked, and many states do not allow for philosophical exemptions.

Currently, religious exemptions are allowed in 45 states as well as Washington D.C., and 15 states allow for exemptions because of the parents' philosophical beliefs. However, all states allow for medical exemptions. Exemption laws generally are hard to enforce. For example, in 2015, California outlawed nonmedical exemptions, such as for religious and philosophical reasons. After the law passed, medical exemptions jumped 250%. One reason was that some healthcare providers began writing medical exemptions for parents who had personal objections to vaccines.

To address this, in November 2021, the American Medical Association (AMA) House of Delegates approved a resolution stating that only licensed physicians should have the medical authority and the power to grant medical exemptions from vaccines. The policy comes in the wake of tens of thousands of people seeking exemptions to state and municipal COVID mandates, contending they have medical reasons for remaining unvaccinated. The definition of "medical authority" varies from state to state, with some states allowing alternative practitioners, such as naturopathic providers, to approve vaccine exemptions. Many naturopathic providers and other alternative medicine providers, such as homeopaths and chiropractors, are less likely to recommend vaccines or even recommend against vaccines despite scientific evidence of safety and efficacy. The AMA already has policy opposing religious, philosophic, or personal belief exemptions from immunizations, since such exemptions endanger the health of the unvaccinated individual and the health of the community at large.

DISCUSSION

In 2015, an outbreak of measles occurred among children in California who visited Disneyland and another theme park. Some parents were believed to be claiming a religious exemption to avoid getting their children vaccinated. Since 2015, five more states have eliminated vaccine exemptions in public schools: Connecticut, Mississippi, Maine, New York, and West Virginia. In 2020, the number of cases of measles in the United States declined for the first time in 6 years.

1. Should there be religious exemptions for any type of vaccine for a disease? How should that be determined?
2. Should public safety take a higher priority than a parental authority? Should parental authority be absolute?
3. How does the elimination of the religious exemption conflict with the Constitution?

COVID-19 VACCINE MANDATE

Although vaccines are not routinely required for adults in most settings, they are often mandated for military service members, new immigrants seeking permanent U.S. residence, college and university students, and healthcare workers. Previous epidemics like the 2018–2019 measles outbreak in New York City were quashed by emergency vaccine mandates for adults in affected zones. Even before President Biden's COVID-19 vaccine mandate announcements, several cities and states, businesses, and institutions of higher education had issued their own vaccine mandates to address the COVID-19 pandemic.

Unlike cities and states, the federal government does not have broad public health authority. The president has only limited public health powers and could not, for example, issue a nationwide vaccine mandate. However, the Biden Administration had strong legal support and can authorize more specific mandates. One of the mandates was for all federal workers and contractors to be vaccinated. As the head of the federal workforce, President Biden has the legal authority to set safety standards, including requiring masks and vaccines. Specifically, the Equal Employment Opportunity Commission and the Department of Justice both advised that governments and businesses can require COVID-19 vaccines as a condition of employment, so long as they provide religious and medical exemptions.

Another mandate the Biden Administration enacted was for all healthcare facilities to require COVID-19 vaccinations as a condition of receiving Medicare and Medicaid funding. In the case of *South Dakota v. Dole* in 1987, the Supreme Court ruled that the federal government can set reasonable conditions in order to receive federal funds.

The Biden Administration's most controversial mandate was requiring businesses with 100 or more employees to either mandate the COVID-19 vaccinations or implement weekly testing for those employees who opt out of receiving the vaccinations. In doing this, President Biden exercised his executive power over the Occupational Safety and Health Act, which empowers the Department of Labor to set uniform national workplace safety standards, including emergency temporary standards in response to workplace hazards. The Administration believes that the exposure to COVID-19 can be just as hazardous as workplace injury risks. The Occupational Safety and Health Administration (OSHA) already set emergency temporary standards for COVID-19 exposures in healthcare settings. Previously, OSHA set bloodborne pathogen standards that included hepatitis B vaccinations. Thus, it would not be a big leap for OSHA to include emergency standards for COVID-10 vaccinations or weekly testing requirements.

In an attempt to stem the rising tide of COVID-19 and its variants, Delta and Omicron, a rapidly growing number of places across the United States are requiring people to show proof they have been inoculated against COVID-19. This has included healthcare professionals, teachers, police officers, and paramedics, and, in some areas, people must provide proof of vaccination to enter businesses or attend events. New York City was one of the earliest cities to require proof of vaccination to enter restaurants, bars, and other indoor settings. New Orleans, San Francisco, Chicago, and Boston soon followed and imposed similar rules.

Legal Challenges to Vaccine Mandate

Since the announcement of the Biden Administration's vaccine mandate, it has met with a series of legal challenges from businesses, organizations, cities, and states. For what is referred to as the Centers for Medicare & Medicaid Services (CMS) mandate, which required all healthcare facilities to require COVID-19 vaccinations as a condition of receiving funding from federally sponsored programs, Florida, Missouri, Louisiana, and Texas sought preliminary injunctions to block the mandate from going into effect. For the OSHA mandate, which required businesses with 100 or more employees to either mandate the COVID-19 vaccinations or implement weekly testing for those employees who opt out of receiving the vaccinations, there were over 40 lawsuits challenging the mandate which went to the U.S. Court of Appeals. Both the CMS and OSHA mandates will go to the Supreme Court to help resolve the different challenges between the states and the federal government.

GENDER, TRANSGENDER, AND NONCONFORMING IDENTITIES

Over the last several years, there has been a growing awareness, discussion, and public consciousness of transgender, gender identity, and what it means to be biologically vs. identifying as male or female or none of the above. There have been great strides in recognizing and improving access to health care for lesbian and gay patients in the last several decades. However, these strides were less inclusive of transgender patients, although they often face similar or even more health disparities due to societal stigma, discrimination, denial of their civil and human rights, and a general lack of visibility in the healthcare system. It is important to understand the changing definitions of gender and how that affects the delivery and access to health care and what are the legal and ethical ramifications.

The concepts of sex and gender have often been used interchangeably. But the term **sex** is generally used to refer to a binary of being either female or male as denoted by attributes that comprise biological sex, such as presence of ovaries or testes. **Gender**, on the other hand, is meant to refer to the various socially constructed roles, behaviors, expressions and identities of girls, women, boys, men, and gender-diverse people. Additionally, other distinct terms are gender identity and gender expression. Gender identity is one's internal knowledge of one's gender—for example, your knowledge that you are a man, a woman, another gender, or neither. Gender expression is how people present their gender on the outside, often through behavior, clothing, hairstyle, voice, or body characteristics.

There are a growing number of people who have reported not feeling that their sex or what they were born as align with how they seem themselves—male, female, or neither. They generally would see themselves as transgender. According to the National Center for Transgender Equality, transgender is a broad term that can be used to describe people whose gender identity is different from the gender they were thought to be when they were born. ("Trans" is often used as shorthand for transgender.) Estimates of the number of transgender adults significantly increased over the past decade, with a current best estimate of 390 per 100,000 adults. That is about 1 in every 250 adults, or almost 1 million Americans, which is most likely an underestimation since many people may not disclose this information for fear of discrimination and stigmatization.

Some transgender people may identify as neither a man nor a woman, or as a combination of male and female, and may use terms like *nonbinary, genderqueer, or* gender nonconforming to describe their gender identity. Gender nonconforming (GNC) can refer to a gender identity—one's personal and subjective sense of gender—that is neither male nor female. It can also refer to a gender expression characterized by mannerisms and behaviors that are not conventionally associated with an assigned gender. People with nonconforming gender identities can identify with more than one gender (e.g., bigender), no gender (e.g., agender), or feel that their gender fluctuates or is undefinable by traditional terms (e.g., genderfluid). Those who are nonbinary or GNC often prefer to be referred to as "they" and "them."

In some cases, transgender people who want to live according to their gender identity, rather than the gender they were thought to be when they were born, may go through a *gender transition*. Possible steps in a gender transition may or may not include changing their clothing, appearance, name, or the pronoun people use to refer to them (like "she," "he," or "they"). If they can, some people change their identification documents, like their driver's license or passport, to better reflect their gender. Some people may also undergo hormone therapy or other medical procedures to change their physical characteristics and make their body match the gender they better identify as. Despite these terms and definitions, they are all evolving, and some people may define themselves entirely differently that these terms.

Expanding Access to Care for Transgender Patients

Many transgender people risk social stigma, discrimination, and harassment when they tell other people who they really are. This includes seeking and receiving medical services. All transgender people are entitled to the same dignity and respect, regardless of whether or not they have been able to take any legal or medical steps in transitioning. It is important for every member of the healthcare team to use respectful terminology and treat transgender and GNC people as they would treat any other person or patient.

When providing patient care, the healthcare team should treat them according to their gender identity, not their sex at birth. For example, someone who lives as a woman today is a transgender woman and should be referred to as "she" and "her." A transgender man lives as a man today and should be referred to as "he" and "him." This also includes using the name they have asked you to call them (not their old name). If the healthcare professional is unsure, it is appropriate to ask politely.

To ensure the highest quality of health care, healthcare providers must have accurate patient information and the patient must have stable access to medical care. Given that there are medical issues related to a patient's sexual history, sexual orientation, and gender identity, it would be difficult to provide good medical care for lesbian, gay, and bisexual, and transgender (LGBT) people without this information.

However, transgender and GNC people often face social, structural, and economic barriers that inhibit their access to health care. For instance, employment-based discrimination may prevent some transgender and GNC populations from obtaining jobs that offer employer-sponsored health insurance. In addition, applying for public health insurance programs, such as Medicare or Medicaid, may present bureaucratic hurdles. Some transgender and GNC individuals may require legal documents and identification that match their current name and gender identity rather than the name and gender assigned at birth.

Expanding Legal Protection

Recent policy changes have, at least theoretically, improved access to care for transgender and GNC individuals. At the state level, twenty-four states and the District of Columbia currently prohibit transgender exclusions in health insurance service coverage. Currently, only Arkansas legally permits insurers to refuse gender-transitioning care.

As part of the passage of the Affordable Care Act (ACA) in 2010, qualified health providers, including physicians, hospitals, and clinics could not discriminate on the basis of gender. In 2014, the ACA prohibited insurers from denying coverage to individuals on the basis of their gender identity, and the Department of Health and Human Services lifted a ban on Medicare coverage for gender reassignment surgery, which had been in place since 1989.

In addition, on June 15, 2020, in the case of *Bostock v. Clayton County*, the Supreme Court affirmed that Title VII of the Civil Rights Act of 1964 prohibited sex discrimination in employment to include sexual orientation and gender identity. At the beginning of his presidency, President Biden signed an executive order directing all agencies to enforce federal laws prohibiting sex discrimination to include discrimination based on sexual orientation and gender identity in areas including employment, housing, health care, education, and credit. Essentially, the executive order implemented the *Bostock v. Clayton County* decision throughout the country's major civil rights law to consistently protect LGBTQ people from discrimination and ensure equal protection under the law.

Despite these laws and policy changes to improve access to health care for transgender and GNC individuals, substantial control is left in the hands of individual healthcare providers and facilities, many of whom may not be experienced or trained to treat this population. For example, decisions about Medicare coverage for gender reassignment surgeries are left to health insurers and healthcare providers who must determine whether gender reassignment surgery and related services are medically necessary.

DISCUSSION

Many transgender and gender nonconforming people are not covered by private or public health insurance. Those that do have health insurance their policies may not cover their gender transition. This may include hormonal therapy and gender reassignment surgery, such as breast or chest surgery, hysterectomy, genital reconstruction, and facial reconstruction. Transitioning adults may not be able to afford the out-of-pocket expenses for these transition-related procedures excluded from coverage, which can cost $100 per month for hormonal therapy to over $100,000 for some comprehensive transition procedures. For many years, federal programs, such as Medicare, did not cover transition-related surgery due to a decades-old policy that categorized such treatment as "experimental." In 2014, it is illegal for Medicare to deny coverage for medically necessary transition-related care. However, some local Medicare contractors have specific policies detailing their coverage for transition-related care, as do some private Medicare Advantage plans.

1. Should these gender transitioning services be included as part of the health insurance coverage?
2. What are the reasons that would make gender-transitioning surgeries and procedures considered *medically necessary*?

CAPTURING GENDER IDENTITY IN EHRS

One area of disparity in the healthcare system that has gained focus over the last several years is improving the data collection of patient information for transgender and GNC patients. Unfortunately, many healthcare providers do not routinely discuss sexual orientation or gender identity with patients, and many healthcare facilities have not developed systems to collect this critical patient information from all patients. Without this information, LGBT patients and their specific healthcare needs cannot be identified, the health disparities they experience cannot be addressed, and important healthcare services may not be delivered. Such services include appropriate preventive screenings, assessments of risk for sexually transmitted diseases and HIV, discussions about parenting, and effective interventions for behavioral health concerns that can be related to the experiences and stigma of being transgender and GNC. This is also an opportunity for transgender people to share information about themselves in a welcoming and patient-centered environment and to develop a more trusting patient–provider relationship.

Collecting accurate gender identity data in electronic health records (EHRs) is essential to providing high-quality, patient-centered care. Including gender identity data collection has been recommended by both the National Academy of Medicine and The Joint Commission as a way to learn about which populations are being served and to measure the quality of care provided to transgender and GNC people. Some patients may question the relevance of being asked about their sex listed at birth or their sexual orientation. However, healthcare providers need this information to recommend appropriate preventive care. It is important to note that a patient's sexual orientation and gender identity may be fluid across time and should be reassessed periodically to ensure the most current information is documented in the patient's medical record. Transgender and GNC patients who are referred to in a healthcare setting using the wrong pronoun or name may suffer distress, ridicule, or even assault by others in the waiting area, and may not return for further care.

Gender ID Data

The U.S. General Accountability Office's Health Information Technology (HIT) Policy Committee has recently recommended that the Office of the National Coordinator for Health Information Technology include the capture of gender identification (ID) data in EHR systems as part of Meaningful Use, which is a federal mandate on the use of EHR systems to improve quality, safety, efficiency, reduce health disparities, and improve population and public health. **Gender ID data** can be defined as gender identification, birth-assigned sex, legal sex, preferred name, and legal name. Special efforts and considerations must be taken to optimize the manner in which gender ID data is collected, stored, and then accessed and displayed in an electronic medical record.

Many clinics and healthcare organizations are already changing their patient registration forms to document their patient's information more accurately. Some forms allow for the collection of gender ID data of both gender ID and birth-assigned sex. This includes the ability for patients to use preferred neutral pronouns as opposed to the traditional binary "he/him" and "she/her." In some cases, the pronouns "they/them" or "zie/hir" are used (pronounced "zee" and "here").

Along with changes to registration forms, many EHR systems are now able to capture birth sex and gender identity. In the EHR, birth sex is an important variable for patients to answer since it is used to facilitate effective patient care that is efficient, equitable, and patient-centered. Knowing the patient's birth sex is often used to trigger recommended health screens, such as mammograms, pap smears, and prostate exams. For example, a transgender man, or a biological female who has transitioned to a man, may still need to have mammograms and pap smears if he has not undergone gender transition surgeries. Gender identity fields in EHR are independently beneficial because healthcare providers can use this information to ensure proper pronoun use and avoid misgendering a patient. Additionally, the gender identity field informs healthcare providers to conduct more frequent or different health screenings to evaluate specific health risks that are more prevalent in gender minority patients.

Two-Step Self-Identification Approach

The American Medical Informatics Association and its members endorsed a two-step self-identification approach when collecting data related to a patient's sexual orientation and gender identity. This method allows individuals to specify both their gender identity—female, male, nonbinary, questioning, not listed, or prefer not to disclose—and their assigned gender at birth, or the gender that appears on their birth certificate. The Center of Excellence for Transgender Health at the University of California, San Francisco created a similar questionnaire to better capture patient information that the CDC recommends (Box 14.3). The gender identity questions have two parts but focuses entirely on identity and not on sexual orientation, although that information is also included in the patient's social history. The first part asks about current gender identity and the second part on the sex listed at birth. These questions replace "Sex: male or female?" on patient information forms and in EHRs. Asking two questions offers a clearer, more clinically relevant representation of transgender patients. For example, asking whether someone is transgender will exclude some transgender people who do not identify as such (e.g., a person who was born male but whose

BOX 14.3 Collecting Sexual Orientation and Gender Identity Information

Sexual Orientation

Do you think of yourself as:

- Straight or heterosexual
- Lesbian or gay
- Bisexual
- Queer, pansexual, and/or questioning
- Something else, please specify: _______
- Don't know
- Decline to answer

Gender Identity

Do you think of yourself as:

- Male
- Female
- Transgender man/transman/female-to-male (FTM)
- Transgender woman/transwoman/male-to-female (MTF)
- Genderqueer/gender nonconforming (neither exclusively male nor female)
- Additional gender category (or other); please specify: _______
- Decline to answer

What sex was originally listed on your birth certificate?

- Male
- Female
- Decline to answer

Name and Pronouns

What is your name as you would like it to appear on your health records?

What are your pronouns?

- He/him
- She/her
- They/them
- Other:______

Source: Collecting Sexual Orientation and Gender Identity Information, April 1, 2020, Centers for Disease Control and Prevention: https://www.cdc.gov/hiv/clinicians/transforming-health/health-care-providers/collecting-sexual-orientation.html

gender identity is female may check "female" rather than "transgender" on a form). The gender identity question also includes options for people who have a nonbinary gender identity (e.g., people who do not identify as male or female).

In addition to collecting gender identity data, asking patients to include the name they want the healthcare team to use as well as the correct pronouns to use is also recommended. Many transgender patients may have insurance records and identification documents that do not accurately reflect their current name and gender identity. Asking these questions and training the whole healthcare team to use an individual's pronouns and name can greatly facilitate patient-centered communication.

DISCUSSION

Some EMR systems only allow patients to select their birth sex information. As a result, transgender and GNC patients may choose to align the "sex" with their gender identity and not birth sex. This change would ensure healthcare providers and staff not misgender them and use respectful, gender-consistent pronouns when speaking with them.

1. What medical issues would arise if patients did not distinguish and report differences between birth sex and gender identity?
2. How would this affect patient care regarding screening tests, lab results, and medication dosages?

CONCLUSION

The healthcare system in the United States is rapidly changing owing to a variety of factors and influences from a variety of sources, including societal, political, legal, and technological. Federal and state governments have a role in protecting the health and well-being of the public and community through public health measure and mandates, such as improving sanitation and recommending vaccines. With infectious diseases, including the COVID-19 pandemic, these public health mandates have faced opposition and conflict with some people's view of autonomy and personal liberty. Another issue is the growing awareness of transgender and gender nonconforming people and the legal and ethical challenges to providing accessible health care and services to a marginalized and vulnerable population.

CHAPTER REVIEW QUESTIONS

1. Which of the following diseases was not considered an epidemic?
   A. Cholera
   B. Plague
   C. Rhinovirus
   D. Smallpox
2. All the following are public health measures to minimize and prevent infectious diseases except:
   A. handwashing.
   B. Increasing one's exposure to improve immunity.
   C. Immunizations.
   D. quarantine.
3. The coronavirus 2019 (COVID-19) is considered a pandemic because
   A. it is believed to originate in China.
   B. a vaccine is effective against the virus.
   C. there is an outbreak that is spread across a few communities.
   D. it affects many people across the world.
4. The landmark ruling in *Jacobson v. Massachusetts* resulted in:
   A. upholding the states' right to require vaccinations.
   B. upholding citizens' right to refuse vaccinations.
   C. allowing religious exemption of vaccines.
   D. forcing infected individuals to be quarantined.
5. The Biden Administration's Centers for Medicare & Medicaid Services (CMS) mandate required which of the following.
   A. It required all healthcare facilities to require COVID-19 vaccinations.
   B. It required all healthcare facilities to require COVID-10 vaccinations as condition of receiving funding from federally sponsored programs.
   C. It required all businesses to have their employees receive COVID-19 vaccinations by January 1st.
   D. It required all businesses with 100 or more employees to either mandate the COVID-19 vaccinations or implement weekly testing.
6. The Latin term *parens patria* means
   A. the state may exempt a child from vaccinations if the parent chooses it.
   B. the state may require vaccine mandates for parents.
   C. the state may act as the parent in the case of no parental authority.
   D. the state can exert its authority over child welfare.
7. The general term used to refer to a binary of being either biologically male or female is
   A. gender.
   B. gender expression.
   C. gender identity.
   D. sex.
8. Wearing a dress if you are a female and pants for male are socially constructed ideas of
   A. gender.
   B. gender expression.
   C. gender identity.
   D. sex.
9. How people present their gender on the outside, often through behavior, clothing, hairstyle, voice, or body characteristic is called
   A. gender.
   B. gender expression.
   C. gender identity.
   D. sex.
10. Gender ID data includes all the following except
    A. birth-assigned sex.
    B. insurer's designated name.
    C. gender identification.
    D. legal sex.

SELF-REFLECTION QUESTIONS

1. One notorious carrier is Mary Mallon, later nicknamed "Typhoid Mary," who was an asymptomatic chronic carrier of *Salmonella Typhi*. As a cook in New York City and New Jersey in the early 1900s, it was proven she unintentionally infected more than 122 people, resulting in 5 deaths until she was placed in isolation on an island in the East River, where she died 23 years later. Mallon was the first known case of a healthy carrier in the United States. Research this case on the Internet. How does this relate the current COVID-19 pandemic and the different measures to control disease transmission?
2. What are some of the reasons a person would refuse a vaccination? How would you explain the importance of vaccinations for someone who refuses them for measles and polio?
3. What if you had a patient who is transgender? How comfortable would you feel caring for them as a patient? How would you examine your own bias?

INTERNET ACTIVITIES

1. Research the concept of "herd immunity" and what that means in reference to immunizations. How does that relate to the COVID-19 pandemic?
2. Research the National Conference of State Legislatures' State Vaccination Policies database at: https://www.ncsl.org/research/health/state-vaccination-policies-requirements-and-exemptions-for-entering-school.aspx. What are your state's requirements?
3. Research the healthcare laws and policies for transgender people at: https://www.lgbtmap.org/equality-maps/healthcare_laws_and_policies. What protections or restrictions does your state have?

ADDITIONAL RESOURCES

Gonzales, G., & Henning-Smith, C. (2017). Barriers to care among transgender and gender nonconforming adults. *The Milbank Quarterly*, *95*(4), 726–748. https://doi.org/10.1111/1468-0009.12297.

Kronk, C. A., Everhart, A. R., Ashley, F., Thompson, H. M., Schall, T. E., Goetz, T. G., et al. (2021). Transgender data collection in the electronic health record: Current concepts and issues. *Journal of the American Medical Informatics Association*, *29*(2), 271–284. https://doi.org/10.1093/jamia/ocab136.

National LGBT Health Education Center. *Focus on forms and policy: Creating an inclusive environment for LGBT patients.* https://www.lgbtqiahealtheducation.org/wp-content/uploads/2017/08/Forms-and-Policy-Brief.pdf.

Stroumsa, D. (2014). The state of transgender health care: policy, law, and medical frameworks. *American Journal of Public Health*, *104*(3), e31–e38. https://doi.org/10.2105/AJPH.2013.301789.

The College of Physicians of Philadelphia. *The history of vaccines.* https://www.historyofvaccines.org/timeline/all.

BIBLIOGRAPHY

Burgess, C., Kauth, M. R., Klemt, C., Shanawani, H., & Shipherd, J. C. (2019). Evolving sex and gender in electronic health records. *Federal Practitioner*, *36*(6), 271–277.

Division of HIV Prevention, National Center for HIV, Viral Hepatitis, STD, and TB Prevention, Centers for Disease Control and Prevention. https://www.cdc.gov/hiv/clinicians/transforming-health/health-care-providers/collecting-sexual-orientation.html.

Gostin, L. O. (2021). COVID-19 vaccine mandates—A wider freedom. *JAMA Health Forum*, *2*(10), e213852. https://doi.org/10.1001/jamahealthforum.2021.3852.

Institute of Medicine (US) Committee for the Study of the Future of Public Health. The Future of Public Health. (1988). Washington (DC): National Academies Press (US). 3, A History of the Public Health System. Available from: https://www.ncbi.nlm.nih.gov/books/NBK218224/.

Institute of Medicine Committee on Quality of Health Care. (2001). *Crossing the quality chasm: A new health system for the 21st century*. Washington, DC: National Academies Press. https://www.ncbi.nlm.nih.gov/books/NBK222274.

Movement Advancement Project. *Equality maps: Healthcare laws and policies.* https://www.lgbtmap.org/equality-maps/healthcare_laws_and_policies. Accessed 12/24/2021.

National Center for Transgender Equality. *Understanding transgender people: The basics.* https://transequality.org/issues/resources/understanding-transgender-people-the-basics.

A APPENDIX

Case Discussions

CASE DISCUSSION 1: PROTECTING THE PUBLIC SAFETY

A female passenger from Nigeria is on a flight to LaGuardia Airport in New York. She asks one of the flight attendants for some cold water because she is not feeling well. Several hours into the flight, the passenger tells the flight attendant that she feels worse and complains of severe headache and muscle pains. The flight attendant asks on the intercom if there is a physician on board, and one offers his assistance. The physician, who is a pediatrician, determines that the passenger is feverish, and she reported having several days of diarrhea and vomiting with some blood before the flight. The physician suggests that the passenger may have Ebola because she is from West Africa. Because the Ebola virus is transmitted through physical contact and bodily fluids, he recommends quarantining the patient and having the plane make an emergency landing. The flight attendant confers with the pilots, who decide to reseat the passenger in the back of the plane. The passenger refuses and is adamant that she does not have Ebola. A scuffle occurs between the passenger and flight attendants, with the passenger being injured after being forcibly removed from her seat.

Case Discussion 1 Questions

1. Could the airline's actions be considered discriminatory toward the passenger?
2. Is the physician or airline liable for the passenger's injury?
3. Does the United States have a responsibility to the general public to screen passengers coming from a country where Ebola is prevalent?

CASE DISCUSSION 2: FAILURE TO PROVIDE CRITICAL DIAGNOSIS

A woman goes to her physician with a very persistent cough. After running a series of tests, the physician determines that she has advanced lung cancer and, in his opinion, there are very few options for treatment. The woman also told the physician that she was about to leave on a cruise for a week for a family reunion.

Case Discussion 2 Questions

1. Should the physician tell the woman that she has an incurable lung cancer? Should he tell her before or after her cruise?
2. What if she passes away before the physician informs her of the diagnosis? Would the physician be found negligent?

CASE DISCUSSION 3: REFUSAL OF ADVANCE DIRECTIVE

An older woman in Maryland with a multitude of medical problems had completed her advance directive. Her husband was aware and gave his consent. The woman's advance directive was also shared with their children, where they understood that she should not be resuscitated if she was admitted into the hospital. Two years later, the woman goes into cardiac and respiratory arrest. When she arrives at the hospital, the hospital staff begin resuscitation efforts. The woman survives but has multiple broken ribs, a lung punctured, and a long path to recovery and rehabilitation that she and her husband cannot afford. Both the woman and her family are outraged and sue the hospital for keeping her alive and disregarding her advance directive.

Case Discussion 3 Questions

1. Do you think it is more important to keep a patient alive or allow him or her to die if that is what the patient requests?
2. Do you think the court will side with the patient or hospital staff? Why?

CASE DISCUSSION 4: REFUSING LIFE-PROLONGING TREATMENT

J. L. is an 80-year-old man living with his wife in a retirement community. He has always valued his independence, but recently he has been having trouble caring for himself. He is having difficulty walking; managing his medications for diabetes, heart disease, and hypertension; and starting to show signs of kidney failure. J. L.'s physician diagnoses depression after noting that he has lost interest in the things he used to enjoy. He refuses medication, and his symptoms have worsened, and he talks of suicide. Several months later, the physician informs J. L. that he will have to start dialysis because of his advancing kidney failure. This would require his going to the dialysis unit three times a week for 3–4 h each session. After the second treatment, J. L. informs his physician that he refuses dialysis treatment and asks to be allowed to die.

Case Discussion 4 Questions

1. Is J. L. competent enough to decide about the right to die?
2. How does his earlier diagnosis of depression affect how you would manage his decision?

CASE DISCUSSION 5: PATIENT CONFIDENTIALITY VS. PATIENT SAFETY

A surgeon on staff at a hospital goes to see a fellow physician as a patient. The surgeon shares that he has been having brief lapses of consciousness related to complex partial seizures, a form of epilepsy that had gone unrecognized during his residency. He admitted to having at least one minor seizure in the operating room, but no one observed it. The surgeon is getting treatment for the seizures but has not disclosed his condition to the hospital for fear of losing his job.

Case Discussion 5 Questions

1. If you were a physician, what would you do?
2. What do you think is more important: patient safety or patient confidentiality?

CASE DISCUSSION 6: PATIENT CONSENT

A 25-year-old man was out drinking with friends when he fell and hit his head on the bar. He was rushed to the hospital, where doctors discovered he had severe swelling and bleeding of the brain. Before the physician declares him legally brain dead, the man's girlfriend arrives and asks for a testicular biopsy: she wants to retrieve his sperm before he dies so she can conceive his child.

Case Discussion 6 Questions

1. Should the physician grant her request?
2. Because the man is unable to consent, would there be anyone that could consent in his place?

CASE DISCUSSION 7: REFUSAL OF TREATMENT

A homeless man enters the hospital with chronic gangrene, osteomyelitis, and diabetes. After the patient intake, the physicians determine that he also had a psychiatric condition. He refuses treatment with medication or to submit to a psychiatric evaluation. He requests simply to be fed, given his insulin, and given a bed for the night. His physicians try to persuade him to accept intravenous antibiotics, but he refuses. The physicians must make a decision: send him back to the street or seek a court order declaring the man incapable of making decisions for himself, essentially forcing him into the physicians' care.

Case Discussion 7 Questions

1. Would it be legal for the hospital staff to restrain the man?
2. Based on his condition, would it be ethical and legal to discharge him?

CASE DISCUSSION 8: PATIENT'S CONSENT FOR LIFE-SAVING SURGERY

A woman enters the emergency room with abdominal pain. She undergoes a CT scan and is diagnosed with an abdominal aortic aneurysm, which is a weakening in the wall of the aorta. The physician informs her that she needs surgery immediately to correct the problem. Otherwise, the aneurysm may rupture, and she would bleed out and die in a matter of minutes. The woman is a swimsuit model, and she worries that the surgery will leave a scar that will negatively affect her ability to work. Therefore, she refuses any surgical treatment. Several days later, the woman arrives in the emergency room for an unrelated condition. She was in a car accident while driving under the influence of alcohol. She is stable but unconscious. The same physician in the emergency room sees her and decides to perform the surgery to repair her aneurysm. After the surgery, she is told of the procedure and that it was done just in time because the aneurysm was most likely to rupture, resulting in death. Regardless, the woman sues the hospital.

Case Discussion 8 Questions

1. Do you believe that the physician's actions are justified because it saved the woman's life?
2. When do you think it is ethically and legally right to take away an individual's autonomy?
3. What do you think a court would decide in this situation?

CASE DISCUSSION 9: CULTURAL COMPETENCE IN HOME REMEDIES

A mother brings in her child for a pediatric visit who is complaining of flu-like symptoms. Upon entering the room, the pediatrician asks the boy to remove his shirt and she notices a pattern of very distinct bruises on the boy's torso. She asks the mother where the bruises came from, and she says they are from a procedure she performed on him known as "cao gio," which is also known as "coining." This is a common ancient remedy commonly practiced in Southeast Asian cultures and involves rubbing warm oil or balm on a person's skin with a coin or other flat metal object. The mother explains that cao gio is used to raise our bad blood and improve circulation and healing. When you touch the boy's back with your stethoscope, he winces in pain from the bruises.

Case Discussion 9 Questions

1. Should the pediatrician contact Child Protective Services and report the mother? What professional duty does the physician have?
2. If the pediatrician believes this treatment is useless, should she tell the mother?
3. Should the pediatrician be concerned about alienating the mother and other people of her ethnicity and culture from modern medicine?

CASE DISCUSSION 10: A WOMAN WITH DEGENERATIVE DISEASE AND HER RIGHT TO LIFE AND DEATH

A woman was diagnosed with amyotrophic lateral sclerosis (ALS), which is a fatal neurodegenerative disease 5 years ago. This is a condition that destroys motor nerves, making control of movement impossible, while the mind is virtually unaffected. The prognosis of people with ALS is poor with death usually within 4 years of diagnosis, often from respiratory failure due to the inability of the inspiratory muscles to contract. The woman's condition has steadily declined, and she is expected not to live past 6 months. She expresses concern about the pain that she will face in her final weeks and hours. She asks her physician to give her a high dose narcotic for pain if she begins to suffocate or choke. This will lessen her pain, but it will also hasten her death. About a week later, she falls very ill, and is having trouble breathing.

Case Discussion 10 Questions

1. What is the woman's right to die? Does she have a right to make this choice, especially considering her diagnosis?
2. Does her prognosis matter? Or the amount of pain she is in?
3. Does the physician have an ethical or legal responsibility to help the patient live or die?

CASE DISCUSSION 11: A SURROGACY GONE WRONG

A woman is about to have a hysterectomy performed due to endometrial cancer. She decides to harvest her eggs for future children. Since she is unable to carry her own children, she and her husband contact a surrogacy company to find a woman to carry the baby for them. The husband's sperm is used to fertilize one of the wife's eggs and is implanted in the surrogate mother. The couple pays the woman's pregnancy-related expenses and an extra $20,000 as compensation for her services as a surrogate. After carrying the pregnancy to term, the surrogate says that she has become too attached to the child and refuses to give it up to the couple. A legal battle ensues.

Case Discussion 11 Questions

1. Does the surrogate have a legal right to the child?
2. Is it legal to provide compensation to a surrogate outside of the necessary medical expenses?
3. Does paying the surrogate harm her and/or the child's dignity?
4. Who do you think should receive the child, and why?

CASE DISCUSSION 12: CALL TO DUTY IN A PANDEMIC

A nurse begins experiencing respiratory symptoms, and she thinks she may have COVID-19. Since she works in the intensive care unit (ICU), which has a high number of patients with COVID, it is likely she has been exposed to it. The nurse gets tested and is awaiting the results. There is already a shortage of healthcare workers in hospitals and she knows her coworkers are exhausted and stressed. She is worried that, if she takes time to wait for the results of the test or needs to quarantine, this will significantly increase her coworker's patient load.

Case Discussion 12 Questions

1. Should she go to work as usual? What are the pros and cons to her doing this?
2. How should she balance her health to her call of duty as a nurse?

B APPENDIX

Case Studies

CASE STUDY 1: NURSE SHARES PATIENT INFORMATION WITH HUSBAND

A licensed practical nurse at a midsize clinic in Arkansas was straightening up the medical charts when she saw the name of the car accident victim who was suing the nurse's husband. The nurse read the patient's medical file and gave the private information to her husband. The husband called the plaintiff and demanded that the lawsuit be dropped based on the patient information provided by his wife. The plaintiff quickly called the clinic and filed a complaint to the state's attorney general.[a]

Case Study 1 Questions

1. What law did the nurse violate? Based on the violation, what should be the penalties?
2. What steps should the nurse's employer take?
3. Besides the employer and state's attorney general, which other organization(s) may investigate the nurse?

CASE STUDY 2: HEALTH INSURER VIOLATES WHISTLEBLOWER ACT

Health Net, California's fourth-largest health insurer, has agreed to pay $340,000 for violating securities laws on whistleblower awards. Since 2010, Health Net used illegal severance agreements to require employees to waive their ability to collect whistleblower awards in their departing severance agreements. This prevented any departing employees from speaking to state and federal officials about company violations. Although Health Net did not admit or deny the findings, it agreed to pay the penalty and contact all employees who had signed the severance agreements between August 12, 2011, and October 22, 2015, to inform them that they were not prohibited from exercising their rights as whistleblowers.[b]

Case Study 2 Questions

1. Which specific law did Health Net violate when it required its departing employees to sign the severance agreement?
2. Why is it important for employees to be able to exercise their right as whistleblowers?
3. What would happen if Health Net terminated a patient who acted as a whistleblower?

CASE STUDY 3: SPINE SURGEON FAILED TO DISCLOSE CONFLICTS OF INTEREST

Jeffrey Wang, an orthopedic surgeon, performed spinal surgery on Jerome Lew, a 52-year-old screenwriter in Orange County, by implanting a controversial bone-growth product. After the surgery, Lew said he had recurring pain and other complications, which required additional surgeries. The bone-growth product was not approved by the Food and Drug Administration (FDA) for the procedure Wang used it in, although physicians are legally allowed to use medications and devices as "off-label." However, Wang failed to inform and obtain consent from Lew. In addition, Wang did not disclose that, from 2004 to 2013, he received more than $450,000 for product royalties, consulting work, and lectures from the company that markets the bone-growth product. The hospital agreed to pay nearly $8.5 million to settle the lawsuit.[c]

[a] https://www.americanmobile.com/nursezone/nursing-news/nurse-pleads-guilty-to-hipaa-violation/.

[b] https://www.sec.gov/litigation/admin/2016/34-78590.pdf.

[c] http://www.allgov.com/usa/ca/news/where-is-the-money-going/uc-regents-settle-whistleblower-lawsuit-by-former-top-ucla-surgeon-for-10-million-140423?news=852980.

Case Study 3 Questions

1. Why was this considered a conflict of interest for the surgeon?
2. What is the meaning of "off-label" as it relates to the FDA?
3. Should a healthcare professional be prohibited from receiving compensation from a drug or device company? Why or why not?

CASE STUDY 4: WOMAN SUED FOR AIDING IN CAR CRASH

In 2004, Lisa Torti and her coworker, Alexandra Van Horn, had been at a bar in Chatsworth, California, with a group of friends. After leaving the bar, the car Van Horn was riding in spun out of control and hit a telephone pole. Torti, who was a passenger in another car, was following them and witnessed the accident. Torti said she thought she had seen smoke and feared the car would explode and offered to help Van Horn from the wreckage. Torti pulled her from the car, allegedly causing injury to Van Horn's vertebrae. Van Horn was taken to the hospital, where she underwent surgery and was found to be permanently paralyzed. Van Horn sued Torti for her injuries. Torti's defense was that she was protected from legal action under California's Good Samaritan laws. However, the California Supreme Court ruled that Van Horn may sue Torti for allegedly causing her friend's paralysis because the state statute immunizing rescuers from liability applies only if the individual is providing medical care in emergency situations.[d]

Case Study 4 Questions

1. How did Torti's action not meet California's Good Samaritan laws?
2. Should both medical and nonmedical actions be covered under the Good Samaritan law?
3. What legal defense would Torti have in this case?

[d] Lisa Torti, Defendant and Respondent. Alexandra Van Horn, Plaintiff and Appellant, v. Anthony Glen Watson et al., Defendants and Respondents. Nos. B188076, B189254 (March 21, 2007).

CASE STUDY 5: DIAGNOSTIC COMPANY OWNER'S FRAUD RESULTED IN PATIENT DEATHS

From 1997 through 2013, Rafael Chikvashvili, owner of Alpha Diagnostics in Baltimore, Maryland, created false radiology, ultrasound, and cardiologic interpretation reports and submitted insurance claims for medical examination interpretations that were never completed by licensed physicians or that were never completed at all. Chikvashvili directed Timothy Emeigh, vice president in charge of operations at the company and who was a licensed radiological technician, to view medical images using his personal laptop and then draft false physician interpretation reports. Chikvashvili would then affix the handwritten signature of an actual physician to the report or forge the physician's signature himself.

As a result of the radiology tests not being interpreted by a qualified radiologist, two patients failed to be properly diagnosed with congestive heart failure. One of the patients had mild congestive heart failure and, because of the misinterpreted x-ray, was cleared for elective surgery and experienced significant bleeding. She died 6 days later. Chikvashvili was convicted of defrauding Medicare and Medicaid of $7.5 million and two counts of healthcare fraud, resulting in death.[e]

Case Study 5 Questions

1. Why is licensure and certification important in this situation?
2. Which laws were violated in this situation?

CASE STUDY 6: MISSED LABORATORY TEST LEADS TO PARALYSIS

On June 28, 2006, Cynthia Adae was taken to Clinton Memorial Hospital with symptoms of right shoulder pain, limited range of motion of her right upper extremity, a cough, and a fever. The attending physician suspected it was an infection or thyroid abnormality. After ordering a series of blood tests, the physician discharged Adae the next day without confirming the results. On July 1, Adae was admitted to another hospital,

[e] https://www.justice.gov/usao-md/pr/maryland-health-care-provider-convicted-patient-deaths.

Middletown Regional Hospital, and was again discharged without a diagnosis and without the hospital getting the blood culture results that were performed at Clinton Memorial Hospital. In fact, the physician at Clinton Memorial Hospital was made aware of the blood culture results on July 2 but failed to advise the patient of those results or take any action to further evaluate or treat her.

Four days later, Adae was readmitted to Middletown Regional Hospital, where she was finally diagnosed with an epidural abscess. By that time, however, Adae had developed progressive paraplegia, weakness of her upper and lower extremities, slurred speech, and acute renal failure. Adae sued Clinton Memorial Hospital and its affiliate teaching university.[f]

Case Study 6 Questions

1. Although Clinton Memorial Hospital was sued, should Middletown Regional Hospital have been included in the lawsuit?
2. Why was the hospital sued and not the physician who misdiagnosed the patient and neglected to confirm the blood culture tests?

CASE STUDY 7: HOSPITAL FINED FOR "PATIENT DUMPING"

On March 30, 2016, Pacifica Hospital of the Valley discharged 38-year-old Kasey Lucious, a patient with a history of mental illness and homelessness, after a 30-day stay. Hospital staff put Lucious in a taxi to Crenshaw Nursing Home without contacting her family and without confirming that the nursing home would admit her. Lucious was dropped off at the nursing home but never checked in. Her family filed a missing person report, and she was found wandering the streets 3 days later. The hospital agreed to a settlement of $1 million to resolve allegations that it failed to follow homeless patient discharge protocols.[g]

Case Study 7 Questions

1. What are the laws that protect patients who arrive at hospitals for medical care?
2. What actions should the hospital have taken before discharging the patient?

CASE STUDY 8: MEDICAL CENTER WRONGFULLY TERMINATES EMPLOYEE

Amanda Perry, a 41-year-old medical biller, was working at Covenant's Visiting Nursing Association Department for several years before being promoted to office coordinator of two physicians' offices in 2012. Perry, who had a history of psychiatric illness, suffered from worsening psychiatric symptoms and requested a leave of absence between July 25 and October 6, 2014. Perry's supervisor allegedly expressed concerns about the amount of time she was taking off from work and told her "to get it together."

On her return to work, Perry was reassigned and, a few weeks later, she received a "step I" discipline for behavioral and performance issues. She subsequently received a "step III" discipline for unprofessional conduct and for crying in front of a patient. Perry was effectively fired when she received a "step IV" discipline for allegedly asking a coworker to provide a false statement. Although the healthcare organization claimed she was fired for the issues identified in the disciplinary warnings, Perry said she was terminated because she requested time off and because of her disability. Perry sued, and the federal jury awarded more than $500,000 to her for violation of the Family and Medical Leave Act (FMLA) and the Disabilities Civil Rights Act.[h]

Case Study 8 Questions

1. What are the conditions that would allow an employee to take FMLA leave?
2. To protect both the employee and employer in this case, what information should be included in an employee handbook?
3. Could this employee be terminated if she worked in a state with employment-at-will laws?

[f] Cynthia A. Adae v. University of Cincinnati, Case No. 2007-08228.

[g] https://www.lacityattorney.org/single-post/2016/06/23/City-Attorney-Mike-Feuer-Secures-1-Million-in-Penalties-Over-Allegations-of-Second-Incident-of-Homeless-Patient-Dumping-By-Pacifica-Hospital-of-the-Valley.

[h] Perry v. Covenant Medical Center, Inc. Case No. 15-cv-11040.

CASE STUDY 9: NURSES CLAIM DISCRIMINATION

Four former healthcare professionals filed separate lawsuits against Capital Health Regional Medical Center in Trenton, New Jersey, claiming they faced months of racial and disability discrimination before they were unjustly fired. One of the lawsuits was filed on behalf of an African American woman who worked at the hospital as a medical assistant. She claims she was subjected to racial slurs from one supervisor and that another supervisor made racist comments around her. In her lawsuit, she claimed she was fired in June 2015 and replaced with a Caucasian employee. Two other former employees—a nurse and a medical assistant—claim they were also subjected to racial discrimination. The nurse was fired in June 2015, and the medical assistant was fired in February 2015, and both claim they were replaced by Caucasian employees.

The fourth lawsuit was brought on behalf of a nurse practitioner working at the hospital. The nurse practitioner began working at the hospital in 2013, but she was left disabled by a car crash in March 2015. Although she could still perform her duties with accommodations for her disability, she was fired in May 2015. She further alleges that the hospital retaliated against her for refusing to prescribe medication to patients when she thought they were abusing drugs and for objecting to racial discrimination that she witnessed.[i]

Case Study 9 Questions

1. How is discrimination in the workplace defined?
2. If the racial comments came from coworkers and not the supervisors, would this still be defined as discrimination?

CASE STUDY 10: INJURED MOTORIST FILES NEGLIGENCE AND *RESPONDEAT SUPERIOR* CASE

A motorist was seriously injured when another car, operated by Christopher Richardson, crossed the center line, causing a head-on collision. Richardson, a longshoreman, fell asleep at the wheel while traveling home after working a 22-h shift at his job site located at the Port of Baltimore. The injured motorist, Sergeant Michael Barclay, and his wife, Robin Barclay, filed a lawsuit against several parties, including Richardson's employer, Ports America Baltimore, Inc.

The lawsuit alleged that the employer was liable for Barclay's injuries under *respondeat superior* and primary negligence by failing to protect the general motoring public from an employee driving home after an unreasonably long shift. The employer contested the lawsuit and asserted that, based on both doctrines, neither requirement was met. The trial court agreed with employer. The Court of Special Appeals affirmed.[j]

Case Study 10 Questions

1. Does the employer have a duty to the public to ensure that an employee's abilities are not impaired after working an extended work schedule?
2. Why did the courts dismiss the lawsuit based on *respondeat superior*?
3. Why did the lawsuit not meet the legal requirement of negligence?

CASE STUDY 11: PHYSICIAN FORCED TO ALLOW SUICIDE

In September 2007, 26-year-old Kerrie Wooltorton ingested a lethal dose of antifreeze. Although her intent was to commit suicide, she called an ambulance and was rushed to the hospital. In the previous 12-month period, Wooltorton had attempted suicide several times by ingesting antifreeze but still accepted lifesaving treatment. Wooltorton had a history of self-harm, depression, and an untreatable personality disorder. However, on this occasion, she declined all treatment. Furthermore, on admission at the hospital, Wooltorton provided an advance directive when she was still conscious. Her physician requested a second opinion and legal advice but ultimately felt obligated to comply with Wooltorton's wishes. Wooltorton did not receive any treatment, except for comfort care, and died the following day.[k]

[i] http://www.nj.com/mercer/index.ssf/2016/06/group_of_nurses_sues_capital_health_over_racial_di.html.

[j] Michael S. BARCLAY, et ux. v. Lena BRISCOE, et al., Lena Briscoe, Personal Representative of the Estate of Christopher Eugene Richardson. v. Ports America Baltimore, Inc. No. 41, Sept. Term, 2011.

[k] https://www.theguardian.com/society/2009/oct/01/living-will-suicide-legal.

Case Study 11 Questions

1. Should her physicians have followed her advance directive or provided lifesaving treatment because she accepted it the previous times?
2. What would be the legal repercussions if her physician acted against her wishes and provided lifesaving treatment?

CASE STUDY 12: PREGNANT NURSING HOME WORKER FORCED ON UNPAID LEAVE

Asia Myers worked as a certified nursing assistant at Hope Healthcare Center, a long-term care facility. Early in her pregnancy, she experienced complications and was told by her physician that she could continue to work but should not do any lifting on the job. Myers requested an accommodation from her employer. Even though the long-term care facility had a history of providing light-duty accommodations to employees with temporary lifting restrictions, including workers who had been injured on the job, Myers was told not to return to work until the restrictions were lifted. She was out of work for 34 days with no wages and no health insurance. Myers was able to return to work after her physician determined the complications had passed, but she suffered significant financial hardship from being out of work for more than a month. Myers sued her employers, and a settlement was reached.[l]

Case Study 12 Questions

1. What law was the employer violating?
2. How was this case based on discrimination?

CASE STUDY 13: INMATE AS AN ORGAN TRANSPLANT RECIPIENT

A 45-year-old inmate is a former alcoholic and drug addict who is serving a life sentence for double homicide and is suffering from hepatitis C and symptoms of end-stage liver disease. The prison physician was asked by the prison staff to evaluate the inmate's eligibility for a liver transplant. Before giving his approval, the physician needs to evaluate the likelihood that the inmate will comply with follow-up treatment and how likely it is that he will remain drug and alcohol free for the rest of his life upon his release from prison.[m]

Case Study 13 Questions

1. Based on his conviction, should the inmate be approved for a transplant over an individual not incarcerated?
2. What other factors must the physician and United Network for Organ Sharing consider before approving an organ for transplantation?

CASE STUDY 14: SEVERELY BURNED VICTIM REFUSED RIGHT TO DIE

In 1973, Dax Cowart, a 25-year-old Air Force Reserve pilot, went with his father to visit a tract of land they were interested in purchasing. Unbeknownst to them, there was a propane gas leak that was filling the area. When they started the car, the propane was ignited, which created a massive explosion. Cowart's father died. Cowart suffered serious burns on two-thirds of his body and loss of both hands, eyes, and ears.

Fearing he would be unable to regain his former function, he refused treatment on the way to the hospital. While hospitalized for 10 months, Cowart repeatedly begged his physicians to end treatment and allow him to die, especially because many of the treatments were excruciatingly painful for him. He was also given only limited painkillers and denied access to legal assistance. Despite his demand to discontinue treatment, wound care was continued, skin grafts performed, and nutritional and fluid support provided. He was discharged after the amputation of several fingers and removal of his right eye and became dependent on others to assist in personal functions.[n]

Case Study 14 Questions

1. Who was liable or negligent that caused the accident?
2. Did Cowart have the right to refuse care? Was he competent enough to make that decision?
3. Did the physician have the right to disregard Cowart's autonomy and patient's rights?

[l] *Myers v. Hope Healthcare Center LLC.*

[m] http://journalofethics.ama-assn.org/2008/02/ccas2-0802.html.

[n] *JAMA*. 1989;262:2613–14. https://doi.org/10.1001/jama.1989.03430180159054.

CASE STUDY 15: MERCY KILLING OF DISABLED DAUGHTER

Tracy Latimer was born November 23, 1980. An interruption in Tracy's supply of oxygen during birth caused cerebral palsy; severe mental and physical disabilities; and violent seizures, which were controlled with seizure medication. She had little or no voluntary control of her muscles, wore diapers, and could not walk or talk. In addition, Latimer was in constant pain with almost every movement. During this time, her family provided her excellent care, and she underwent several surgeries, including surgeries to lengthen tendons, release muscles, and correct scoliosis in which rods were inserted into her back. However, Latimer still suffered constant pain.

On October 24, 1993, Latimer's mother found her dead while in the care of her father. After autopsy results showed Latimer died of carbon monoxide poisoning, her father confessed that he had killed her by placing her in his truck and connecting a hose from the truck's exhaust pipe to the cab. He said he did it out of love and compassion and not wanting to see his daughter in constant pain and having to endure multiple surgeries. Latimer's father was convicted of second-degree murder and sentenced to life imprisonment with no possibility of parole for 10 years.[o]

Case Study 15 Questions

1. Does this meet the conditions of euthanasia because Latimer was unable to consent?
2. Was the conviction and sentence of Latimer's father appropriate?

CASE STUDY 16: MISDIAGNOSIS RESULTS IN DISABILITY

Bryan Mejia was born with only one leg and no arms. His parents, Ana Mejia and Rodolfo Santana, have accused Marie Morel, MD, and OB/GYN Specialists of the Palm Beaches and Perinatal Specialists of the Palm Beaches of negligence for not properly detecting their son's defect and disability through ultrasound scans before he was born. They said they would have aborted their son if they had known he would have only one limb. The parents sued the physician and the clinic. The defendant's attorney argued that Morel is not to blame because the parents opted to not undergo amniocentesis, which might have detected any abnormalities. The parents rejected it because they were told that there was a small risk that performing the test would cause a miscarriage. The parents decided they would rather risk the chance of having a child with mental retardation than to risk a miscarriage. The court awarded the parents $4.5 million for a wrongful birth lawsuit.[p]

Case Study 16 Questions

1. Should Mejia's parents be held responsible because they declined the amniocentesis that might have detected their son's defect?
2. Would this be a case of eugenics? Does it promote aborting unborn children when diagnosed with physical or mental disability?

CASE STUDY 17: DISCLOSURE OF PATIENT INFORMATION

In July 2011, Kimberly White requested Tufts Medical Center in Boston to send a form for a disability claim. Instead, the hospital sent four pages of medical records about her hysterectomy to a shared fax machine at her workplace, which her colleagues read. White felt embarrassed and that she "can't go back there [work]" and that she "couldn't live with knowing what these people knew about me." White filed a complaint in Plymouth County Superior Court. However, the hospital denied any wrongdoing, stating that, "In this matter, we complied with a patient's request to share information. We firmly believe we responded to the patient's request appropriately."[q]

Case Study 17 Questions

1. Did the hospital violate HIPAA?
2. What damages could White request in this situation?

[o] http://www.yorku.ca/rweisman/courses/sosc3992/pdf/Latimer-timelineandsupplement-PopularTrials.pdf.

[p] http://www.palmbeachpost.com/news/jury-awards-west-palm-beach-parents-child-born-with-arms-one-leg-million/E4pWBxRxQqGsj0wtzkPYsI/.

[q] https://www.bostonglobe.com/metro/2011/10/28/kimberly-white-drops-privacy-breach-suit-against-tufts-medical-center/oORZkGGb5DiifYLRYlVWyI/story.html.

CASE STUDY 18: CONSCIENTIOUS CLAUSE IN PROVIDING CONTRACEPTIVES

On July 6, 2002, a University of Wisconsin–Stout student went to the Kmart in Menomonie, Wisconsin, to fill her prescription for birth control pills. The only pharmacist on duty, Neil Noesen, asked if she intended to use the prescription for contraception. When she replied "yes," Noesen, a Catholic, refused to fill the prescription, explaining that to do so would be against his religious beliefs. He also refused to transfer the prescription or tell her how or where she could get the prescription filled because, in his view, it would constitute participating in wrongful behavior. Before employment at Kmart, Noesen had informed the district manager that he would not dispense contraceptives; however, he did not mention that he would refuse to refer or to transfer prescriptions.

The woman filed a complaint with the Wisconsin Department of Regulation and Licensing's Pharmacy Examining Board. The administrative law judge who heard the complaint found that the ordinary standard of care "requires that a pharmacist who exercises a conscientious objection to dispensing of a prescription must ensure that there is an alternative mechanism for the patient to receive his or her medication, including informing the patient of their options to obtain their prescription." Furthermore, he found that Noesen's conduct constituted "a danger to the health, welfare, or safety of a patient and was practiced in a manner that substantially departs from the standard of care ordinarily exercised by a pharmacist and which harmed or could have harmed a patient." His ruling also limited Noesen's license, requiring him to notify any pharmacy where he worked of any practices he would refuse to perform and how he would ensure patient access to prescriptions that he declined to fill. Noesen appealed, but the judge's decision was upheld.[r]

Case Study 18 Questions

1. Did Noesen have the right to refuse based on the conscientious clause and his religious freedom?
2. Would Noesen's actions be considered discriminatory? How so?
3. Does Noesen's employer, Kmart, have any liability in this case?

CASE STUDY 19: PARENTAL AUTHORITY RESULTS IN BABY'S DEATH

Rachel Joy Piland, 30, and her husband, Joshua Barry Piland, 36, gave birth to a newborn baby girl. The baby was delivered by a midwife, who did not see any problems at the delivery. The midwife returned the next day as a follow-up and saw that the baby was severely jaundiced. The midwife urged the parents to take the baby to a physician or the hospital, warning that the baby could suffer brain damage or die if she did not receive proper medical attention. The parents did not, with Rachel Piland stating, "God doesn't make mistakes." The Pilands began to pray over their infant. Despite the midwife continuing to urge them to get medical attention for the baby, the Pilands did not and eventually stopped going to their appointments with the midwife. Three days later, the infant was dead. Rachel's brother notified the authorities, and, when the police arrived at the couple's home, they found people from the Pilands' church praying over the baby.[s]

Case Study 19 Questions

1. Do physicians and authorities have the right to override parental authority or religious freedom?
2. Is the midwife negligent for not reporting this to the authorities?

CASE STUDY 20: TERMINAL BABY USED FOR ORGAN DONATION

At 19 weeks pregnant, Royce Young and his wife, Keri, found out that their unborn daughter had a rare birth defect called *anencephaly,* a condition in which the baby will be born with an underdeveloped brain and an incomplete skull. Their options were either to terminate the pregnancy or to give birth and the baby would soon die. The

[r] Neil NOESEN, Petitioner-Appellant v. STATE of Wisconsin DEPARTMENT OF REGULATION AND LICENSING, PHARMACY EXAMINING BOARD, Respondent-Respondent. No. 2006AP1110 (March 25, 2008).

[s] http://www.lansingstatejournal.com/story/news/local/2017/10/03/lansing-couple-newborn-death-refused-order-banning-physical-discipline/722940001/.

Youngs decided to continue with the pregnancy and, once the baby was born, donate her organs. The baby would not be able to survive on her own once born and would be dependent on life-sustaining equipment until her organs could be donated. The baby was unexpectedly stillborn, and none of her organs could be used for donation.[t]

Case Study 20 Questions

1. Owing to the shortage of organs, did the Youngs make the most moral and ethical decision in planning on donating their terminally ill daughter's organs?
2. Is it unethical to artificially sustain the baby's life for the purpose of organ donation?

Case Study 21: Death in Pregnancy

Marlise Muñoz was found unconscious on the floor by her husband at their family home on November 26, 2013. She had suffered a massive pulmonary embolism. When paramedics arrived, she was alive but not breathing. She was rushed to John Peter Smith Hospital in Fort Worth, Texas, where she was pronounced brain dead 2 days later. She and her husband, 33 years old, both veteran paramedics, had discussed end-of-life issues, and Muñoz made it clear that she did not want to be kept alive by life support under any circumstances. Her other family members agreed, and they requested withdrawal of ventilation and other measures sustaining her body's function.

However, Muñoz was 14 weeks pregnant. The hospital refused, citing the Texas Advance Directive Act that prohibits the discontinuation of life-sustaining treatment if a woman is pregnant. The physicians and the hospital explained that it did not matter what Muñoz, her husband, or her family wanted—it was a law of the state. She would be required by law to stay on the ventilator until her 14-week-old fetus was delivered or died. The hospital kept Muñoz alive for 2 months despite Muñoz being declared brain dead and the fetus not being viable. Muñoz's husband sued the hospital.[u]

[t] https://www.washingtonpost.com/news/parenting/wp/2017/04/29/they-knew-their-unborn-baby-would-die-just-not-like-this/?utm_term=.a74bcfb96043.

[u] https://www.npr.org/sections/health-shots/2014/01/28/267759687/the-strange-case-of-marlise-Muñoz-and-john-peter-smith-hospital.

CASE STUDY 21 QUESTIONS

1. Do you think a mother's rights should supersede the rights of an unborn child?
2. Although when she was alive, Muñoz requested to refuse life-sustaining treatment; do you think her decision would have been different knowing she was pregnant?
3. What do you think the court decided?

CASE STUDY 22: MEDICATION ERROR IN ACTOR'S NEWBORN TWINS

In November 2007, Dennis Quaid, the actor, and his wife Kimberly gave birth to their twin children, Zoe Grace and Thomas Boone. When the newborns were just 2 weeks old, they developed a bacterial infection, which required treatment with antibiotics and heparin, a blood thinning medication. However, the Quaid twins were administered 1000 times more heparin than prescribed. The hospital said a pharmacy technician took the heparin from the pharmacy's supply without having a second technician verify the drug's concentration, as hospital policy required. Then, when the heparin was delivered to a satellite pharmacy that serves the pediatrics unit, a different pharmacy technician there did not verify the concentration, as required. Finally, the nurses who administered the heparin to the twins violated policy by neglecting to verify that it was the correct medication and dose before administering. The medication error was only identified only after one of the twins started to seep blood from a puncture site.

After almost 2 weeks in intensive care, the twins made a full recovery. The Quaids filed a lawsuit against Baxter Healthcare Corporation, the makers of heparin, and the hospital. The case against Baxter was dismissed, but the case with the hospital was settled for $750,000.[v]

Case Study 22 Questions

1. What are the four conditions of negligence? Which one(s) did the healthcare professions violate?

[v] Dennis Quaid and Kimberly Quaid, Parents and Next Friends of Zoe Grace Quaid and Thomas Boone Quaid, Plaintiffs-Appellants, v. Baxter Healthcare Corporation, Defendant-Appellee, No. 1-08-2727 (June 2009).

2. Who would ultimately be liable for the malpractice lawsuit?
3. Which types of damages did the Quaids receive?

CASE STUDY 23: SURGERY PERFORMED ON THE WRONG SIDE

In 2007, on three different occasions, three surgeons at Rhode Island Hospital started operating on the wrong side of the brain. For two of the surgeries, the patients were able to make a full recovery. The third patient died a few weeks later after having the surgery. That surgery prompted the state to order the hospital to develop a neurosurgery checklist that includes information about the location of the surgery and a patient's medical history, and to train staff on the new checklist. In addition, the hospital said it was reevaluating its training and policies, providing more oversight, and giving nursing staff the power to ensure proper procedures are followed. The Board of Medical Licensure and Discipline and Board of Nursing also investigated, with the surgeon receiving a 2-month suspension of his license before returning to work.[w]

Case Study 23 Questions

1. Was the 2-month suspension of the surgeon appropriate and fair?
2. What kind of crime could the surgeon be charged with?
3. Besides crimes, what other penalties could the surgeon face?

CASE STUDY 24: NEGLIGENCE DURING SURGICAL ANESTHESIA RESULTS IN SUICIDE

In January 2006, Sherman Sizemore, a former coal miner and minister, was admitted to Raleigh General Hospital for exploratory surgery for abdominal pain. Sizemore was administered paralytic drugs to prevent muscle movement as an anesthesia during surgery. However, 16 min into the surgery, Sizemore was found to still be awake. The surgery team realized that a second general anesthetic drug, which would make Sizemore lose consciousness and prevent him from feeling the pain of the surgery, was not administered. Sizemore experienced nearly a half hour of surgery, complete with pain, while fully conscious. Sizemore was never told what happened but, since the surgery, was experiencing panic attacks, insomnia, nightmares, and thoughts that people were trying to bury him. With no prior history of psychiatric or psychological conditions, Sizemore committed suicide. Sizemore's two daughters filed a lawsuit against the Raleigh Anesthesia Associates after a physician mentioned the possibility of the connection, prompting a closer look at his medical records. The lawsuit was settled.[x]

Case Study 24 Questions

1. What kind of damages or compensation could the patient receive?
2. Does the surgeon have a duty to disclose to the patient what happened during the surgery even though the patient made it through the surgery?
3. What concerns should physicians have in providing too much information, especially if an indent was minor and had no impact on the surgery?

CASE STUDY 25: TRANSPLANT PATIENT RECEIVES INCOMPATIBLE ORGANS

In 2003, 17-year-old Jesica Santillan came to the United States from Mexico to receive treatment for a life-threatening heart and lung condition. Her parents illegally smuggled her into the country. They moved to North Carolina and lived in a trailer until they could raise enough money for the surgery. Once a heart and lung were made available, the organs were transplanted into Santillan. The surgeon had almost completed the operation when he learned that the organs came from a donor with type A blood, incompatible with Santillan's type O blood. Santillan's body rejected the organs and her condition quickly deteriorated. A second transplant with compatible organs was performed but, by this time, Santillan had suffered irreversible brain damage and organ failure.

[w]http://news.legalexaminer.com/rhode-island-hospital-reprimanded-for-wrong-site-surgeries.aspx?googleid=28640.

[x]http://www.timeswv.com/news/local_news/update-settlement-reached-in-suit-over-anesthesia/article_6dfa728e-b878-51e9-921b-e175de90d3fb.html.

Two weeks later, Santillan was taken off life support. It was discovered that more than a dozen staff members at the hospital and at the two organizations responsible for getting the new heart and lungs to Santillan failed to cross-check her blood type before the surgery to see if it was a match with the blood type of the donor. The surgeon, who had performed more than one hundred heart transplants, took responsibility for the error, and the hospital implemented a new system to double-check transplants to prevent similar errors from occurring.[y]

Case Study 25 Questions

1. Although the surgeon took responsibility for the error, which other party or parties could be liable for this negligence?
2. What are the factors when allocating an organ? Should immigration status be a factor?

CASE STUDY 26: SURGEON ILLEGALLY ACCESSES MEDICAL RECORDS

Huping Zhou, a former cardiothoracic surgeon and a researcher at the UCLA School of Medicine, began accessing patient medical records after being terminated for performance issues. Zhou illegally accessed the UCLA medical records system more than 300 times, viewing the health records of his immediate supervisor, his coworkers, and several celebrities, including Arnold Schwarzenegger, Drew Barrymore, Leonardo DiCaprio, and Tom Hanks. Zhou was sentenced to 4 months in jail and a $2000 fine.[z]

Case Study 26 Questions

1. What law(s) did Dr. Zhou commit?
2. What are the fines and penalties for violating this law? Was the sentence and fine appropriate?

CASE STUDY 27: FERTILITY PHYSICIAN USES OWN SPERM FOR INSEMINATION

Donald Cline, a retired Indianapolis fertility physician, was accused of inseminating patients with his own sperm. Cline allegedly told six adults who believed they were his children that he had donated his own sperm about 50 times starting in the 1970s, according to court documents when he was charged. He had told his patients they were receiving sperm from medical or dental residents or medical students, and that no single donor's sperm was used more than three times. However, paternity tests indicate Cline is likely the biological father of at least two of his patients' children, and online genetic tests show he may be the father of more than 20 other children. No charges were filed against Cline because Indiana law does not prohibit fertility physicians from using their own sperm.[aa]

Case Study 27 Questions

1. What laws could Dr. Cline be charged with?
2. What lawsuit could the patients file against Dr. Cline?
3. Could the children of the patients that were born from Dr. Cline's sperm file lawsuits? What could they be based on?

CASE STUDY 28: DYING PATIENT DENIED CPR

On March 2013, Lorraine Bayless, 87, collapsed in a dining room at Glenwood Gardens, an elderly living facility. A staff member called 911 and a fire department dispatcher urged a nurse, who had CPR training, to start CPR on Bayless. The nurse refused to perform the procedure on Bayless, saying it was against the facility's policy. Based on the facility's policy, staff members are prohibited from performing CPR or other medical interventions. Bayless was later pronounced dead at the hospital. No criminal charges were filed, but the facility was conducting a company-wide review of its policies.[ab]

Case Study 28 Questions

1. Why did the nurse face any criminal charges or negligent charges?
2. Should the hospital have faced any penalties?
3. Based on the concept of scope of practice, should the nurse or other healthcare professionals at the facility performed CPR?

[y] https://www.ncbi.nlm.nih.gov/pmc/articles/PMC1125622/.
[z] United States of America, Plaintiff–Appellee, v. Huping Zhou, Defendant–Appellant. No. 10-50231 (May 2012).

[aa] https://www.washingtontimes.com/news/2017/dec/14/donald-cline-retired-fertility-doctor-faces-judge-/.
[ab] http://www.cnn.com/2013/03/04/health/california-cpr-death/index.html.

CASE STUDY 29: DERMATOLOGY PRACTICE PENALIZED FOR HIPAA VIOLATIONS

A thumb drive was stolen from an employee at Adult & Pediatric Dermatology, P.C., of Concord, Massachusetts, and never recovered. The lost thumb drive was unencrypted and contained the electronic protected health information of about 2200 patients. The incident was reported to the U.S. Department of Health and Human Services' Office for Civil Rights (OCR), who fined the medical practice a $150,000 penalty. In addition, the OCR required the practice to implement a corrective action plan for losing confidential patient information and for not identifying the theft and managing the risk in a HIPAA risk analysis.[ac]

Case Study 29 Questions

1. Should the dermatology clinic have been penalized since the patient information was stolen?
2. What corrective actions should the clinic take to prevent this situation from occurring again?

CASE STUDY 30: NURSE OUTS STD PATIENT TO MAN'S GIRLFRIEND

A registered nurse employed by a New York clinic learned of the sexually transmitted disease of a patient who happened to also be her sister-in-law's boyfriend. The nurse sent several text messages to the sister-in-law about the patient's condition. The sister-in-law forwarded the text messages to the patient, who filed a complaint to the clinic. The patient then sued the clinic, despite the clinic having already terminated the nurse's employment. The patient claimed that the clinic and several related entities had breached their responsibility under the law to keep his medical information confidential. The trial court judge dismissed the claim on the grounds that the nurse's actions were both unforeseeable and based on personal reasons. In January 2014, the U.S. Court of Appeals for the Second Circuit upheld the dismissal by the lower court because, under New York law, there is no liability for the employer when an employee acts outside the scope of his or her responsibility.[ad]

Case Study 30 Questions

1. What laws did the nurse violate?
2. The nurse was still an employee of the clinic when she sent the texts to her sister-in-law. Do you agree or disagree with the courts' dismissal of the case?

CASE STUDY 31: SURROGATE GIVES BIRTH TO TRIPLETS FOR UNFIT PARENT

In the court case of *C.M. v. M.C.*, Melissa Cook was hired through a surrogacy broker to carry the embryos from Chester Moore, Jr., and a 20-year-old donor's eggs. Cook was paid $30,000 for one child and $6000 for each additional child. Three embryos were implanted, and all proved to be viable. Moore requested that one or two embryos be aborted because he wanted only one or two children and could not afford to support three children. When Cook refused and did not accept payment of more than half of the money still owed to her, she was threatened with a lawsuit. The triplets were born premature in February 2016 and spent 10 weeks in the NICU.

Once discharged from the hospital, custody of the three babies was given custody to Moore, who was then a 50-year-old, deaf, mute Georgia postal worker living in his disabled, elderly parents' basement. In addition, Moore was reported to suffer from depression, anxiety, a paranoid personality disorder, and irrational anger fits that occasionally turned violent. There was no home visit or inquiry into Moore's parental fitness before he entered into the contract, as would be required for an adoption. After an appeal was denied by California's supreme court, on September 20, 2017, a petition was filed with the U.S. Supreme Court to hear California's enforcement of surrogacy contracts under the state's statute. On October 2, 2017, the U.S. Supreme Court refused to hear the case.[ae]

[ac] https://www.hhs.gov/hipaa/for-professionals/compliance-enforcement/examples/APDerm/index.html.

[ad] http://ceas.uc.edu/content/dam/aero/docs/fire/Clinic.pdf.

[ae] Court of Appeal, Second District, Division 1, California. C. M., Plaintiff and Respondent, v. M.C., Defendant and Appellant. B270525 (January 2017).

Case Study 31 Questions

1. Based on Moore's current mental condition and living situation, should he have been prevented from having a child through surrogacy?
2. Does Cook, the surrogate, have any legal right to the baby that she carried? How about the 20-year-old donor?

CASE STUDY 32: BIRTH CONTROL UNDER THE AFFORDABLE CARE ACT

Under the Affordable Care Act (ACA), insurers must cover preventative services, which includes providing birth control. However, in 2014, religious nonprofit organizations, such as universities and charities, said providing birth control violates their religious beliefs. The U.S. Supreme Court ruled that closely held private companies can object to the ACA mandate, but employers' insurers may provide coverage instead of the employer. In 2015, the Little Sisters of the Poor Home for the Aged and its affiliates filed a petition requesting an exemption that would keep employees from getting birth control at all under the employer's health plan.[af]

Case Study 32 Questions

1. On what conditions can organizations, such as the Little Sisters of the Poor Home for the Aged, petition to be exempt for specific mandates?
2. What other exemptions can organizations or individuals file to avoid specific requirements and mandates?

CASE STUDY 33: FILE CONVERSION LEADS TO BREACH IN PATIENT CONFIDENTIALITY

In 2016, an orthopedic clinic hired an outside vendor to convert all x-ray films on file to digital form. However, as required by HIPAA guidelines, the clinic did not first sign a business associate agreement with the vendor. The OCR ordered the clinic to pay $750,000 and implement a Corrective Action Plan.[ag]

[af]Little Sisters of the Poor v. Burwell, No. 13-1540 (10th Cir. 2015).
[ag]https://www.hhs.gov/hipaa/for-professionals/compliance-enforcement/agreements/raleigh-orthopaedic-clinic-bulletin/index.html.

Case Study 33 Questions

1. According to HIPAA, what crime(s) was violated?
2. Why is it important for the clinic to have the business sign an associate agreement?

CASE STUDY 34: HOME-HEALTH AGENCY FILES FALSE CLAIMS TO MEDICARE

From February 2006 to June 2015, Marie Neba and her husband, Ebong Tilong, were co-owners of Fiango Home Healthcare and defrauded Medicare of almost $13 million. Neba paid illegal kickbacks to several physician and medical groups in exchange for authorizing home-health services for Medicare beneficiaries that were not needed. They also paid illegal kickbacks to patient recruiters for referring Medicare beneficiaries for those services and paid Medicare beneficiaries for allowing them to use their Medicare information to bill the agency for home-health services that were either not needed or never provided. In addition, Neba falsified medical records to make it appear that the Medicare beneficiaries qualified for and received home-health services. In November 2016, Neba was convicted, and Tilong pled guilty. Four others have pleaded guilty based on their roles in the fraudulent scheme, including the former medical director and two patient recruiters.[ah]

Case Study 34 Questions

1. What law does kickbacks violate? Are they civil or criminal?
2. What penalties could Neba, Tilong, the medical director, and the patient recruiters face?

CASE STUDY 35: WORKPLACE VIOLENCE

Employees of Brookdale University Hospital and Medical Center in Brooklyn were exposed to head, eye, face, and groin injuries and intimidation and threats during routine interactions with patients and visitors. The U.S. Department of Labor's Occupational Safety

[ah]https://www.justice.gov/opa/pr/owner-home-health-agency-sentenced-75-years-prison-involvement-13-million-medicare-fraud.

and Health Administration (OSHA) found approximately 40 incidents of workplace violence reported between February 7 and April 12, 2014, where employees were threatened and physically or verbally assaulted by patients and visitors or when breaking up altercations between patients. The most serious incident was on February 7, when a nurse was assaulted while working and sustained severe brain injuries. As a result, OSHA cited Brookdale for one willful violation and a proposed fine of $70,000 for failing to develop and implement adequate measures to reduce or eliminate the likelihood of physical violence and assaults against employees by patients or visitors.[ai]

Case Study 35 Questions

1. What are the responsibilities of Brookdale as an employer to safety?
2. What actions can Brookdale take to address workplace violence? What role does risk management have?

[ai] https://www.osha.gov/ooc/citations/Brookdale.pdf.

APPENDIX C

State Medical Record Laws

State Medical Record Laws: Minimum Medical Record Retention Periods for Records Held by Medical Doctors and Hospitals

State	Medical Doctors	Hospitals
Alabama	As long as may be necessary to treat the patient and for medical/legal purposes. Ala. Admin. Code r. 545-X-4-.08 (2007).[a]	5 years Ala. Admin. Code § 420-5-7.10 (adopting 42 C.F.R. § 482.24).
Alaska	N/A	**Adult patients** 7 years after the discharge of the patient. **Minor patients (under 19)** 7 years after discharge or until patient reaches the age of 21, whichever is longer. Alaska Stat. § 18.20.085(a) (2008).
Arizona	**Adult patients** 6 years after the last date of services from the provider. **Minor patients** 6 years after the last date of services from the provider or until patient reaches the age of 21, whichever is longer. Ariz. Rev. Stat. § 12-2297 (2008).	**Adult patients** 6 years after the last date of services from the provider. **Minor patients** 6 years after the last date of services from the provider or until patient reaches the age of 21, whichever is longer. Ariz. Rev. Stat. § 12-2297 (2008).
Arkansas	N/A	**Adult patients** 10 years after the last discharge, but master patient index data must be kept permanently. **Minor patients** Complete medical records must be retained 2 years after the age of majority (i.e., until patient turns 20). 016 24 Code Ark. Rules and Regs. 007 § 14(19) (2008).
California	N/A[a]	**Adult patients** 7 years after discharge of the patient. **Minor patients** 7 years after discharge or 1 years after the patient reaches the age of 18 (i.e., until patient turns 19), whichever is longer. Cal. Code Regs. tit. 22, § 70751(c) (2008).

Continued

State Medical Record Laws: Minimum Medical Record Retention Periods for Records Held by Medical Doctors and Hospitals—cont'd

State	Medical Doctors	Hospitals
Colorado	N/A[a]	**Adult patients** 10 years after the most recent patient care usage. **Minor patients** 10 years after the patient reaches the age of majority (i.e., until patient turns 28). 6 Colo. Code Regs. § 1011-1, chap. IV, 8.102 (2008).
Connecticut	7 years from the last date of treatment or upon the death of the patient, for 3 years Conn. Agencies Regs. § 19a-14-42 (2008).	10 years after the patient has been discharged. Conn. Agencies Regs. §§ 19-13-D3(d)(6) (2008).
Delaware	7 years from the last entry date on the patient's record. Del. Code Ann. tit. 24, §§ 1761 and 1702 (2008).	N/A
District of Columbia	**Adult patients** 3 years after last seeing the patient. **Minor patients** 3 years after last seeing the patient or 3 years after patient reaches the age of 18 (i.e., until patient turns 21). D.C. Mun. Regs. tit. 17, § 4612.1 (2008).	10 years after the date of discharge of the patient. D.C. Mun. Regs. tit. 22, § 2216 (2008).
Florida	5 years from the last patient contact. Fla. Admin. Code Ann. 64B8-10.002(3) (2008).	Public hospitals: 7 years after the last entry. Florida Department of State, General Records Schedule GS4 for Public Hospitals, Health Care Facilities and Medical Providers, (2007), http://dlis.dos.state.fl.us/barm/genschedules/GS04.pdf (accessed September 12, 2008).
Georgia	10 years from the date the record item was created. See Ga. Code Ann. § 31-33- 2(a)(1)(A) and (B)(i) (2008).	**Adult patients** 5 years after the date of discharge. **Minor patients** 5 years past the age of majority (i.e., until patient turns 23). See Ga. Code Ann. §§ 31-33-2(a)(1)(B)(ii) (2008); 31-7-2 (2008) (granting the department regulatory authority over hospitals) and Ga. Comp. R. & Regs. 290- 9-7-.18 (2008).
Guam	N/A	N/A

State Medical Record Laws: Minimum Medical Record Retention Periods for Records Held by Medical Doctors and Hospitals—cont'd

State	Medical Doctors	Hospitals
Hawaii	**Adult patients** Full medical records: 7 years after last data entry. Basic information (i.e., patient's name, birthdate, diagnoses, drugs prescribed, x-ray interpretations): 25 years after the last record entry. **Minor patients** Full medical records: 7 years after the patient reaches the age of majority (i.e., until patient turns 25). Basic information: 25 years after the minor reaches the age of majority (i.e., until patient turns 43). Haw. Rev. Stat. § 622-58 (2008).	**Adult patients** Full medical records: 7 years after last data entry. Basic information (i.e., patient's name, birth date, diagnoses, drugs prescribed, x-ray interpretations): 25 years after the last record entry. **Minor patients** Full medical records: 7 years after the minor reaches the age of majority (i.e., until patient turns 25). Basic information: 25 years after the minor reaches the age of majority (i.e., until patient turns 43). Haw. Rev. Stat. § 622-58 (2008).
Idaho	N/A	Clinical laboratory test records and reports: 5 years after the date of the test. Idaho Code Ann. § 39-1394 (2008).
Illinois	N/A	10 years See 210 Ill. Comp. Stat. 85/6.17(c) (2008).
Indiana	7 years Burns Ind. Code Ann. § 16-39-7-1 (2008).	7 years Burns Ind. Code Ann. § 16-39-7-1 (2008).
Iowa	**Adult patients** 7 years from the last date of service. **Minor patients** 1 years after the minor attains the age of majority (i.e., until patient turns 19). See Iowa Admin. Code r. 653-13.7(8) (2008); Iowa Code § 614.8 (2008).	N/A
Kansas	10 years from when professional service was provided. Kan. Admin. Regs. § 100-24-2 (a) (2008).	**Adult patients** Full records: 10 years after the last discharge of the patient. **Minor patients** Full records: 10 years or 1 year beyond the date that the patient reaches the age of majority (i.e., until patient turns 19), whichever is longer. Summary of destroyed records for both adults and minors—25 years Kan. Admin. Regs. § 28-34-9a (d)(1) (2008).

Continued

State Medical Record Laws: Minimum Medical Record Retention Periods for Records Held by Medical Doctors and Hospitals—cont'd

State	Medical Doctors	Hospitals
Kentucky	N/A	**Adult patients** 5 years from date of discharge. **Minor patients** 5 years from date of discharge or 3 years after the patient reaches the age of majority (i.e., until patient turns 21), whichever is longer. 902 Ky. Admin. Regs. 20:016 (2007).
Louisiana	6 years from the date a patient is last treated. La. Rev. Stat. Ann. § 40:1299.96(A)(3)(a) (2008).	10 years from the date a patient is discharged. La. Rev. Stat. Ann. § 40:2144(F)(1) (2008).
Maine	N/A	**Adult patients** 7 years **Minor patients** 6 years past the age of majority (i.e., until patient turns 24). See 10-144 Me. Code R. Ch. 112, § XII.B.1 (2008). Patient logs and written x-ray reports—permanently. 10-144 Me. Code R. Ch. 112, § XV.C.5 (2008).
Maryland	**Adult patients** 5 years after the record or report was made. **Minor patients** 5 years after the report or record was made or until the patient reaches the age of majority plus 3 years (i.e., until patient turns 21), whichever date is later. MD. Code Ann., Health–Gen. §§ 4-403(a)–(c) (2008).	**Adult patients** 5 years after the record or report was made. **Minor patients** 5 years after the report or record was made or until the patient reaches the age of majority plus 3 years (i.e., until patient turns 21), whichever date is later. MD. Code Ann., Health–Gen. §§ 4-403(a)–(c) (2008).
Massachusetts	**Adult patients** 7 years from the date of the last patient encounter. **Minor patients** 7 years from date of last patient encounter or until the patient reaches the age of 9, whichever is longer. 243 Mass. Code Regs. 2.07(13)(a) (2008).	30 years after the discharge or the final treatment of the patient. Mass. Gen. Laws ch. 111, § 70 (2008).
Michigan	7 years from the date of service. Mich. Comp. Laws § 333.16213 (2008).	7 years from the date of service. Mich. Comp. Laws § 333.20175 (2008).

State Medical Record Laws: Minimum Medical Record Retention Periods for Records Held by Medical Doctors and Hospitals—cont'd

State	Medical Doctors	Hospitals
Minnesota	N/A	Most medical records: Permanently (in microfilm). Miscellaneous documents: **Adult patients** 7 years **Minor patients** 7 years after the age of majority (i.e., until the patient turns 25). Minn. Stat. § 145.32 (2007) and Minn. R. 4642.1000 (2007).
Mississippi	N/A	**Adult patients** Discharged in sound mind: 10 years. Discharged at death: 7 years[b] **Minor patients** For the period of minority plus 7 years.[c] Miss. Code Ann. § 41-9-69(1) (2008).
Missouri	7 years from the date the last professional service was provided. Mo. Rev. Stat. § 334.097(2) (2008).	**Adult patients** 10 years **Minor patients** 10 years or until patient's 23rd birthday, whichever occurs later. Mo. Code Reg. tit. 19, § 30-094(15) (2008).
Montana	N/A[a]	**Adult patients** Entire medical record—10 years after the date of a patient's discharge or death. **Minor patients** Entire medical record—10 years after the date the patient either attains the age of majority (i.e., until patient is 28) or dies, whichever is earlier. Core medical record must be maintained at least an additional 10 years beyond the periods provided earlier. Mont. Admin. R. 37.106.402(1) and (4) (2007).
Nebraska	N/A	**Adult patients** 10 years after a patient's discharge. **Minor patients (under 19)** 10 years or until 3 years after the patient reaches age of majority (i.e., until patient turns 22), whichever is longer. Neb. Admin. Code 175 § 9-006.07A5 (2008).
Nevada	5 years after receipt or production of healthcare record. Nev. Rev. Stat. § 629.051 (2007).	5 years after receipt or production of healthcare record. Nev. Rev. Stat. § 629.051 (2007).
New Hampshire	7 years from the date of the patient's last contact with the physician, unless the patient has requested that the records be transferred to another healthcare provider. N.H. Code Admin. R. Ann. Med 501.02(f)(8) (2008).	**Adult patients** 7 years after a patient's discharge. **Minor patients** 7 years or until the minor reaches age 19, whichever is longer. N.H. Code Admin. R. Ann. He-P 802.06(h) (1994).[d]

Continued

State Medical Record Laws: Minimum Medical Record Retention Periods for Records Held by Medical Doctors and Hospitals—cont'd

State	Medical Doctors	Hospitals
New Jersey	7 years from the date of the most recent entry. N.J. Admin. Code § 13:35-6.5(b) (2008).	**Adult patients** 10 years after the most recent discharge. **Minor patients** 10 years after the most recent discharge or until the patient is 23 years of age, whichever is longer. **Discharge summary sheets (all)** 20 years after discharge. N.J. Stat. Ann. § 26:8-5 (2008).
New Mexico	**Adult patients** 2 years beyond what is required by state insurance laws and by Medicare and Medicaid requirements. **Minor patients** 2 years beyond the date the patient is 18 (i.e., until the patient turns 20). N.M. Code R. § 16.10.17.10 (C) (2008).	**Adult patients** 10 years after the last treatment date of the patient. **Minor patients** Age of majority plus 1 year (i.e., until the patient turns 19). N.M. Stat. Ann. § 14-6-2 (2008); N.M. Code R. § 7.7.2.30 (2008).
New York	**Adult patients** 6 years **Minor patients** 6 years and until 1 years after the minor reaches the age of 18 (i.e., until the patient turns 19). N.Y. Education § 6530 (2008) (providing retention requirements in the definitions for professional misconduct of physicians).	**Adult patients** 6 years from the date of discharge. **Minor patients** 6 years from the date of discharge or 3 years after the patient reaches 18 years (i.e., until patient turns 21), whichever is longer. **Deceased patients** At least 6 years after death. N.Y. Comp. Codes R. & Regs. tit. 10, § 405.10(a)(4) (2008).
North Carolina	N/A	**Adult patients** 11 years after discharge. **Minor patients** Until the patient's 30th birthday. 10 A N.C. Admin. Code 13B.3903(a), (b) (2008).
North Dakota	N/A	**Adult patients** 10 years after the last treatment date. **Minor patients** 10 years after the last treatment date or until the patient's 21st birthday, whichever is later. N.D. Admin. Code 33-07-01.1-20(1)(b) (2007).
Ohio	N/A	N/A

State Medical Record Laws: Minimum Medical Record Retention Periods for Records Held by Medical Doctors and Hospitals—cont'd

State	Medical Doctors	Hospitals
Oklahoma	N/A	**Adult patients** 5 years beyond the date the patient was last seen. **Minor patients** 3 years past the age of majority (i.e., until the patient turns 21). **Deceased patients** 3 years beyond the date of death. Okla. Admin. Code § 310:667-19-14 (2008).
Oregon	N/A[a]	10 years after the date of last discharge. Master patient index—permanently. Or. Admin. R. 333-505-0050(9) and (15) (2008).
Pennsylvania	**Adult patients** At least 7 years after the date of the last medical service. **Minor patients** 7 years after the date of the last medical service or 1 year after the patient reaches age 21 (i.e., until patient turns 22), whichever is the longer period. 49 Pa. Code § 16.95(e) (2008).	**Adult patients** 7 years after discharge. **Minor patients** 7 years after the patient attains majority[e] or as long as adult records would be maintained. 28 Pa. Code § 115.23 (2008).
Puerto Rico	N/A	N/A[f]
Rhode Island	5 years unless otherwise required by law or regulation. R.I. Code R.14-140-031, § 11.3 (2008).	**Adult patients** 5 years after discharge of the patient. R.I. Code R. 14 090 007 § 27.10 (2008). **Minor patients** 5 years after patient reaches the age of 18 years (i.e., until patient turns 23). R.I. Code R. 14 090 007 § 27.10.1 (2008).
South Carolina	**Adult patients** 10 years from the date of last treatment. **Minor patients** 13 years from the date of last treatment. S.C. Code Ann. § 44-115-120 (2007).	**Adult patients** 10 years. **Minor patients** Until the minor reaches age 18 and the "period of election" expires, which is usually 1 year after the minor reaches the age of majority (i.e., usually until patient turns 19). S.C. Code Ann. Regs. 61-16 § 601.7(A) (2007). See S.C. Code Ann. § 15-3-545 (2007).[g]
South Dakota	When records have become inactive or for which the whereabouts of the patients are unknown to the physician. S.D. Codified Laws § 36-4-38 (2008).	**Adult patients** 10 years from the actual visit date of service or resident care. **Minor patients** 10 years from the actual visit date of service or resident care or until the minor reaches age of majority plus 2 years (i.e., until patient turns 20), whichever is later. See S.D. Admin. R. 44:04:09:08 (2008).

Continued

State Medical Record Laws: Minimum Medical Record Retention Periods for Records Held by Medical Doctors and Hospitals—cont'd

State	Medical Doctors	Hospitals
Tennessee	**Adult patients** 10 years from the provider's last professional contact with the patient. **Minor patients** 10 years from the provider's last professional contact with the patient or 1 year after the minor reaches the age of majority (i.e., until patient turns 19), whichever is longer. Tenn. Comp. R. & Regs. 0880-2-.15 (2008).	**Adult patients** 10 years after the discharge of the patient or the patient's death during the patient's period of treatment within the hospital. Tenn. Code Ann. § 68-11-305(a)(1) (2008). **Minor patients** 10 years after discharge or for the period of minority plus at least 1 year (i.e., until patient turns 19), whichever is longer. Tenn. Code Ann. § 68-11-305(a)(2) (2008).
Texas	**Adult patients** 7 years from the date of the last treatment. **Minor patients** 7 years after the date of the last treatment or until the patient reaches age 21, whichever date is later. 22 Tex. Admin. Code § 165.1(b) (2008).[h]	**Adult patients** 10 years after the patient was last treated in the hospital. **Minor patients** 10 years after the patient was last treated in the hospital or until the patient reaches age 20, whichever date is later. Tex. Health & Safety Code Ann. § 241.103 (2007); 25 Tex. Admin. Code § 133.41(j)(8) (2008).[h]
Utah	N/A	**Adult patients** 7 years **Minor patients** 7 years or until the minor reaches the age of 18 plus 4 years (i.e., patient turns 22), whichever is longer. Utah Admin. Code r. 432-100-33(4)(c) (2008).
Vermont	N/A[a]	10 years Vt. Stat. Ann. tit. 18, § 1905(8) (2007).
Virginia	**Adult patients** 6 years after the last patient contact. **Minor patients** 6 years after the last patient contact or until the patient reaches age 18 (or becomes emancipated), whichever time period is longer. 18 Va. Admin. Code § 85-20-26(D) (2008).	**Adult patients** 5 years after patient's discharge. **Minor patients** 5 years after patient has reached the age of 18 (i.e., until the patient reaches age 23). 12 Va. Admin. Code § 5-410-370 (2008).
Washington	N/A	**Adult patients** 10 years after the patient's most recent hospital discharge. **Minor patients** 10 years after the patient's most recent hospital discharge or 3 years after the patient reaches the age of 18 (i.e., until the patient turns 21), whichever is longer. Wash. Rev. Code § 70.41.190 (2008).[i]

State Medical Record Laws: Minimum Medical Record Retention Periods for Records Held by Medical Doctors and Hospitals—cont'd

State	Medical Doctors	Hospitals
West Virginia	N/A	N/A
Wisconsin	5 years from the date of the last entry in the record. Wis. Admin. Code Med. § 21.03 (2008).	5 years Wis. Admin. Code Health & Family Services §§ 124.14(2)(c), 124.18(1)(e) (2008).
Wyoming	N/A	N/A[i]

All years are minimum periods (e.g., "at least" 7 years). Chart does not address retention of original X-rays or tracings, which may be subject to other requirements.

Minor = Person under 18 years old unless otherwise noted. N/A = No statute or regulation found.

[a]No statutory or regulatory requirement but state medical board or medical association recommends as follows:

Alabama: At least 10 years. *See* "Medical Records," available on the website of the Medical Association of the State of Alabama (MASA) at: http://www.masalink.org/uploadedFiles/Practice_Management/policy_Medicalrecords.pdf.

California: Indefinitely, if possible. See CMA ON-CALL: The California Medical Association's Information-On-Demand Service, available at http://www.thedocuteam.com/docs/retention_medicalrecords.pdf (accessed August 14, 2008).

Colorado: Adult patients 7 years after the last date of treatment and the records of minor patients 7 years after the last date of treatment or 7 years after the patient reaches the age of 18, whichever is later. See Colorado Board of Medical Examiners, Policy 40-7: "Guidelines Pertaining to the Release and Retention of Medical Records." Available at: http://www.dora.state.co.us/Medical/policies/40- 07.pdf (accessed September 16, 2008).

Montana: Seven years from the date of last contact with the patient. Birth and immunization records: Until the patient's 25th birthday. See Montana Board of Medical Examiners, Statement on Physician Obligation to Retain Medical Records (2004), available at http://www.mt.gov/dli/bsd/license/bsd_boards/med_board/pdf/patient_medrec.pdf (accessed July 17, 2008).

Oregon: In accordance with Oregon's statute of limitations, at least 10 years after the patient's last contact with the physician. If space permits, indefinitely for all living patients. See Oregon Medical Board, available at http://www.oregon.gov/OMB (accessed August 8, 2008).

Vermont: Patient's lifetime if possible. Minor's records: at least until the child reaches age 21 and decedent's records at least 3 years after the patient's death. *See Vermont Guide to Health Care Law,* available at http://www.vtmd.org/ (accessed September 16, 2008).

[b]If a patient dies in the hospital or within 30 days of discharge and is survived by one or more minors who are or claim to be entitled to damages for the patient's wrongful death, the hospital must retain the patient's hospital record until the youngest minor reaches age 28. Miss. Code Ann. § 41-9-69(1) (2008).

[c]A person under the age of 21 is generally considered a "minor" in Mississippi. However, for purposes of consenting to healthcare, an "adult" is a person aged 18 or older. See Miss. Code Ann. §§ 1-3-27 and 41-41-203(a) (2008).

[d]Hospital licensure rules have expired, but, as of June 2008, they were still in current use by the state Bureau of Licensing & Certification, which licenses healthcare facilities.

[e]The age of majority in Pennsylvania is 21. *See* 1 Pa. Cons. Stat. § 1991 (2008). However, minors over 18 may consent to health services in their own right. See 35 Pa. Cons. Stat. § 10101 (2008).

[f]Based only on statutes, not on regulations, which currently are published only in Spanish.

[g]The period of election is the time during which a person may elect to bring a lawsuit for malpractice that occurred while the patient was a minor, generally a maximum of 1 year after the minor reaches the age of majority. See S.C. Code Ann. § 15-3-545 (2007).

[h]The physician may not destroy medical records that relate to any civil, criminal, or administrative proceedings unless the physician knows the proceeding has been finally resolved. 22 Tex. Admin. Code § 165.1(b) (2008); Tex. Health & Safety Code Ann. § 241.103 (2007); 25 Tex. Admin. Code § 133.41(j)(8) (2008).

[i]Must maintain a record of a patient's healthcare information: for at least 1 year after receipt of authorization to disclose that healthcare information; and during the pendency of a request for examination, copying, correction, or amendment of that healthcare information. Wash. Rev. Code § 70.02.160 (2008); Wyo. Stat. Ann. § 35-2-615 (2008).

From https://www.HealthIT.gov: http://www.healthit.gov/sites/default/files/appa7-1.pdf

GLOSSARY

A

Abortion A procedure to end a pregnancy by a medical or surgical procedure to remove the embryo or fetus and placenta from the uterus.

Abuse A misuse or a maltreatment. In relationships, it is the pattern of misuse or inappropriate treatment systematically to gain control and power over another individual.

Accommodating Conflict behavior style in which an individual allows the needs of a group or team to supersede the individual's own needs. Also known as "smoothing."

Accreditation Process of officially recognizing a person or organization for meeting the standards in an area based on preestablished industry criteria.

Active euthanasia The active acceleration of death by use of drugs, for example, whether by oneself or with the aid of a physician.

Active patient files Files of patients who are being actively seen within the specific healthcare facility.

Addiction Habit or a compulsive behavior in which a person engages in a habit or action despite its negative consequences and effect.

Administrative law Establishes laws between citizens and government agencies and provides power to the agencies to enforce these laws and regulations.

Admissions of fact Discovery technique that asks the opposing party (in writing) to admit or deny any material fact or the authenticity of documents to be introduced into evidence at trial.

Adoption The legal action that bestows parental rights on a person who was not the child's legal parent before the proceeding.

Advance directive The treatment preferences and designation of an alternate decision maker in the event that a person should become unable to make medical decisions on his or her own behalf.

Affirmative defense A defense strategy that allows the defendant (usually provider or facility) to present the argument that the patient's condition was the result of factors other than negligence on the defendant's part.

Aggregate limit The maximum dollar amount your insurer will pay in total to settle your claims over the entire period of coverage.

Allied health professional A large and varied group of health care related professions and personnel whose functions include assisting, facilitating, or complementing the work of physicians and other healthcare providers in the healthcare system.

Alternative dispute resolution (ADR) The procedure for settling disputes by means other than litigation.

Amendment An official or formal change made to a law, contract, constitution, or other legal document.

Americans with Disabilities Act of 1990 (ADA) Laws enacted in 1990 to protect citizens with disabilities from discrimination.

Anti-Kickback Statute A federal law that prohibits the exchange or offer to exchange anything of value in an effort to induce or reward the referral of business.

Appellate court A court that hears appeals from lower court decisions; sometimes called court of appeals.

Arbitration The process to resolve a dispute outside the courts with a person or persons assigned by the court to mediate in a civil suit and then decide the outcome of the dispute.

Artificial insemination (AI) Injection into the female vagina of seminal fluid, which contains male sperm from a husband, partner, or other donor, to aid in conception.

Assault A threat or attempt to inflict offensive physical contact or bodily harm on a person who puts the person in immediate danger of or in apprehension of such harm or contact.

Associate practice A legal agreement in which physicians share staff and overhead expenses of operation but do not share in the legal responsibility or in the profits of business.

Assumption of risk A legal defense that asserts that the plaintiff was aware of and accepted the risks associated with the activity involved.

Avoiding Conflict behavior style in which the issue is not addressed at all or ignored.

B

Battery Bodily harm or unlawful touching of another. In the medical field, treating the patient without consent is considered battery.

Bias A preference of one thing over another, usually unfairly favoring one over another.

Bioethicists Specialists who study the ethical dilemmas resulting from advances in medical research and in science.

Bioethics Ethical dilemmas and issues that arise attributable to advances in medicine.

Birth certificate An official record declaring a live birth of the baby.

Brain death The irreversible loss of function of the brain, including the brainstem.

Breach of confidentiality The public revelation of confidential or privileged information without an individual's consent.

Burden of proof The legal responsibility and requirement to prove a claim is true.

C

Case investigation The process of identifying and investigating individuals with confirmed and probable diagnoses of a reportable communicable disease.

Centers for Medicare and Medicaid Services (CMS) The federal agency that oversees most of the regulations related to the healthcare system and provides government-subsidized medical coverage, such as Medicare, Medicaid, and State Children's Health Insurance Program (SCHIP).

Certification A process that verifies the qualifications of professionals and assesses their background and their ability to legally and/or competently work in their field

Certificate of live birth An unofficial record of a live birth that is signed by the healthcare provider in attendance at the birth and includes information of the baby, parents, and the events at the time of the birth.

CHAMPVA Acronym denoting Civilian Health and Medical Program of the Department of Veterans Affairs. Coverage designed specifically for disabled veterans and their dependents. Also known as *Veterans Health Administration*.

CHEDDAR A type of organization of medical record documentation that breaks down information into chief complaint, history, examination, details, drugs, assessment, and return visit plan.

Chief complaint (CC) The main reason that the patient is being seen by the healthcare provider.

Chromosomes Threadlike structures in the center of the cell (nucleus) that transmit the genetic information about the person.

Civil lawsuit A noncriminal lawsuit for damages, usually based in tort, contract, labor, or privacy.

Civil Rights Act of 1964 Law that made it illegal to discriminate against someone for his or her color, sex, race, religion, or national origin with regard to voting and public access.

Claims-made policy Insurance policy in which coverage is triggered on the date that the insured first becomes aware of the possibility of a claim and notifies the insurer.

Clearinghouse An entity that processes electronic transactions into HIPAA-standardized transactions for billing submission.

Clinical Laboratory Improvement Act of 1988 (CLIA) Regulates all laboratory facilities for safety and handling of specimens to ensure accuracy and timeliness of testing regardless of where the test is performed.

Clinical trials A type of medical research that involves patients or human subjects.

Closed-ended questions Types of questions that can be answered by a simple "yes" or "no."

Clone Duplicate cell reproduced artificially from a natural, original single cell.

Code of ethics Standards of behavior, initiated by an employer or organization, defining the acceptable conduct of its members/employees (also called *code of conduct*).

Coinsurance The percentage of payment that is agreed on by the insured as their portion of any claims; cost-sharing.

Collaborating Conflict behavior style in which the needs and goals of the individuals are combined to meet a common goal.

Common ethics Also called group ethics, a system of principles and rules of conduct accepted by a group or culture.

Common law Law of precedents built on a case-by-case basis and established by citing interpretation of existing laws by judges in previous suits. Also known as "judge-made law."

Communicable disease Specific disease or illness that can cause an epidemic or pandemic to the general public.

Comparative negligence A legal defense that proves the plaintiff's own actions, or lack of action, contributed to the damages done.

Compensatory damages The awarded amount given to the plaintiff in a court case to reimburse the plaintiff for loss of income or for pain and suffering.

Competing Conflict behavior style in which an individual's own needs are advocated over the needs of others.

Compliance Adherence to guidelines and regulations set forth by an organization and/or a governing body.

Compliance officer The individual in an organization or practice who is designated to maintain and inspect the adherence of all areas of regulations and guidelines. (In healthcare organizations, these officers perform audits and use established checks and balances to prevent fraud and abuse.)

Compliance plan Policies and procedures used to ensure that guidelines and regulations are obeyed, including auditing, monitoring, and protocol for taking action when infractions (whether deliberate or unintentional) are discovered.

Compromising Conflict behavior style in which people give and receive in a series of tradeoffs.

Confidentiality Keeping private all personal information regarding the patient.

Conflict The mental struggle resulting from incompatible or opposing needs, drives, wishes, or external or internal demands.

Conflict management The long-term management of disputes and conflicts, which may or may not lead to resolution.

Conflict of interest An occurrence when self-interest affects an individual's professional obligations to one's patients, organization, and/or profession.

Conflict resolution The process of ending a disagreement between two or more people in a constructive fashion for all parties involved.

Congressional Budget Office (CBO) A federal agency that manages the budget.

Conscience protection The refusal to perform a legal role or duty based on personal beliefs, sometimes called conscience clause.

Consent The acknowledgment of a person (usually the patient) regarding the risks and alternatives involved in a treatment, as well as permission for the treatment to be performed. This can be in some cases a verbal consent but in the medical field is usually a written document.

Consumer Credit Protection Act Law that requires providers to be up front about fees and finance charges when offering credit.

Contact tracing The process to identify, monitor, and support individuals who may have been exposed to a person with a communicable disease, often follows case investigation.

Continuity of Care Record (CCR) A patient's medical health record is accurate to ensure continuity of care when a patient is transferred to another healthcare provider or to a medical specialist.

Contraception The intentional prevention of conception through the use of various devices, sexual practices, chemicals, drugs, or surgical procedures, also commonly called birth control methods.

Contract An agreement voluntarily joined by two parties. These can be verbal or written and can be expressed or implied.

Contributory negligence A defense strategy that allows the defendant to present the argument that the patient's condition was the result of factors other than negligence on the defendant's part.

Control group Group of subjects in a research study who do not receive any treatment or, in some cases, are given a placebo. In testing, it is the principle of the constant that remains the same to evaluate the changes of a given experiment.

Controlled Substances Act Federal drug policy regulating the manufacture, importation, possession, use, and distribution of certain substances.

Copay A fixed amount that is determined by the health insurance policy that is paid for services to offset premiums paid by the insured.

Coroner An elected or appointed position, often not a physician, to perform autopsies and testing to determine cause of death and time of death in suspicious deaths or under circumstances when no person was in attendance of the death.

Corporation A company that is established legally and is managed by a board of directors.

Covered entity (CE) Health plans, healthcare clearinghouses, and healthcare providers under HIPAA who electronically transmit any health information.

Credentialing The process of verifying an individual's professional qualifications

Criminal law State or federal government law covering violations of written criminal code or statute.

D

Damages The actual injury or loss suffered by a defendant in a suit; usually given a monetary award by the court based on the extent of the loss or injury.

Death The permanent cessation of all biological functions that sustain a living organism.

Deductible An amount of money that is paid by the insured before the insurance company pays for services, usually a fixed amount paid annually.

Defamation Any intentional false communication, either written or spoken, that harms a person's reputation; decreases the respect, regard, or confidence in which a person is held; or induces disparaging, hostile, or disagreeable opinions or feelings against a person.

Defendant Person or entity sued.

Defensive medicine The practice of ordering unnecessary tests, treatments, and other procedures to protect against medical malpractice.

Denial Legal assertion of innocence; made only if all four elements of negligence are false.

Dereliction (of duty) A neglect or negligence of one's duty.

Differential diagnosis A list of possible diagnoses that may likely be the cause of the presenting symptoms.

Direct cause In a negligence case, the correspondence between the dereliction of duty and the actual damage sustained by the plaintiff.

Discovery Process of gathering information in preparation for trial.

Discovery rule Law or statute that states the statute of limitations does not begin until the discovery of the diagnosis or injury.

Discrimination Treatment of a person or thing, either unsupportive or supportive, based on bias or prejudice.

Disruptive behavior Personal conduct, whether verbal or physical, that affects or that potentially may affect patient care negatively.

Domestic violence Any abusive act between family members, ex-spouses, intimate cohabitants, former intimate cohabitants, dating couples and former dating couples in which one party seeks to gain/maintain power and control over the other partner.

Do-not-resuscitate order (DNR order) Sometimes called a "No Code," is a legal order written either in the hospital or on a legal form to communicate the wishes of a patient to not undergo CPR or advanced cardiac life support if the patient's heart stops or the patient stops breathing.

Double-blind study In testing, one group receives the placebo, and the other group receives the new agent, which prevents either group from knowing who is receiving the real drug or the placebo.

Double-lock system A safeguard that requires passing through two systems of security to access any confidential patient information.

Due process Procedures or actions followed to safeguard individual rights. In the workplace, the process to safeguard an employee if he or she feels his or her rights are in jeopardy.

Durable power of attorney A type of advance medical directive in which legal documents provide the power of attorney to another person in the case of an incapacitating medical condition.

Duty In a malpractice suit, the proof of responsibility of the parties involved.

Duty-based ethics (deontology) Philosophy of ethics that focuses on performing one's duty to a group, individual, or organization.

E

Electronic medical record (EMR) Electronic medical records that contain medical and health records of individual patients, maintaining the HIPAA standards for privacy and security.

Electronic health record (EHR) Electronic medical records that can be shared, created, managed, and consulted by authorized healthcare providers, professionals, and staff across more than one healthcare organization.

Emancipation The legal process of a minor achieving independence from his or her parents.

Emergency Medical Treatment and Active Labor Act (EMTALA) of 1986 Federal law that any hospital emergency room that receives payments from federal healthcare programs to provide medical screening and treat and stabilize any patient regardless of insurance status.

Emotional intelligence (EI) An individual's skill to perceive, understand, reason with, and manage his or her emotions and the emotions and behaviors of others.

Emotional quotient (EQ) A measurement of emotional intelligence.

Employee assistance program (EAP) Program designed to help employees receive counseling for substance abuse or other issues of abuse, without fear of losing their jobs; may offer legal and financial counseling as well.

Employment-at-will The employment contract that allows an employer to fire or discharge an employee without showing just cause for the termination.

Epidemic An outbreak that affects many people at one time and can spread through one or several communities.

Equal Employment Opportunity Act of 1972 Act that prohibits employment discrimination on the basis of race, color, national origin, sex, religion, age, disability, political beliefs, and marital or familial status.

Equal Pay Act of 1963 Act that prohibited wage differentials based on sex.

Ethics Branch of philosophy that relates to morals and moral principles.

Eugenics The study of all agencies under human control which can improve or impair the racial quality of future generations.

Euthanasia Termination of a life to eliminate pain and suffering related to a terminal illness, usually performed by giving a drug or agent to induce cessation of bodily functions. Also known as *assisted suicide.*

Executive branch President of the United States or governor of an individual state. Can propose laws, veto laws proposed by the legislature, enforce laws, and establish agencies.

Experimental group In testing, the group that receives the new, researched treatment agent.

Explicit consent Also known as *express* or *direct consent*, it means that an individual is clearly presented with an option to agree or disagree or to express a preference or choice, often verbally or in writing.

F

Facilitation The process in which a third party (facilitator) assists in the resolution of a dispute.

Fair Credit Billing Act Law that requires businesses to provide prompt written response to billing complaints and investigation of possible billing errors.

Fair Credit Reporting Act Law that protects patients from inaccurate information on their credit reports.

Fair Debt Collection Practices Act Law that prohibits debt collectors, including physician office staff, from using deceptive or abusive practices in the collection of consumer debts.

False Claims Act Federal law that prevents an individual or organization from knowingly creating a false record or submitting a false claim to any federal government payer.

False imprisonment Restraint of a person so as to impede his or her liberty without justification or consent.

Family Medical Leave Act (1993) Law that requires employers with 50 or more employees to allow eligible employees to take unpaid leave to help care for a family member's illness or to stay at home after the birth or adoption of a child.

Federal court Court having jurisdiction over cases in which the U.S. Constitution and federal statutes apply; these can be federal district courts (trial courts), district courts of appeals, or the U.S. Supreme Court.

Felony Serious crime punishable by relatively large fines and/or imprisonment for more than 1 year and, in extreme cases, death.

Fertilization Assistance in conception, most commonly performed either as artificial insemination or as in vitro fertilization to produce pregnancy.

Firewall A network security device that monitors incoming and outgoing network traffic and decides whether to allow or block specific traffic based on a defined set of security rules.

Fraud Wrongful or criminal deception intended to result in financial or personal gain.

G

Gatekeeper A person, such as the primary care physician, or an organization that is appointed by a managed care carrier to maintain and approve services to reduce costs and unnecessary spending.

Gender Refers to the various socially constructed roles, behaviors, expressions and identities of girls, women, boys, men, and gender-diverse people.

Gender expression Refers to how people present their gender on the outside, often through behavior, clothing, hairstyle, voice, or body characteristics.

Gender ID data Information that includes gender identification, birth-assigned sex, legal sex, preferred name, and legal name.

Gender identity Refers to one's internal knowledge of one's gender, such as being a man, a woman, or another gender.

Gender nonconforming (GNC) Refers to a gender identity—one's personal and subjective sense of gender—that is neither male nor female. It can also refer to a gender expression characterized by mannerisms and behaviors that are not conventionally associated with an assigned gender.

Gene therapy Process of splicing or infusing genes to replace malfunctioning genes. Alteration of the DNA of body cells to control production of a particular substance.

Genetic discrimination A type of discrimination when people treat others differently because of their genetic information.

Genetic testing A type of medical test that identifies changes in genes, chromosomes, or proteins.

Good Samaritan Law Law providing immunity for those who render healthcare for an emergency or disaster without reimbursement.

Group practice A medical practice with three or more physicians of the same or similar specialty, who share the same overhead and staff and practice medicine together.

H

Healthcare proxy A legal document in which an individual designates another person to make healthcare decisions if he or she is rendered incapable of making his or her wishes known.

Health Information Technology for Economic and Clinical Health (HITECH) Act An Act that provides the authority to establish programs to improve health care quality, safety, and efficiency through the promotion of health information technology.

Health Insurance Portability and Accountability Act of 1996 (HIPAA) Federal legislation that provides data privacy and security provisions for safeguarding medical information.

Health Maintenance Organization (HMO) A type of managed care company that serves participating patients by offering services at a fixed rate within the group of participating providers and facilities. A fixed fee schedule is negotiated with the providers as well.

Hospice Organization or program involving a multidisciplinary group of medical professionals available to aid in support of the terminally ill and their families.

Human Genome Project Medical research program, sponsored by the federal government, established to map and sequence the number of genes that are within the 23 pairs of chromosomes (i.e., the 46 chromosomes) with the goal of advanced lifesaving or disease-preventing treatments.

I

Implied consent Consent that is not expressly granted by a person, but rather inferred from a person's actions and the facts and circumstances in a specific situation.

Inactive patient files Files of patients who have not been seen within the specific healthcare facility over the preceding 3 years.

Incident to billing A method of billing outpatient services provided by a nonphysician provider when working under the direct supervision of a physician.

Indemnity plans Fee-for-service plans that allow the patient to direct his or her healthcare. Typically require the patient to pay deductible and a percentage (cost-share) of the allowed charge. Allows both in-network and out-of-network coverage.

Informed consent A process when a detailed, listing and covering all possible risks and potential prognoses to patients or participants for having a treatment or procedure performed and the alternatives available.

***In personam* jurisdiction** A court's power to adjudicate cases filed against a specific individual, as opposed to *in rem* jurisdiction, which concerns property disputes.

***In rem* jurisdiction** A term that delineates the court's jurisdiction over property or things, including marriage, rather than over persons.

***In vitro* fertilization** Process to assist in conception by harvesting an ovum from a woman and combining it with the male's sperm outside of the uterus and then implanting the fertilized embryo back into the woman's uterus.

Integrity Unwavering adherence to an individual's values and principles with dedication to high standards.

Intent The willful decision to bring about a prohibited consequence.

Intentional infliction of emotional distress Type of conduct that deliberately causes severe emotional trauma to the victim.

Intentional tort A category of torts that describes a civil wrong resulting from an intentional act on the part of another person or entity.

Interface The ability for two or more systems to communicate and function together.

Interrogatory Pretrial set of written questions that must be answered in writing under oath and returned within a given timeframe.

Intimate partner violence (IPV) A form of domestic violence or abuse resulting in physical, sexual, or psychological harm caused by a current or former partner or spouse; can occur among either heterosexual or same-sex couples.

Invasion of privacy The wrongful intrusion into private affairs with which the perpetrator or the public has no concern.

Involuntary euthanasia The active effort to end the life of a patient who has not explicitly requested aid in dying. This term is most often used with respect to patients who are in a persistent vegetative state and who probably will never recover consciousness.

J

Judicial branch Federal constitutional court system; one of the three parts of the U.S. federal government; interprets legislation and determines its constitutionality, applying it to specific cases. May overrule cases presented on appeal from lower courts.

Jurisdiction Authority given by law to a court to try cases and rule on legal matters within a particular geographical area and/or over certain types of legal cases.

Justice-based ethics Ethical philosophy based on all individuals having equal rights.

L

Law The foundation of statutes, rules, and regulations that govern people, relationships, behaviors, and interactions with the state, society, and federal government.

Legislative branch The U.S. House of Representatives and Senate and any similar state legislature that develops statutory law.

Liability Legal responsibility and accountability for all health and financial patient care.

Liable Legal responsibility for a person's own actions.

Libel Written, printed, or other visual communication that harms another person's reputation.

Licensing An official permission to perform certain duties

Limited Liability Company (LLC) A legally structured company in which the members of the corporation cannot be held personally liable for the debts or actions of the company or another party in the company.

Litigious Highly inclined to sue.

Living will A document in which the patient states his or her wishes regarding medical treatment, especially treatment that sustains or prolongs life by extraordinary means, in the event that the patient becomes mentally incompetent or unable to communicate.

M

Malfeasance The performance of an illegal act.

Malpractice Improper, illegal, or negligent professional activity or treatment by a medical practitioner.

Managed Care Organization (MCO) Provides healthcare plans that balance healthcare delivery while controlling costs by limiting the providers who can be seen by the patient and discounting payments to those providers.

Mandate An order or requirement an executive body given by the legislature in a state of emergency.

Mandatory reporting The legal responsibility of healthcare professionals to report vital information and incidence to the appropriate agencies for the protection and welfare of the general public and specific vulnerable populations.

Mediation The process by which a neutral third party who is trained in mediation techniques facilitates and assists in resolving a dispute.

Medicaid Federal program administered by each individual state that provides healthcare coverage for the indigent and/or medically needy patients.

Medical ethics Principles based on the medical profession that determine moral behavior.

Medical examiner An elected or appointed position to perform autopsies and testing to determine cause of death and time of death, often a physician with training in forensic pathology.

Medical exemptions A request to not receive a state mandated vaccine due to believing that the vaccine would not be safe for themselves or their child.

Medical law Laws that are prescribed specifically pertaining to the medical field.

Medical practice acts Laws defined by each of the states that regulate the licensing and medical laws for that state and define the scope of practice for licensed and unlicensed individuals in the healthcare field.

Medicare Federal program that provides medical insurance coverage to members older than age 65 or to those who are deemed permanently disabled.

Medicare fraud Providing false information to claim medical reimbursements beyond the scope of payment for actual healthcare services rendered.

Minor A person who does not have the legal rights of an adult and has not yet reached the age of majority.

Misdemeanor Lesser crime punishable by usually modest fines or penalties established by the state or federal government and/or imprisonment of less than 1 year.

Misfeasance Poor performance of a duty or action, causing damage.

Morals Standards of right and wrong. Moral values that govern behavior and thinking based on principles of what is right and wrong. The norms of measuring right from wrong.

N

Negative conflict Conflict that has devolved into disruptive behaviors or violence.

Negligence The failure to use such care as a reasonably prudent and careful person would use under similar circumstances; an act of omission or failure to do what a person of ordinary prudence would have done under similar circumstances.

Negotiation Any communication used in an attempt to achieve a goal, approval, or action by another.

Nominal damages A small payment or award given by the court.

Nonfeasance A failure to perform an action when needed.

Nonintimate partner violence A form of domestic violence between individuals who are not intimate partners, but have a familial relationship, such as mother/adult son, or brother/sister.

Nonphysician providers Also called *midlevel providers,* providers that are educated and skilled to perform similar medical services and procedures to physicians.

Nontherapeutic research Medical research in which the test subjects are not necessarily suffering from a disease or the particular disease that the study is researching, and therefore, the subjects are not receiving a direct medical benefit from participating in the study.

Nonvoluntary euthanasia Euthanasia conducted when the consent of the patient is unavailable, such as the patient is in a coma, is a young child or infant, has dementia, is severely mentally retarded, or has severe brain damage.

O

Occupational Safety and Health Act of 1970 Act that defines and enforces safety regulations for the health and protection of employees in the workplace.

Occupational Safety and Health Administration (OSHA) Federal agency within the Department of Labor that designs, regulates, and monitors standards for employee safety.

Occurrence-basis policy An insurance policy that covers claims taking place during the policy period, regardless of when claims are made.

Office for Civil Rights (OCR) Federal office established to uphold the rights of individuals, regarding rights to privacy and standards of care. Enforces the HIPAA regulations.

Office of Inspector General (OIG) Independent agency that functions under the Department of Justice to investigate and protect the integrity of the Department of Health and Human Services (HHS) and their recipients, as well as welfare programs.

Office of the National Coordinator for Health IT (ONCHIT) The principal federal entity charged with coordination of nationwide efforts to implement health information technology and facilitating the exchange of electronic health information

Older Americans Act of 1987 (OAA) Legislation passed to protect adults older than the age 60 from abuse, neglect, abandonment, and exploitation.

Open-ended questions Types of questions that require more thought and more than a simple one-word answer.

Ordinance Statutory law passed by local or city governments or councils.

P

Palliative care Literally meaning to ease or comfort; the care provided to terminally ill patients to alleviate symptoms and discomfort suffered while dying.

Pandemic An outbreak that affects many people at one time and the spread is global.

Parens patriae The doctrine in which the state exerts authority over child welfare.

Passive euthanasia The act of allowing a patient to die without medical intervention.

Patient abandonment A legal claim that occurs when a healthcare provider terminates the professional relationship with a patient without reasonable notice and when continued care is medically necessary.

Patient's Bill of Rights Basic rules of conduct between patients and medical caregivers.

Patient Self-Determination Act Federal law that requires all healthcare institutions receiving Medicare or Medicaid funds to provide patients with written information about their right under state law to execute advance directives. The written information must clearly state the institution's policies on withholding or withdrawing life-sustaining treatment.

Persistent vegetative state (PVS) Condition characterized by the irreversible cessation of higher brain functions, usually as a result of damage to the cerebral cortex.

Personal ethics A type of ethics determined by what an individual believes about morality and right and wrong.

Philosophical exemptions Also called personal exemptions, an exemption based on individuals or parents' personal beliefs about vaccines, such as vaccine safety.

Placebo Nontherapeutic drug or agent given to a control group. (Commonly referred to as a "sugar pill.")

Plaintiff The person or entity bringing a suit or claim.

Physician-assisted suicide The practice whereby a physician provides a potentially lethal medication to a terminally ill patient at his or her request to end life.

Physician orders for life-sustaining treatment (POLST) An approach to encourage healthcare providers to speak with patients to help create specific medical orders to be honored by healthcare professionals during a medical crisis.

Point of Service Plan (POS) Insurance plans that combine some elements of HMO and PPO plans; allows members to choose a primary care provider that will directly refer to in-network providers when needed.

Positive conflict The idea that healthy discussion can happen in the face of a disagreement, regardless of differing personalities, education levels, or responsibilities.

Postmortem Examination that is performed on an individual after death.

Preferred provider organization (PPO) A type of managed care organization that allows members to see any in-network provider without first obtaining a referral from the patient's primary care provider.

Premium The amount of money an insurer charges to provide the coverage described in the policy.

Primary care physician (PCP) A designated provider who oversees the care and manages the healthcare services for an individual.

Prior acts coverage Insurance coverage for incidents that occur before the start of the policy but whose claims are made during the policy period.

Professional corporation (PC) A specific legal company structure that is designed for individuals providing professional services to their clients, such as lawyers, physicians, or architects.

Professionalism An individual's conduct in the workplace.

Protected health information (PHI) Any information about a patient's health status, provision of healthcare, or payment for healthcare that is created or collected by a covered entity (or a business associate of a covered entity) and can be linked to a specific individual.

Public health The science of protecting and improving the health of people and their communities, achieved by promoting healthy lifestyles; researching disease and injury prevention; and detecting, preventing, and responding to infectious diseases.

Punitive damages An award granted by the courts to punish the defendant for the damages done based on a malicious or intentional act.

Q

Quarantine A state, period, or place of isolation in which people or animals that have arrived from elsewhere or been exposed to infectious or contagious disease are placed.

Quasi-intentional tort A voluntary act that directly causes damage to a person's privacy or emotional well-being, but without the intent to injure or to cause distress.

***Qui tam* (whistleblower)** In Latin meaning "who as well"; this is the term used for a private citizen who exposes and sues a company or organization that is violating a law and/or breaching a contract with the government. In such cases, the whistleblower may be entitled to a percentage amount or settlement reward for the uncovering of the illegal action.

R

Registration A professional organization in a specific healthcare field administers examinations and/or maintains a list of qualified individuals

Release of tortfeasor Law that asserts that once the person causing damage (the tortfeasor) is released from further liability in a previous suit's settlement, he or she cannot be held liable in a subsequent suit.

Religious exemption laws Also called "Religious Freedom Restoration Acts" or RFRAs, permit people, churches, nonprofit organizations, and sometimes corporations to seek exemptions from state laws that burden their religious beliefs.

Request for production of documents A discovery tool whereby requests are submitted to the opposing party to produce specific documents or items that are pertinent to the issues of the case.

Res ipsa loquitur In Latin: "The thing speaks for itself." Legal indication that there is clear proof that the defendant had the responsibility (duty) to the patient and that the injury would not and could not have occurred without the negligence of the defendant.

Res judicata Law that forbids suing for a subsequent time for the same damages once a case has already been resolved.

Respondeat superior Legal doctrine that states in many circumstances an employer is responsible for the actions of employees performed within the course of their employment.

Rider An add-on provision to a basic liability insurance policy that provides additional benefits to the policyholder at an additional cost.

Right of contribution When there are others, although not named in the claim, who bear some responsibility for an incident that resulted in a claim.

Rights-based ethics Philosophy of ethics based on theory of the rights of each individual (autonomy).

Risk management The process of identifying threats that could harm the organization, its patients, staff, or anyone else within the organization.

S

Sanctions Penalties that can be levied on an individual for violating a policy or rule. (Can also mean permission or agreement in other contexts.)

Scope of practice Officially sanctioned description of the specific procedures, actions, and processes that are permitted for a licensed or nonlicensed professional; based on the specific state's laws for education and experience requirements, plus demonstrated competency. Established by the state's laws, licensing board, and/or agency regulations.

Settlement Legal agreement that is reached between two parties in a civil matter.

Sexual assault Any type of sexual activity to which a person does not agree.

Sexual harassment Use of power or intimidation over an individual for sexual favors; unwanted or unwelcomed sexual advances and actions or behaviors with sexual implications or innuendoes, leading another individual to feel uncomfortable or offended.

Slander Spoken or verbal communication in which one person discusses another in terms that harm that person's reputation.

SOAP An acronym used to document in patient's medical chart meaning: **S**ubjective, **O**bjective, **A**ssessment, and **P**lan.

Sole proprietorship A single professional-owned business in which an individual employs other professionals in the same field. In medical practice, single physician-owned practice that employs other physicians to work for the practice.

Solo practice Single owner/operator of the company or business. In the medical field, this would represent a single-physician practice.

Specialist In the medical field, an individual who has undergone further specific training in a certain discipline and practices medicine in that discipline, such as dermatology or endocrinology.

Standard of care The degree of caution with which a similarly qualified healthcare professional would have managed the patient's care under the same or similar circumstances.

Standards of practice Basic skill and care expected of healthcare professionals in the same or similar branch of medicine; based on what another medical professional would deem to be appropriate in similar circumstances.

Stare decisis In Latin: "to stand by the things decided" or to adhere to a decided case; condition in which, once a court rules, that decision becomes law for other cases. Also known as *precedent.*

Stark laws Laws designed to maintain the integrity of the medical field; include antitrust and antikickback laws to prevent physicians from gaining financially from solicitation of services or monopolization of services.

State supreme court Highest court in any given state in the U.S. court system.

Statute Written laws enacted by the state or federal legislative branch

Statute of limitations A law that sets out the maximum time that parties must initiate legal proceedings from the date of an alleged offense.

Statutory law Written laws, usually enacted by a legislative body, that include regulatory.

Statutory reporting The legal responsibility of healthcare professionals to report vital information and incidence to the appropriate agencies for the protection and welfare of the general public and specific vulnerable populations.

Stem cells Cells of the body that can control the production of specialized cells by becoming other types of cells as needed during growth or healing.

Sterilization Any procedure performed to permanently prevent reproduction.

Strict liability A person places another person in danger, even in the absence of negligence, simply because he is in possession of a dangerous product, animal, or weapon.

Surrogacy A method of assisted reproduction that helps a party start a family when that party otherwise could not.

T

Terminally ill Relating to an illness where the patient has an expected survival of less than 6 months.

Thanatology The study of the effects of death and dying, especially the investigation of ways to lessen the suffering and address the needs of the terminally ill and their survivors.

The Joint Commission The organization that accredits hospitals and other healthcare organizations.

Therapeutic research Medical research performed on chronically or terminally ill patients who may benefit from the agent being tested.

Third-party payer Usually refers to the insurance company but can be any other person or organization that is responsible for the medical care coverage of a patient.

Tort A civil case that results in injury to another's person, property, reputation, or the like, and for which the injured party is entitled to compensation.

Transgender A broad term that can be used to describe people whose gender identity is different from the gender they were thought to be when they were born; "trans" is often used as shorthand for transgender.

Trespass An unlawful intrusion that interferes with one's person, property (called "chattels"), or land.

TRICARE Government medical program for active-duty military and their dependents, as well as coverage for military retirees (after 20 or more years of service).

U

Umbrella policy Liability insurance policy that provides protection against claims that are not covered, or are in excess of the amount covered, under a basic liability insurance policy.

Uniform Anatomical Gift Act Legislation that allows a person to make an anatomical gift at the time of death by the use of a signed document such as a will or driver's license—the person can donate all or part of his or her body for medical education, scientific research, or organ transplantation.

Uniform Determination of Death Act (UDDA) Model state legislation that has since been adopted by most U.S. states and is intended "to provide a comprehensive and medically sound basis for determining death in all situations."

Uniform Rights of the Terminally Ill Act Legislation that allows a person to declare a living will specifying that he or she does not wish to be kept alive through life support if terminally ill or in a coma.

United States Supreme Court Highest court in the United States, having ultimate judicial authority within the United States to interpret and decide questions of federal law. It is head of the judicial branch of the U.S. government.

Utilitarianism Ethical theory based on the greatest good for the greatest number (also known as *cost/benefit analysis*).

V

Values Principles that individuals choose to follow in their lives.

Vicarious liability The liability of an employer for the actions of its designated agents.

Virtue-based ethics Ethical theory or philosophy that relies on the principle that individuals share and will hold as their governing principle values of moral behavior and character.

Vital statistics Community-wide recording of individual key human events such as births, deaths, marriages, or divorces.

Voluntary euthanasia Conscious medical act that results in the death of a patient who has given consent.

W

Whistleblower An individual, usually an employee, who turns in his or her employer for potential fraud and abuse.

Workers' compensation A form of mandated insurance program that covers medical costs and wage replacement for employees injured on the job.

Workplace violence Any act or threat of physical violence, harassment, intimidation, or other disruptive behavior that causes fear for personal safety in the workplace.

Writ of certiorari Order a higher court issue to review the decision and proceedings in a lower court and determine whether there were any irregularities.

INDEX

Note: Page numbers followed by *f* indicate figures, *t* indicate tables, and *b* indicate boxes.

E

F